The U.S. Navy SEAL Guide to Fitness and Nutrition

The U.S. Navy SEAL Guide to
Fitness and Nutrition

Forewords by

Don Mann

Skyhorse Publishing

Skyhorse Publishing books may be purchased in bulk at special discounts for sales promotion,
corporate gifts, fund-raising, or educational purposes. Special editions can also be created to specifications.
For details, contact the Special Sales Department, Skyhorse Publishing, 307 West 36th Street, 11th Floor,
New York, NY 10018 or info@skyhorsepublishing.com.

Skyhorse® and Skyhorse Publishing® are registered trademarks of Skyhorse Publishing, Inc.®,
a Delaware corporation.

www.skyhorsepublishing.com

10 9 8 7 6 5 4 3 2 1

Library of Congress Cataloging-in-Publication Data is available on file.

ISBN: 978-1-62914-326-2

Printed in China

Part I — Table of Contents

Physical Fitness

Part I — List of Tables

Part I — List of Figures

Part II — Table of Contents

The U.S. Navy SEAL Guide to Nutrition

Part II — List of Tables

Part II — List of Worksheets

Part I — Physical Fitness

Acknowledgments

The authors would like to recognize the invaluable contributions to the development of this guide by the following individuals. CAPT Kenneth Long participated in both panel reviews and provided useful suggestions and comments. His meticulous work was greatly appreciated by all. CAPT Peter Toennies reviewed and provided substantive comments about the chapter "Swimming for Fitness." Mr. Jeremy Levine and Ms. Brandi Schoeber provided information about strength training.

Importantly, we were extremely fortunate to receive valuable input from several SEALs throughout the development of this guide. ENS Frances Franky and BM1 George Vernia participated in the first panel review and their suggestions were incorporated in the second draft of the manual. BM1 Vernia helped organize and participated in the second and final panel review. Other SEAL panel reviewers included CW03 John Shellnut, Master Chief Bob Bender, LCDR Pat Butler, and BMCS Duane Noel. Each one of these SEALs provided suggestions and practical recommendations which were instrumental in the finalization of the *The Navy SEAL Physical Fitness Guide*.

About the Authors

The Navy SEAL Physical Fitness Guide

CAPT Frank K. Butler, Jr., M.D., developed the chapter "SEAL Mission-Related Activities." He is currently the Biomedical Research Director for the Naval Special Warfare Command, Chairman of the U.S. Special Operations Command Biomedical Initiatives Steering Committee, and a Staff Ophthalmologist at the Naval Hospital, Pensacola, Florida. He obtained his undergraduate degree from Georgia Institute of Technology in 1971, with high honors. His medical degree is from Medical College of Georgia, 1980. Dr. Butler's Family Practice Internship was at the Navy Regional Medical Center, Jacksonville, Florida (1980-1981) and his Ophthalmology Residency was at the National Naval Medical Center, Bethesda, MD. where he was Chief Resident (1988-1989). He completed his Undersea Medical Officer Training from the Undersea Medical Institute, Groton, Ct., 1981. CAPT Butler has been a platoon Commander for Underwater Demolition Team TWELVE and SEAL Team ONE, and a Diving Medical Research Officer at the Navy Experimental Diving Unit. He has published extensively and been a frequent guest lecturer on the subject of closed-circuit diving and Special Warfare.

CAPT John S. Hughes, M.D., developed the chapter "Swimming for Fitness" and contributed to "Other Training-Related Issues." He is a Navy Reserve Undersea Medical Officer who resides near Littleton, Colorado. A graduate of the University of Colorado School of Medicine, Dr. Hughes has a Naval Reserve assignment to NAVSEA in Crystal City, Virginia, where he is assigned to the Supervisor of Diving and Salvage. Dr. Hughes has been involved with Navy diving medicine since 1981. He is Board Certified in Occupational Medicine and his civilian medical practice in Colorado and Wyoming involves operation of clinics and health facilities covering a wide range of high risk industries including commercial diving.

Special qualifications allow Dr. Hughes to participate in the development of the Navy SEAL Physical Fitness Guide. He swam freestyle in the NCAA Championships and won the 1976 Big 8 Conference Championship in the 1650 yd freestyle for the University of Colorado and has remained active as a competitive swimmer. As a mountaineer and cross country skier he has organized and participated in numerous climbs, including two on Denali and Denali North Peak in Alaska. His instrumental work with the SEAL team in developing a winter warfare program during 1982 led him to participate as a staff member of the SEAL winter warfare Greenland operation in 1983. For this involvement, Dr. Hughes received a letter of appreciation from the CO of SEAL Team TWO, CDR Rick Woolard. With the theme of Dr. Hughes' career being medical support of high risk military and industrial operations, he feels that work for the SEALs is at the head of the list.

CDR Joseph Moore, M.D., developed the chapter "Training and Sports-Related Injuries. He completed his undergraduate degree in 1978, and medical degree in 1982 from the University of Virginia after which he was commissioned as a Lieutenant in the Naval Medical Corps. CDR Moore completed his internship at Naval Medical Center, Oakland, California, in June 1983, and received orders to the 1st Marine Division, Camp Pendleton, California. He served as Battalion Surgeon, 2nd Battalion, 9th Marines from July 1983 to October 1985, deploying to Okinawa, Korea and Panama. He also served as 5th Marines Regimental Surgeon during this time period. He completed a Family Practice residency at the Naval Hospital, Camp Pendleton in 1987, followed by a tour as Senior Medical Officer on the island of La Maddalena, Italy. CDR Moore was the first Navy physician selected for a primary care Sports Medicine fellowship, and trained at the San Diego Sports Medicine Center and San Diego State University from December 1989 through January 1991.

CDR Moore is currently the Department Head and Fellowship Director for the Navy's Sports Medicine program at the Naval Hospital and Marine Corps Base, Camp Pendleton. In addition to his duties as Specialty Leader to the Surgeon General, Dr. Moore serves as chairman of the Sports Medicine Advisory Panel to the U.S. Naval Special Warfare Command, Coronado, and advisor to Marine Corps Combat Development Command, Quantico. His work with the civilian community has earned him an appointment by the Governor of California to the Governor's Council on Physical Fitness and Sports. He also holds an appointment to the United States Olympic Committee Team Physician Development Program, Colorado Springs, CO. He is co-chairman of the American Academy of Family Physicians' Review Course for Sports Medicine.

CDR Brad L. Bennett, Ph.D., developed the Chapter "Load Bearing" and he has written a technical report "Load Carriage: Are You Preparing Correctly? Naval Medical Research Institute, Technical Memo 96-71, 1991." He is a research physiologist currently assigned to the Department of Military and Emergency Medicine, School of Medicine, Uniformed Services University of the Health Sciences, Bethesda, MD. He serves as an Assistant Professor and Director of the Basic Sciences Division. He is a graduate of Wilderness Medicine and Tactical Emergency Medical Technician courses, and is a department faculty member in the Counter Narcotics Tactical Operations Medical Support (CONTOMS) course as sponsored by the Department of Defense. He earned a Bachelor and Masters Degrees in Exercise Science from San Diego State University and a Ph.D. in Kinesiology from the University of Maryland.

He has completed the Navy's diving medicine course and became designated as a Navy Medical Department Deep Sea Diving Officer. He has conducted biomedical research on the impact of environmental stressors on human performance of Navy Special Warfare (SEAL) personnel, U.S. Marine Corps personnel, and Navy damage control personnel. Dr. Bennett currently serves as the Special Advisor to Navy Surgeon General for Physiology.

Dr. Bennett has enjoyed long distance running (10k, half marathons and marathons) for over twenty years. Other hobbies of interest are hiking, kayaking, camping, weight training, target, and skeet shooting.

LCDR Lisa Thorson, M.D., wrote the Chapters on Flexibility, Calisthenics and Plyometrics. She earned her B.S. in psychology at the University of Oklahoma in Norman, Oklahoma, and her M.D. from the University of Oklahoma School of Medicine. She has completed the Undersea Medical Officer course and had a tour of duty at the Diver Second Class Training Department, Naval Amphibious School, Naval Amphibious Base, Coronado. LCDR Thorson been involved with the Exercise-Related Injury Program, and all aspects of injury prevention for the Special Forces Community. Projects have included the development of injury tracking software used by the Special Forces community. She also organized the first Naval Special Warfare Sports Medicine conference held May 1994. Recommendations from this conference are documented in Naval Health Research Center Technical Document Number 95-4D, "Naval Special Warfare Sports Medicine Conference Proceedings," and Number 95-5D, "Expert Panel Review of the Naval Special Warfare Calisthenics Sports Medicine Conference Summary."

Currently she is in Residency training in Preventive Medicine at the Uniformed Services University of the Health Sciences, Bethesda, Maryland, where her work documenting injuries in the Special Forces community will continue. She has 13 years of ballet training, has taught and competed in aerobic dance competitions, and spends her time weight-training.

Patricia Deuster, Ph.D., M.P.H., the editor of this guide, wrote "Cardio-respiratory Conditioning" and "Strength Training" and contributed to "Other Training-Related Issues." She compiled the group's recommendations and wrote the chapter "Physical Fitness and Training Recommendations." She is an Associate Professor and Director of the Human Performance Laboratory in the Department of Military and Emergency Medicine at the Uniformed Services University of the Health Sciences, School of Medicine in Bethesda, Maryland. She has an undergraduate degree in Mathematics, and graduate degrees in Physical Education (M.A.), Nutritional Sciences (Ph.D.), and Public Health (M.P.H.). Her credentials for editing this book are many. She has been conducting research in the area of sports nutrition and exercise physiology for over 14 years, has published numerous papers on the nutritional needs of U.S. Navy SEALs, and has given many sports nutrition seminars to high school, college, and professional athletes, recreational athletes, SWAT teams, dietitians, and other health professionals. She is also an athlete herself. She was a tennis professional for five years and has competed in several triathlons and over 20 marathons; her best marathon time was a 2:48 in the Boston

Marathon. Dr. Deuster was a nationally ranked runner for several years and a qualifier for the First Women's Olympic Marathon Trials. She is an avid sportswoman and a former skydiver who has logged in over 100 jumps.

Anita Singh, Ph.D., wrote "Overview of Physical Fitness" and "Running for Fitness" and assisted Dr. Deuster with the editing of this guide. She is an Assistant Professor in the Department of Military and Emergency Medicine at the Uniformed Services University of the Health Sciences, Bethesda, Maryland. Dr. Singh has a Ph.D. in Nutrition from the University of Maryland and she has been working in the area of Sports Nutrition and Exercise Physiology for over 10 years. In addition to looking at nutritional needs of U.S. Navy SEAL trainees, she has studied marathoners, ultramarathoners, and recreational athletes. She has presented her research work at various national and international meetings. Dr. Singh has published extensively in scientific journals and she co-authored *The Navy SEAL Nutrition Guide.* She runs and plays tennis.

LDCR Kevin C. Walters, M.D., developed the chapter "Training for Specific Environments." He is a Diving Medical Officer at the Naval Special Warfare Center in Coronado, CA. Dr. Walters enlisted in the Navy in 1974 and graduated from BUD/S in 1976 (class 87) and served five and a half years at SEAL Team ONE. He left active duty in 1983 to return to college and graduate school. He received his M.D. degree in 1993 from the Uniformed Services University of the Health and subsequently completed a Transitional Internship at the Naval Medical Center, San Diego, CA.

CDR Steve Giebner, M.D., contributed to the chapter "Harmful Substances that Affect Performance." He is currently the Force Medical Officer for Commander, Naval Special Warfare Command. His association with the Naval Special Warfare community goes back to 1982 when he took his first operational assignment as the Diving Medical Officer for the Naval Special Warfare Training Department of the Naval Amphibious School, Coronado. He is also plank owner at Naval Special Warfare Center as the first Medical Officer assigned to that command.

Dr. Giebner specialized in Sport and Exercise Preventive Medicine and Health Promotion, having earned the Master of Public Health degree in the Preventive Medicine residency at the University of California at San Diego and San Diego State University. He has long been an active proponent of Sports Medicine in the Navy, and especially within Naval Special Warfare Training Department. His long association with Navy SEALs and his professional training uniquely qualify him to contribute to this manual.

In addition to recreational tennis, golf, and in-line skating, Dr. Giebner has consistently participated in command endorsed physical training programs throughout his Naval career. This year marks his first entry in the San Diego Marathon and a Superfrog Triathlon relay team.

HMC Denise E. Becker, USNR, developed "Appendix A—Weight Lifting Techniques" and assisted in the editing of this guide. She has a B.S. in Occupational Education and is pursuing a Masters degree in Exercise Physiology. She has served as the

Training Chief and is currently assigned to Assault Craft Unit-4 Det 1 as Division Officer and the Medical Department Representative. An avid sportswoman, she has participated in several half marathons, 10 and 5K races, and triathlons. She competed in the Tidewater All-Navy Tennis Tournament. Chief Becker is married to a SEAL, A1 Becker, LCDR, USN-RET and they have five children. The whole family has participated in the UDT/ SEAL Reunion Family Fun Run the past 10 years.

Foreword to Part I

The U.S. Navy SEAL Guide to Fitness was written specifically for the SEAL community by a team of Navy SEALs, physicians, and physiologists. The objectives of the guide are: to create a definitive instructional guide on SEAL physical fitness and cardiovascular health requirements; to enhance the physical abilities required to perform SEAL mission-related physical tasks; to promote long-term cardiovascular health and physical fitness; to prevent injuries and accelerate return to duty; and to maintain physical readiness under deployed or embarked environments.

The U.S. Navy SEALs are considered not only the toughest but also the most versatile and fittest warriors on the planet. SEAL is the acronym for Sea, Air, and Land. Navy SEALs train and operate in every environment the planet has to offer from parachuting into enemy and hostile terrain to swimming in rough seas, diving in icy waters, and conducting maritime operations launching from submarines, small craft, ships, fixed wing aircraft, and helicopters. They operate in arctic, mountain, desert, and jungle terrain. A Navy SEAL can operate efficiently anywhere in this world and can insert or extract from the area of operation (AO) in every possible means the military has to offer. Navy SEALs not only have to be incredibly fit, but also must be able to operate under any condition and in any environment.

From its early beginnings, SEALs and their predecessors faced some of the most physically challenging operations in the history of the U.S. military. The Navy has always required its operators to be in top physical condition to meet the rigorous demands placed on them.

Navy SEALs origins go back to the Scouts and Raiders, whose historical mission was to conduct the pre-invasion recon of the Normandy beaches and to guide the assault waves onto the beaches. Among the earliest of the Navy SEAL predecessors were the Operational Swimmers of the Office of Strategic Services (OSS). Many of the early SEAL missions were assigned to the OSS prior to the establishment of the Underwater Demolition Teams (UDTs). These Navy frogmen, or "naked warriors," wore only swim suits, fins, and dive masks on combat operations. They saw action in every major amphibious landing of the war. During the Korean War, the UDTs conducted demolition raids on railroad tunnels and bridges along the Korean coast, supported mine-clearing operations, conducted beach and river reconnaissance, and infiltrated guerrillas behind enemy lines.

In 1962, the SEAL Teams were established and composed of men from the UDTs. The SEAL mission was to conduct counter guerilla warfare and clandestine operations in maritime and riverine environments. SEAL involvement in Vietnam began immediately after the teams were commissioned. In 1983, all UDTs were re-designated as SEAL Teams or Swimmer Delivery Vehicle Teams.

Naval Special Warfare (NSW) forces have since participated in: Grenada 1983; Persian Gulf 1987–1990; Panama 1989–1990; and Middle East/Persian Gulf 1990–199. Forces have conducted countless missions in Afghanistan, Bosnia, Haiti, Iraq, Liberia Somalia, and elsewhere.

During Operation Iraqi Freedom, Naval Special Warfare deployed the largest number of SEALs in its history. The SEALs were instrumental in numerous special reconnaissance and direct action missions, including the securing of the southern oil infrastructures; clearing waterways; the capture of high value targets; raids on suspected chemical, biological, and radiological sites; and the first POW rescue since World War II.

The Navy Special Warfare (NACSPECWAR) Community remains very focused on the objective of keeping it's personnel as physically fit as possible. NAVSPECWAR spends a great deal of time, money, and research on constantly finding methods to improve the fitness level of the SEALs.

The U.S. Navy SEAL Guide to Fitness provides a detailed, extensively researched report on the following topics:

◆ sports related injuries,
◆ prevention and treatment of injuries,
◆ exercise physiology,
◆ muscle structure and function,
◆ principles of physical training,
◆ energy systems,
◆ and methods of physical training.

It also includes information regarding training in various environments, altitudes, and climate, as well as lessons on how and when to stretch, calisthenics, plyometrics, swimming, and running. In addition to these areas, this book will also help with gear selection. And most importantly—and unlike any other book of its kind— *The U.S. Navy SEAL Guide to Fitness* describes the physical requirements specific to SEAL training and missions.

The U.S. Navy SEAL Guide to Fitness has been a tremendous resource to the Naval Special Warfare Community throughout the years. This edition includes research on training principles as they apply to the SEAL community. If you are interested in a comprehensive guide on training, preventing injuries, and applying your training to the Navy SEAL mission, this guide is for you.

Don Mann
CWO3/SEAL/ret

An Introduction by RADM Raymond C. Smith

Membership in the Naval Special Warfare (NSW) community requires an extraordinarily high level of total body physical fitness. A combination of muscular strength, flexibility and cardiovascular fitness is essential to carry out assigned missions.

To train most effectively for these physically demanding tasks, SEALs and others within the NSW community need clear, concise, and authoritative guidance on physical fitness training regimens. This manual, *The Navy SEAL Fitness Guide*, has been written to meet this need.

The authors of this comprehensive guide, physicians and physiologists, were chosen because of their special qualifications in the area of physical fitness and their knowledge of the NSW and SEAL community. Their expertise ensured the guide would be written with the unique requirements of the NSW community in mind, and that our goal of expanding the individual Navy SEAL's knowledge of attaining and retaining a high level of fitness would be achieved.

I commend *The Navy SEAL Fitness Guide* as a superb source of information. Following the advice in this guide will enable SEALs and other members of the NSW community to prepare for the physically demanding missions to which they are assigned in the future.

Introduction to Part I
Physical Fitness

***The U.S. Navy SEAL Guide to Fitness* has been prepared** for the SEAL community with several goals in mind. Our objective is to provide you, the operator, with information to help:

◆ Enhance the physical abilities required to perform Special Operations mission-related physical tasks;

◆ Promote long-term cardiovascular health and physical fitness;

◆ Prevent injuries and accelerate return to duty;

◆ Maintain physical readiness under deployed or embarked environments.

If this guide is able to achieve those goals, it will be a major success. Being a SEAL is a tough job and requires enormous physical strength and stamina. Injuries, both chronic and acute are occupational hazards, but there are training measures and precautions that can be used to decrease the incidence of these injuries. Understanding the basics of physical fitness can go a long way to achieving these goals.

Physical fitness is typically considered a set of characteristics that people gain through various physical efforts. In fact, physical fitness consists of a variety of **measurable** components, some of which are skill-related and others which are health-related. The components of physical fitness are presented in Table I-1.

Table I-1. Skill- and Health-Related Components of Physical Fitness

Skill-Related	Health-Related
Agility	Cardiorespiratory endurance
Balance	Muscular endurance
Coordination	Muscular strength
Speed	Body composition
Power	Flexibility
Reaction time	

Definitions for each of these components/terms are provided in Chapter 1: Overview of Physical Fitness; all are extremely important in SEAL training. Because these components are measurable, it is clear that there are levels of physical fitness which can range from very low to exceptionally high. Moreover, a wide range may exist across particular components within an individual. For example, a person may have exceptional cardiorespiratory endurance but have very poor flexibility. Thus, a high level in one component does not translate into high physical fitness. A highly fit person should achieve a high level in each of the health-related components for protection of health. However, for SEAL training, components of both skill and health-related groups are requisite. This guide should help you achieve a more favorable balance among the various components, and serve as a resource for you in the future.

Chapter 1
Overview of Physical Fitness

This chapter will introduce terms and definitions commonly used to measure or define fitness levels and other terms associated with athletic training. Terms such as aerobic and anaerobic will be appearing throughout this fitness guide and various training techniques to optimize fitness will be discussed in greater detail in subsequent chapters. We suggest that you take some time to familiarize yourself with the terms and concepts in this chapter as this will greatly enhance your ability to apply the information provided in the remaining chapters.

Exercise Physiology

Exercise physiology is a branch of science which studies how the body responds and adapts physically to exercise training or to an acute bout of physical exertion. Such information is used for designing physical education, fitness and athletic programs. Physical fitness includes cardiopulmonary endurance, body composition, muscular strength and endurance, and flexibility.

Definitions and Terminology

Following are some commonly used exercise physiology terms and their definitions. You will come across many of these terms in subsequent chapters.

Aerobic: A process of producing energy that requires oxygen.

Aerobic Capacity: Total or maximal amount of aerobic work that can be done.

Aerobic Metabolism: Most of the energy needed to support exercise that goes beyond 3 minutes is provided by aerobic or oxidative energy metabolism. In other words oxygen is required to produce energy.

Agility: Ability to change physical position with speed and accuracy.

Anaerobic: A process of producing energy that does not require the presence of oxygen.

Anaerobic Capacity: Total or maximal amount of anaerobic work that can be done.

Anaerobic Glycolysis: A process of breaking down glycogen stores without oxygen; lactate (lactic acid) is the by-product of this process.

Anaerobic Metabolism: A type of energy metabolism that does not require oxygen.

Anaerobic Threshold: Transition point when aerobic metabolism can no longer meet the energetic demands, and energy from sources independent of oxygen are required. This is also the work rate at which blood lactate concentrations start to increase during graded exercise.

Adenosine Triphosphate (ATP): Energy released from food is stored in the muscle in the form of ATP. When ATP is broken down energy is released.

Balance: Ability to maintain equilibrium when stationary or while moving.

Cardiorespiratory Fitness: Ability of the heart, lung, and blood vessels to transport oxygen and to remove waste products from the exercising muscle.

Concentric Contraction: Shortening of the muscle as it develops tension. This type of exercise is sometimes also known as "positive exercise."

Coordination: Ability to use the senses, such as sight, along with the functioning of a set of muscle groups to complete an activity accurately. For example: hand-eye coordination during rifle shooting.

Dynamic Exercise: Alternate contraction and relaxation of a skeletal muscle or muscles causing partial or complete range of movement through a joint.

Eccentric Contraction: Involves the lengthening of a muscle as it develops tension and is also known as "negative exercise." Eccentric contractions are used when resisting gravity as is the case in walking down hill or down stairs.

Electrocardiogram (ECG): A tracing that shows the electrical activity of the heart.

Ergometer: Instrument used to measure work and power.

Ergometry: Measurement of work and power during exercise.

Exercise: Planned, structured, and repetitive movements performed to improve or maintain components of physical fitness. The components include cardiorespiratory fitness, muscle strength and endurance, flexibility and body composition (see Introduction).

Fartlek Training: An unstructured type of interval training for speed-work.

Flexibility: Controlled range of motion of a specific joint. The range is a function of elasticity of the tendons, ligaments, and surrounding soft tissue. Control is a function of strength at each degree of motion, especially at the end ranges.

Glycogen: A form of carbohydrates that is stored in the liver and in muscles for energy.

Glycolysis: Breaking down of simple sugars into simpler compounds (chiefly pyruvate and lactate) for energy. This process is anaerobic.

Glycolytic: Pertaining to or promoting glycolysis.

Heart Rate: Number of heart beats per minute.

Interval Training: Very intense exercise bouts are alternated with rest or periods of low intensity exercise. Exercise during intervals is typically anaerobic.

Isokinetic: Contraction of a muscle or muscle group which results in joint movement at a constant angular velocity. For example: the arm stroke during free style swimming.

Isometric (Static): Muscle contracts without shortening or lengthening such that tension is developed but no muscular work is performed; energy is lost as heat. There is no joint movement during this type of exercise.

Isotonic (Dynamic): Muscle contracts and maintains constant tension by lengthening or shortening.

Lactic Acid (lactate): A by-product of anaerobic metabolism.

Ligament: A band of fibrous tissue that connects bone to bone or bone to cartilage so as to strengthen joints.

Maximal Oxygen Uptake (VO2max): A measure of aerobic fitness: the maximal rate of oxygen uptake, and therefore aerobic energy utilization during exercise. Typically expressed as liters per minute or milliliters per kilogram (kg) of body weight per minute (ml/min/kg).

MET (Metabolic Equivalent Unit): A unit used to estimate the metabolic cost of physical activity. One MET is the energy used by an individual at rest. This is equivalent to 3.5 ml of oxygen consumed per kg body weight per minute.

Metabolism: Physical and chemical processes that maintain life.

Minute Ventilation: Volume of air breathed per minute.

Muscular Endurance: Ability of a muscle or muscle group to contract at a submaximal force, usually against 50 to 60% of maximal resistance, over a period of time. Measured as the number of repetitions completed.

Muscular Strength: Maximal force or tension generated by a muscle or muscle group.

Myoglobin: An iron containing muscle protein that is responsible for the reddish color of various muscle fiber types.

Physical Activity: Movement by skeletal muscles that results in energy expenditure.

Physical Fitness: Ability to perform physical activity.

Plyometrics: Also known as explosive jump training. Muscles are rapidly stretched prior to contraction. Examples include standing jumps, multiple jumps, etc.

Power: Ability of a muscle to quickly generate force over a very short period of time. Examples include sprint starts, vertical jumps, lunges, and throwing a punch.

Rating of Perceived Exertion (RPE): Measured using the Borg Category RPE Scale. As exercise intensity increases, the RPE increases and in general it is closely associated with physiological measures such as heart rate and oxygen consumption.

Reaction Time: Time taken between receiving a signal and reacting to it.

Respiratory Exchange Ratio: Ratio of carbon dioxide produced to oxygen consumed. An indication of the primary energy source used during exercise.

Speed: Ability to perform a movement in a short period of time.

Strength: Ability of a muscle to contract against resistance and provide control throughout the full range of motion.

Stroke Volume: Volume of blood pumped from the heart with each beat.

Tendon: A fibrous cord in which the fibers of a muscle end and by which the muscle is attached to a bone or other structure.

Tidal Volume: Volume of air moved during one breathing cycle while inhaling or exhaling.

Muscle Structure and Function

The three major types of muscle are:

◆ Cardiac muscle
◆ Skeletal muscle
◆ Smooth muscle

This discussion will be limited to skeletal muscles which, by converting chemical energy to mechanical energy, produce movement. We will present a description of the subtypes of skeletal muscles, including their characteristics and distribution. Although there may be many new subtypes of skeletal muscle fibers, generally skeletal muscle can be characterized into three basic types:

◆ Slow Twitch Oxidative (Type I)
◆ Fast Twitch Oxidative-Glycolytic (Type IIa)
◆ Fast Twitch Glycolytic (Type IIb)

Type I Muscle Fibers

Type I muscle fibers are involved in endurance activities. These fibers, also called **slow twitch fibers**, are noted for their ability to produce energy in the presence of oxygen. Thus, they are primarily aerobic. The main fuel source for this fiber is **fats (fatty acids)**, which allow the muscle to work at a steady rate with noticeable resistance to fatigue. Their color is typically quite red, a result of the high content of "myoglobin", an iron-containing protein that stores and delivers oxygen. Slow twitch fibers are not noted for their speed, their anaerobic capacity, or their ability to contract at a fast rate repeatedly, but rather their indefatigability and aerobic capacity.

Type II Muscle Fibers

Type II fibers can be categorized into at least two types: Type IIa and Type IIb. These fibers are adapted for strength and power activities. The **Type IIa fiber** is a cross between a slow twitch and a fast twitch fiber in that it is both aerobic (oxidative) and anaerobic (glycolytic). Whereas, it is "faster" than the slow twitch fiber, it is not as well suited for endurance activities. Its color is also reddish, a result of the myoglobin content.

In contrast, the **Type IIb fiber** is truly a fast twitch fiber, with very high contraction speeds. These fibers are almost exclusively anaerobic and have minimal capacity for aerobic production of energy. They rely primarily on glycogen within the muscle for energy and are therefore very susceptible to fatigue. Their color is pale, and some consider it "white" because it lacks myoglobin. Type IIb fibers tend to accumulate lactate, which ultimately leads to rapid fatigue if the lactate is not removed.

It should be noted that each of the fiber types has different recruitment patterns, and typically the Type IIb fiber is only recruited for use during maximal effort. The other fibers contract during light as well as moderate activity. **Moreover, physical training can lead to changes in the characteristics of the fibers.** Thus, endurance training would lead to changes in the Type IIa fiber such that they take on more characteristics of the Type I, or slow twitch fiber. Table 1-1 presents the distinguishing characteristics of the various fiber types.

Table 1-1. Distinguishing Characteristics of Major Muscle Fiber Types

Fiber Characteristic	Slow Twitch	Type II a Fast Twitch	Type II b Fast Twitch
Aerobic Capacity	High	Moderate/High	Low
Anaerobic Capacity	Low	High	High
Contraction Speed	Slow	Fast	Fast
Fatigue Resistance	High	Moderate/High	Low
Myoglobin Content	High	High	Low
Glycogen Content	Low	Moderate	High
Color	Red	Reddish-white	White

Distribution of Fiber Types

The amount of Type I and Type II muscle fibers in an individual is genetically pre-determined, and all normal skeletal muscle contains all fiber types. However, the proportion or distribution of these fiber types within and across individuals differs. Moreover, within an individual, the distribution of fibers in various muscles can vary widely. **Physical training may transform muscle fiber type, and the metabolic capacity of both type I and type II muscle fibers can be modified by endurance and power training.** It should be noted that performance depends not only on your fiber type composition, but also on the interplay between a variety of factors such as training, and diet, etc. Figure 1-1 represents the average percentage of slow twitch (Type I) fibers found in various subgroups of the population. As can be seen, persons whose activities are primarily endurance-related have a higher proportion of Type I fibers as compared to sprinters or wrestlers. Also in Figure 1-1 are the maximal aerobic capacities of these groups: the greater the proportion of Type I fibers, the higher the maximal aerobic capacity. Note the wide variability in the group of "recreational athletes." Specific types of training can induce changes in muscle fiber composition and characteristics.

Figure 1-1. Muscle Fiber Composition and Maximal Oxygen Uptake Values for Various Athletes by Sport

Figure adapted from: *Exercise Physiology: Energy Nutrition and Human Performance*, McArdle WD, FI Katch, VL Katch. 4th edition. 1996. Williams and Wilkins Publishers.

Principles of Physical Training

The goal of any training program is to improve performance. You are unique in terms of your excellent physical condition and your dedication to further enhancing your fitness. The four principles that apply to all physical training programs are discussed below.

Overload

According to this principle, exercise must be done at a higher level than usual to bring about various training adaptations. Once the body has adapted to the higher level of exercise it will function more effectively and efficiently. **The overload can be obtained by manipulating various combinations of exercise frequency, intensity, duration and type of exercise.** Increasing intensity, duration and frequency can be helpful for running, cycling or swimming, and increasing resistance and repetitions can improve strength training.

Specificity of Training

This principle refers to the training-induced adaptations in metabolic and physiologic systems which are specific to the type of exercise. For example, running will increase physical fitness but it will not increase swimming performance and vice versa. Thus, it is important to train muscles involved in a specific type of exercise to realize greater performance benefits.

Individual Differences

Responses to a particular training program can vary from one individual to another. According to this principle, exercise programs should be individualized to meet the training requirements and physical capacity of each person.

Detraining

Regular exercise is necessary to maintain fitness. Beneficial effects of exercise are gradually lost or reversed after a few weeks off from training. This deconditioning or detraining effect will be discussed later in this chapter.

Because of the nature of your missions it is imperative that you develop all aspects of physical fitness: strength, speed, flexibility, and endurance. Therefore, it is important for you to consider your training in terms of the FITT principle.

FITT = Frequency, Intensity, Time & Type

All four aspects of the **FITT** principle must be included to achieve the most benefit from your training program. Number and intensity of workouts is important as is the time spent exercising and cross training (see Chapter 3). Information on how to determine your training intensity is provided next.

Determining Your Training Heart Rate

When reading the training methods presented in this chapter and throughout this guide, you will come across references to exercise intensity. **Intensity is the rate at which exercise is performed.** If you work out in a gym you may have used an exercise machine that monitors exercise intensity. A quick and easy method for measuring the intensity of your workout is by measuring your heart rate and checking to see if you are within your target training zone (see below).

Measure your heart rate by taking your pulse at the carotid artery (neck) or the radial artery (wrist) for 15 seconds; multiply this value by four to get your heart rate in beats per minute. Compare this heart rate value to your target training intensity. If your heart rate is too low, increase the intensity of your workout. If it is too high, reduce the intensity slightly.

Your target training heart rate can be calculated as follows:

To maintain aerobic conditioning, exercise should be performed at a heart rate between 70% and 90% of your **maximal heart rate (Max HR).**

Remember, this is only an estimate of your maximal heart rate.

Depending on your particular "physiology" and physical conditioning, your Max HR could be higher than what you derive from this equation. However, this is the way it is routinely estimated.

Max HR in beats per minute = 220 - your age (years)

To calculate 70% and 90% of your Max HR, multiply Max HR by 0.70 and 0.90, respectively. This is your target training intensity zone or the range within which your heart rate should be while working out. Figure 1-2 presents an example of how to calculate your desired training heart rate by this method.

Figure 1-2. An Example for Determining Your Target Training Heart Rate

Determining Your Target Heart Rate

A SEAL is 22 years old

Max HR = 220 - 22 = 198 bpm

Lower Target HR = 0.7 X 198 = 139 bpm

Upper Target HR = 0.9 X 198 = 178 bpm

Calculate your target training heart rate zone using the formula provided above or use the chart shown in Figure 1-3. It is important to note that maximal heart rates tend to be lower during swimming and arm exercises. For these activities you should subtract 13 from your maximal heart rate before obtaining your training heart rate. An example of this is shown in Figure 1-4.

Figure 1-3. Target Training Heart Rate Zone

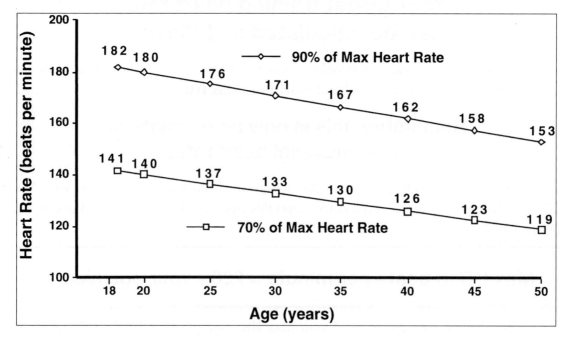

Figure 1-4. An Example for Determining Your Target Training Heart Rate for Swimming

> **A 22 year old SEAL wants to swim at 70% of Max HR**
>
> **Then his Max HR = 220 - 22 = 198 -13 = 185 bpm**
>
> **70% of Max HR = 0.7 X 185 = 130 bpm**

Energy Systems Used by Exercising Muscle

Before describing the methods used for physical training, it is important to understand the three systems that provide energy to the exercising muscle. All three systems are important. Depending on the activity, there may be a greater reliance on one system over the others.

ATP-CP System for Speed Work

Adenosine triphosphate (ATP) is the immediate source of energy within all cells of our body for activities such as sprinting. There are small stores of ATP within skeletal muscle, and these energy stores provide immediate energy to sustain physical activities for a short time. Once the ATP is used, it breaks down into adenosine diphosphate (ADP). For regeneration of ADP into ATP for more energy, creatine phosphate (CP) is needed. It is the CP that regenerates the ATP. Without CP, ATP could provide energy for only a few seconds. With CP, the ATP-PC system can provide energy for about 30 seconds before other energy systems must take over. Thus, this ATP-CP system, sometimes referred to as the phosphate pool or reservoir, provides immediate anaerobic energy for muscle contraction.

$$ATP \longrightarrow ADP + Phosphate + Energy$$

$$ADP + CP \longrightarrow ATP + Creatine$$

Lactic Acid and ATP-CP System for Anaerobic Work

This is a transitional system. When all-out exercise continues beyond 30 seconds, the only way to continue providing ATP to the exercising muscle is by using sugar (glucose) in the muscle. Sugar in the muscle is obtained from glycogen, and the process of breaking down sugar for energy is called glycolysis. However, in the process of generating ATP from glucose, lactic acid (also known as lactate) is formed. Normally there is a only a small amount of lactate in blood and muscle. When lactate begins to accumulate in muscle and then blood, you will begin to experience muscular fatigue, unless it is cleared by the body. Lactate is cleared from the muscle if the intensity of the exercise is moderate. This happens because after a few minutes the aerobic or oxygen system which supplies energy for sustained work kicks in. If an all out effort is sustained, fatigue is inevitable within three to five minutes.

Oxygen System for Aerobic Energy

The oxygen, or aerobic, system provides energy to support long-term steady state exercise, such as long distance running or swimming. **Muscles can use both glucose and fatty acids for energy.** These fuel sources can be taken from the circulating blood and from stores within the muscle. Glucose is stored as glycogen and fatty acids are stored as "triglycerides" in the muscle. When long duration activities are performed at a slow pace more "fat" in the form of fatty acids is used for energy than muscle glycogen.

During many types of exercise, all three energy transfer systems are used at various times. The amount that each system contributes to energy metabolism is related to the duration, intensity and type of activity. In general, high intensity, short duration exercises rely mainly on anaerobic energy. Other examples specific to various activities are provided in Table 1-2.

Table 1-2. Percentage Contributed by Each Energy System to Overall Energy Needs of Various Activities

Physical Activity	ATP-CP System (%)	Lactic Acid and ATP-CP System (%)	Oxygen Aerobic System (%)
Marathon	-	5	95
Rowing	20	30	50
Running - 100 m	98	2	-
Running - 1 mile	20	55	25
Running - 3 miles	10	20	70
Running - 6 miles	5	15	80
Skiing Downhill - Racing	80	20	-
Skiing - Cross-Country	-	5	95
Swimming - 50 m	98	2	-
Swimming - 100 m	80	15	5
Swimming - 200 m	30	65	5
Swimming - 400 m	20	40	40
Swimming - 1500 m	10	20	70

Methods of Physical Training

Most people think of exercise as being either aerobic or anaerobic. However, in most types of exercise, a blend of both aerobic and anaerobic exercise is involved. For example, during a 1500 m run, energy is provided by anaerobic metabolism at the beginning and the end of the run whereas aerobic metabolism supports the middle or the *steady state* part of the run. Aerobic and anaerobic capacity can be improved by using appropriate physical training techniques. The contribution of the three energy systems to the various training methods is shown in Table 1-3. The various physical training techniques are presented below and can be used for enhancing performance during various physical activities.

Table 1-3. Contribution of the Various Energy Systems According to Training Methods

Training Method	ATP-CP System (%)	Lactic Acid and ATP-CP System (%)	Oxygen Aerobic System (%)
Interval Training*	10-80	10-80	10-80
Sprint Training	90	6	4
Acceleration Sprints	90	5	5
Interval Sprints	20	10	70
Fartlek Training	20	40	40
Continuous Running	2	5-8	90-93
Repetition Running	10	50	40

*Depends on rate and distance of exercise interval, type of relief interval and number of repetitions.

Interval Training

Exercise bouts are alternated with rest or relief periods. Relief periods usually involve mild to light exercise. Generally, in swimming no exercise is performed during the relief periods. The duration, intensity, and number (repetitions) of exercise bouts and the length and type of relief intervals are chosen to suit specific exercise performance requirements. Interval training allows you to exercise at a higher intensity than you could if you were exercising continuously. This type of training helps to develop the muscle ATP-PC energy system. Both aerobic and anaerobic metabolism can be improved by interval training.

Sprint Training

Sprint training helps develop speed and increase muscle strength. Individuals are required to sprint repeatedly at maximum speed while allowing for complete recovery between sprints. In general, 6 seconds are needed to go from a stationary position to maximum speed. For a runner this would mean running 55 to 60 meters to reach that maximum speed.

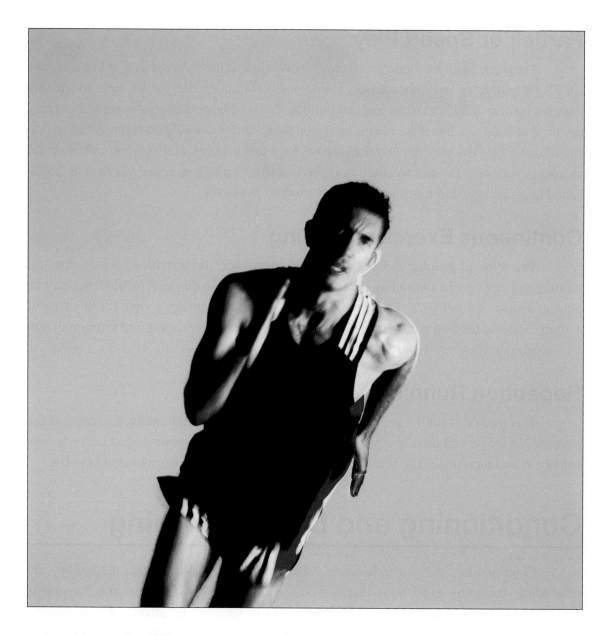

Interval Sprints

This method involves alternately sprinting for 45 to 50 meters and jogging for 55 to 60 meters while covering a distance of about 3 miles. Interval sprinting helps to develop aerobic capacity.

Acceleration Sprints

Acceleration sprint training develops speed and strength. Running speed is gradually increased from jogging to striding to sprinting, followed by a recovery walk. This sequence is repeated. Intervals may range from 50 to 100 meters each. For example: 50 meters jogging, 50 meters striding, 50 meters sprinting and 50 meters walking.

Fartlek or Speed Play

The work *Fartlek* means "speed play" in Swedish. It involves running at fast and slow speeds on both level and hilly courses. Unlike interval training, the *fartlek* form of training does not involve specific exercise and rest periods; you do it as desired. For example, you may say to your buddy, "I'll race you to the next stop sign," and you would both run as fast as you can to that point. You may run at a slower pace for a few minutes, and then run fast again for as long as you want. In other words, it is a speed workout without structure. As such, it is well suited to general conditioning and provides variety to workouts.

Continuous Exercise Training

This type of training is needed to build endurance for activities such as distance running and open ocean swimming. Exercise is performed with distance in mind and may be done at a slow or a fast pace. The aerobic system is the main energy source for this type of activity. Specific training requirements for endurance training in running and swimming will be discussed in Chapters 4 and 5.

Repetition Running

This method is similar to interval training, but unlike interval training, the length of the intervals are longer and usually range from 0.5 to 2.0 miles. Recovery between intervals lasts until the heart rate is under 120 beats per minute, or within 60% of your estimated Max HR.

Conditioning and Deconditioning

Conditioning and deconditioning, also known as training and detraining, are responsible for gains and losses, respectively, in fitness levels. Whereas conditioning is a gradual process and may take six or more weeks to see specific effects, deconditioning occurs relatively quickly. Some of the various metabolic and cardiorespiratory effects of conditioning are presented in Table 1-4.

Table 1-4. Various Effects of Physical Conditioning

Metabolic Changes	Cardiorespiratory Changes
⇑ levels of ATP, CP, glycogen	⇑ in blood volume
⇑ levels of anaerobic enzymes	⇓ heart rate at given workload
⇑ capacity to tolerate blood lactate	⇑ stroke volume
⇑ levels of oxygen within muscle	⇑ ability to take oxygen from blood
⇑ levels of aerobic enzymes	improvement in blood pressure
⇑ capacity to use fat as fuel	⇑ ability to handle heat load

Effects of deconditioning will be noticed within one to four weeks. Deconditioning reverses the positive metabolic, cardiac, respiratory and muscle enzyme effects that result from conditioning. Some major effects of deconditioning include:

◆ Decrease in maximal aerobic capacity—heart rate for a given exercise workload is higher and the amount of blood pumped by the heart with each beat is reduced.

◆ More rapid build up of lactic acid during exercise which leads to earlier fatigue.

◆ Reduction in levels of key muscle enzymes which regulate the muscle's ability to generate energy from various sources.

◆ Reduced ability to store glycogen in muscle between workouts.

◆ Reduced breathing volume which will decrease the amount of oxygen being taken to the exercising muscle.

◆ Decreased endurance capacity—time to fatigue is shortened.

◆ Decreased ability to dissipate body heat during exercise: the ability to exercise in adverse environments, such as in the heat, is reduced due to all factors mentioned above.

Retraining is necessary to reverse the performance reducing effects of deconditioning. **However, deconditioning can be prevented or minimized by maintaining usual exercise intensity during endurance and strength workouts, when the number or length of work outs is decreased.** Aerobic capacity and decreased lactic acid accumulation during exercise can be maintained by training at least two to three times per week at your usual training intensity. Strength gains can be maintained by including one to two strength training workouts sessions per week. Specific training methods for maintaining fitness under deployed conditions and while overcoming an injury will be discussed in other chapters (see Chapters 11 and 12).

Active Recovery

This type of recovery means that you continue to exercise at a low to moderate (30% to 50% of your maximal heart rate) intensity for several minutes after your regular workout. For example, walk for 5 to 10 minutes after completing a run. The benefits of active recovery and additional information about this type of recovery are provided in Chapter 3: Cardiorespiratory Conditioning.

Chapter 2
SEAL Mission-Related Physical Activities

The primary goal of SEAL physical fitness training is to maximize mission-related performance. SEALs need a physical training program which encompasses all of the various mission-related tasks that need to be performed. Thus, before deciding on a physical fitness training regimen, the specific types of athletic activities involved in your missions must be clearly defined. It is important for you to establish specific goals. An athlete training for a marathon will want to train such that he will finish the race in the shortest possible time. Everything else in your program will be secondary to the primary objective of maximizing lower extremity aerobic performance. Likewise, a kayaker will maximize his aerobic performance by focusing on upper extremity conditioning. A competitive weight lifter, in contrast, will strive to maximize the amount of weight that he can lift, with little or no emphasis on endurance training.

What are "mission-related tasks"?

As an illustration, let's consider bicycling. Cycling is a superb way to obtain an intense aerobic (or anaerobic) workout and is very useful in promoting general cardiovascular fitness, but SEALs do not cycle during missions. No mission scenarios require you to hop on your bike and ride 25 miles. In contrast, a two mile swim in fins also provides an excellent cardiovascular workout, and more closely approximates activities required on Special Warfare missions.

Although a good cardiovascular workout on a bike will confer a training benefit for SEALs, cycling is not the preferred substitute for mission-related training. Being in shape for one activity does not necessarily translate into being in shape for another activity which uses entirely different muscle groups. Training by running or biking to perform a long distance swim will result in a high incidence of muscle fatigue and leg cramps on the mission. Some swimming must be incorporated into a training program. Moreover, swimming with fins on a regular basis will ensure that the operator is comfortable in his fins and wet suit booties and prevent the development of painful blisters on the mission. Thus, there are many reasons for specificity of training.

Swimming is not the only mission-related task. The goal of this chapter is to present mission-specific activities and determine the physical tasks associated with these missions. **The doctrine that you should train as you fight is also true for physical fitness training.**

Mission-Specific Activities

What sort of physical activities will SEALs be required to perform in the course of their missions? To answer this question, the types of missions that you perform need to be examined. A partial list of these missions is shown in Table 2-1, and a brief description of these missions is provided below.

Table 2-1. A Summary of Various SEAL Missions

Types of SEAL Missions

Small Unit Patrolling

High Speed Boat Operations

Combat Swimmer Operations

SDV and Dry Deck Shelter Operations

Urban Warfare

Winter Warfare Operations

Small Unit Patrolling

One capability that will be needed in almost all SEAL land warfare operations is the ability to carry a substantial amount of weight over long distances. You will typically carry two weapons and a supply of ammunition. There is no good way to know exactly how much ammunition you will be required to carry for a particular mission and SEAL operators tend to pack heavy in this category. In addition, your loads will often include explosives and specialized items. Water needs to be carried in the loadout, and if the mission is a sustained one, rations must also be included. Loads of 70-80 pounds are standard in the community and much heavier loads are not uncommon. How far must you carry this load? There is no one distance that can accurately be used as an upper limit, but certainly 10-20 miles in a

24 hour period, depending on the difficulty of the terrain, may be required for some operations. Walking long distances with a heavy load is a significant challenge in itself, but you may also be required to run and scramble over terrain features, walls, and fences.

Load-carrying is one of the most important physical activities a SEAL can practice.

The ability to carry a wounded fellow operator on your back or shoulders is also important. Buddy shoulder carries are critical in that they are currently the anticipated mode of transporting a wounded SEAL to a secure area where medical care can be rendered. These carries are somewhat different than long distance hikes with equipment because the load is distributed quite differently on the body and in some cases, the weight of the wounded operator may be in addition to the basic load.

How do you train for these activities? Long distance runs with shorts and running shoes are useful in promoting cardiovascular fitness, but do not adequately simulate load-bearing activities. Similarly, the number of bench presses you can do at a given weight does not ensure your being able to walk long distances with a heavy load. Moreover, some of the problems associated with load-carrying are musculoskeletal injuries and blisters. These can only be avoided (or minimized) by practicing the specific activity.

High Speed Boat Operations

The Special Boat Environment imposes unique physical demands. Such missions typically include extended periods in transit, often at high speeds in stormy seas. This type of activity requires extraordinary stability of the knee, elbow, shoulder, and ankle joints. Since maintaining a slight bend in the knees, elbows, and ankles is essential for minimizing musculoskeletal injuries, training to improve muscle strength and endurance is critical.

Combat Swimmer Operations

With the current-day SEAL teams having had their origin in the Scouts and Raiders, Naval Combat Demolition Units, and Underwater Demolition Teams of World War II, it is not surprising that combat swimmer operations are still an important part of the Naval Special Warfare mission. These operations may last as little as one or two hours in some situations, and as long as eight to 10 hours in others. You may be swimming on the surface or swimming underwater compass courses with the Draeger LAR V or MK 16 closed-circuit underwater breathing apparatuses. These operations are often carried out in very cold water; thus, hypothermia is a constant concern. In many instances, you will be towing something in the water (usually something with a very rapid rate of combustion), thereby increasing the effort needed to accomplish the mission. Some missions involve exiting the water and climbing up the side of a ship using a caving ladder or other climbing apparatus. These are difficult maneuvers under any circumstances, but much more so when your hands are numb from cold exposure and you are climbing with weapons, ammunition, and explosives. **Regular exposure to cold water immersion will help to develop physiological adaptations so that you will fare better when subjected to cold water on a mission.** In addition, both upper body and leg strength are important for shipboarding techniques. **Grip strength, in particular, is critical for maintaining a firm hold on the rope or ladder.** Caving ladder or rope climbs are very important to develop the muscle groups that will be used for shipboarding; you should do these climbs with gear whenever possible.

Swimming with fins is an activity basic to all SEAL combat swimmer missions and should be done on a regular basis in team physical training evolutions. Swimming without fins, while a very good activity for promoting cardiovascular fitness, is not typically required for SEAL missions. It is important to mention that encouraging speed on combat swimmer operations is fine for surface swims, but should not be done on underwater swims because of the reduction in the LAR V operating range and increased risk of central nervous system oxygen toxicity.

High exercise rates under water increase the diver's chance of having an oxygen convulsion.

SDV and Dry Deck Shelter Operations

These operations are basically combat swimmer operations, but ones in which the SDV does the majority of the work. They are typically longer than operations in which free-swimming divers are used, but this is not always the case. As SDV operators, you need to be able to accomplish the same physical tasks noted for combat swimmers above. In addition, these operations may require significant upper body strength to handle the heavy equipment required for the mission both in the Dry Deck Shelter and later at the objective.

Urban Warfare

Some SEAL missions call for direct action operations in an urban setting. Although it is difficult to generalize, these missions might be expected to require less of a load-bearing challenge because some form of transportation will often be available. In addition, the distance to be covered on foot will typically be less than many remote missions. Generally, you will need to carry less food and water than with other types of land warfare missions. Your need for weapons and ammunition, however, will not be reduced, so significant gear loads are still a possibility. Additionally, you may need to perform demanding physical tasks, such as sprints and rapid stair climbs, in the urban warfare setting. Moreover, there is the potential of having to accomplish these maneuvers while carrying or dragging a wounded buddy or hostage.

Winter Warfare Operations

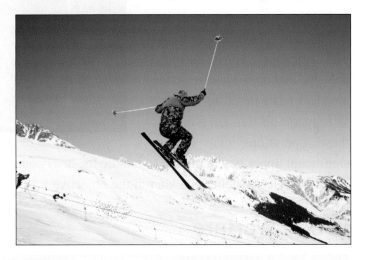

Winter Warfare operations often require long distance cross-country skiing or snowshoeing which will usually have to be done with a heavy equipment load. This activity requires the use of a different set of muscles than walking and running. Not all SEAL units have a primary mission area that requires the ability to operate in winter warfare environments, but those that do should consider cross-country skiing with equipment when designing their workout programs (see Chapter 14).

Specific Mission-Related Physical Tasks

In order to identify the physical demands of direct action SEAL operations, a study was undertaken in early 1990 by the Naval Health Research Center. Missions and the physical requirements (i.e., aerobic and anaerobic components) necessary to complete each mission and mission segment were evaluated. In brief, a total of 82 SEALs, averaging 11 years of experience, participated in the study. Subject matter experts from operational platoons were interviewed regarding missions they had conducted as SEALs. Information obtained during these interviews provided the basis for a questionnaire which was developed and given to the study participants. The questionnaire was composed of a list of missions and mission segments such as "fast rope to the deck of a ship from a height of 40 feet, carrying a 50- pound pack." Each SEAL participant ranked mission and mission segments on scales to rank: difficulty of performance, frequency of performance, and importance to mission success. The individual scores for each scale were then summed to obtain a "composite score". Mission tasks that received the highest composite scores are provided below.

- Walk (i.e., hump) 15 km over uneven terrain at night carrying a 125 lb pack to objective in 70°F, then retrace steps to extraction point.
- Serve as point person for an element, walking a distance of 42 km through dense jungle in tropical heat and humidity over a 3- day period carrying a 60 lb pack and weapons.
- Swim a distance of 2,000 meters in 56°F carrying a limpet mine and using a Draeger; return to Zodiac without limpet, then travel 6 km to extraction point.
- Swim for 3 hours underwater (temperature: 70°F), wearing a wet-suit, mask and fins, and using a Draeger UBA and attack board.
- Drag a fully-loaded F470 Zodiac 50 meters onto a rocky beach with five other SEALs, then, with three of the boat crew, quickly move all equipment and supplies across 200 meters of rocky beach and stage/cache gear in preparation for the overland phase of the mission.
- Perform a rescue drag of a wounded comrade weighing 170 lbs, dragging him by the web gear a distance of 75 meters, with the assistance of one other SEAL.

Given the above list of missions tasks, the question **"what are the physical fitness requirements necessary to complete each task?"** was asked. A summary of the physical tasks data is presented in Table 2-2 and Table 2-3. Table 2-3 presents the numerous physical tasks associated with the missions and the physical characteristics demanded of the SEAL. Table 2-3 extends these characteristics by delineating specific training plans to improve performance on the physical tasks.

Table 2-2. Physical Requirements for Specific Missions and Mission Elements

Mission	Physical Tasks	Physical Requirements
Small Unit Patrolling	Sprint with gear Fast roping Load bearing Long distance hike "Over the beach" Buddy carry Rock climbing	Leg endurance Shoulder/arm strength Shoulder/arm endurance Upper back strength Grip strength
Combat Swimmer	Caving ladder climbs Underwater swimming Surface swimming	Shoulder/arm strength Leg endurance Grip strength
SDV/Dry Deck Shelter	Underwater swimming Heavy equipment handling	Leg strength/endurance Shoulder/arm strength
Urban Warfare	Buddy shoulder carry Climbing buildings Running/sprinting with gear Stair climbing	Shoulder/arm strength Leg strength/endurance Grip strength
High Speed Boats	Maintain joint stability at high speeds Extended periods in transit	Shoulder/arm strength Shoulder/arm endurance Leg strength/endurance Grip strength
Winter Warfare	Snow shoeing with gear Skiing with gear	Upper back strength Upper back endurance Leg strength/endurance Shoulder/arm strength Shoulder/arm endurance Grip strength

Table 2-3. Specific Physical Task-Related Training

Physical Tasks	Task-Related Training
Run/sprint with gear	Running/intervals
Load bearing Long distance hike	Weight training
"Over the beach"	Plyometrics
Buddy shoulder carry	Load-bearing hikes
Obstacle negotiation with gear	Grip strength
Fast roping	Grip strength
Caving ladder	Rope climbs
Rock climbing	Squeezing tennis balls
Climbing buildings	Weight training
	O'course
Swim with fins	Surface swims
Underwater swimming	Underwater swims
Swimming with load	
Snow shoeing	Cross-country skiing
Skiing with gear	Distance running
	Load-bearing hikes
	Weight training
Maintain joint stability at high speeds	Weight training
	Grip strength

The critical point in these tables is that your physical training program must be a whole body conditioning program with upper and lower body endurance, flexibility, and strength activities. Most missions involve multiple physical tasks, therefore, an effective training program must address the physical requirements of all these tasks. The training program provided in the last chapter has been designed with this goal in mind.

SEAL training must be whole body conditioning with upper and lower body endurance, flexibility, and strength activities.

Summary

The most important types of SEAL mission-related athletic activities are listed below. Each of these activities should be incorporated into a training program, ideally on a weekly basis. For other/substitute activities, please refer to Chapter 15: Physical Fitness and Training Recommendations.

◆ Long distance hikes with heavy equipment loads

◆ Cross-country skiing with equipment

◆ Caving ladder climbs with gear

◆ Swimming with fins

◆ Sprints with gear

◆ Obstacle negotiation with gear

◆ Fast-roping

For more information you may wish to consult the Navy Technical Report: No. 95-24 entitled: "Physical Demands of U.S. Navy Sea-Air-Land (SEAL) Operations," WK Prusaczyk, JW Stuster, HW Goforth, Jr., T Sopchick Smith, and LT Meyer.

Chapter 3
Cardiorespiratory Conditioning

The American College of Sports Medicine (ACSM) and the Centers for Disease Control and Prevention recently formulated new guidelines for the American public with respect to exercise. The new recommendations state that *"Every U.S. adult should accumulate 30 minutes or more of moderate intensity physical activity on most, preferably all, days of the week."* They defined moderate intensity physical activity as "activity performed at an intensity of 3 to 6 METS, or the equivalent of brisk walking at 3 to 4 m.p.h. for most healthy adults." Whereas the previous recommendations for the U.S. population emphasized the importance of extended periods of strenuous exercise, these new guidelines state that short, intermittent bouts of moderate exercise are important and sufficient for health benefits. The overall goal of these organizations is to promote cardiorespiratory conditioning, an important aspect of overall fitness, health, and disease prevention. However, activity above and beyond the recommendations for the public is necessary for SEALs and other highly competitive athletes. In this chapter we will discuss:

◆ Basic concepts of cardiorespiratory conditioning
◆ How to estimate your maximal aerobic capacity
◆ Types of aerobic activities and basic workouts

Many of the definitions and terminology associated with cardiorespiratory conditioning have been presented in Chapter 1. However, other terms are used interchangeably to reflect cardiorespiratory conditioning; these include cardiovascular, cardiopulmonary, and aerobic conditioning. The important point is that this form of conditioning improves health and work capacity by enhancing the circulation and overall functioning of the heart and lungs.

Basics Concepts of Cardiorespiratory Exercise

Cardiorespiratory conditioning consists of both aerobic exercise, which requires oxygen to sustain muscle activity, and anaerobic exercise, which does not use oxygen for the short bursts of highly intense activity. Most daily work and activities are aerobic in nature, and thus, improving the delivery of oxygen to the working skeletal muscle will improve work performance. Your ability to utilize oxygen for exercise depends on a variety of processes including:

◆ Functioning of vyour muscles of respiration or pulmonary ventilation
◆ Ability of oxygen to diffuse across lungs into your blood
◆ Ability of heart to increase rate of beating and amount of blood pumped with each beat
◆ Ability of blood vessels in and surrounding skeletal muscle to regulate blood flow
◆ Ability of contracting skeletal muscle to extract and use oxygen in blood

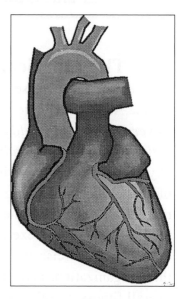

All of these factors are important in determining your ability to sustain a submaximal workload and your maximal aerobic capacity. Two other factors which help determine maximal aerobic capacity are your percentage of specific muscle fiber types and your genetic makeup. Some persons are endowed with a high aerobic capacity, whereas others are not. However, everyone can and will improve if a cardiorespiratory conditioning program is followed.

Terms Related to Conditioning

Many terms are used to define or describe exercise conditioning and work rate, also referred to as exercise intensity or work load. The two terms used throughout this chapter for describing how to gauge your work rate will be maximal oxygen uptake and energy expenditure as calories/hour or kcal/ hr. Other terms to describe work rate and their interrelationships will be discussed at the end of this chapter.

Maximal Oxygen Uptake

The primary measure or predictors of one's capacity to sustain work performance is maximal oxygen uptake (VO_{2max}) or maximal aerobic (cardiorespiratory) capacity. VO_{2max} is measured in **milliliters per minute** (ml/min), **Liters/min**, or after adjusting for body weight in kilograms, as **ml/ kg/min**; a higher value indicates a higher level of cardiorespiratory fitness.

Your maximal aerobic capacity or oxygen uptake is the best indicator of how much work you can sustain without fatigue.

Typical VO_{2max} values range from 30 ml (of oxygen)/kg/min for an unfit person up to 80 ml/kg/min for an exceptionally fit, endurance athlete. If the unfit and highly fit persons both weighed 70 kg (155 lb) then their respective absolute maximal aerobic capacities would be 2.1 liters (of oxygen)/ min and 5.6 liters (of oxygen)/min.

Using 1 liter of oxygen/min is equivalent to expending 5 kcal/min

As such, the unfit person can only work at a rate of up to 10 kcal/min (2.1 L x 5) whereas the highly fit could work at up to 25 kcal/min (5.6 L x 5 kcal) if needed. If a specific task required 2 L/min, then this would amount to 10 kcal/min of energy. Resting energy expenditure requires less than one kcal/min, or about 0.200 to 0.250 L (of oxygen)/min. In order to account for different body sizes, resting energy expenditure for an individual is usually defined as:

3.5 ml of oxygen/kg body weight/minute.

Thus, for a 70 kg (155 lb) SEAL, resting energy expenditure would be approximately 245 ml/min or 0.245 L/min (3.5 x 70). This is equivalent to expending around 1 to 1.25 kcal/min.

Anaerobic Power

How much strenuous work can you sustain without oxygen? Most people can do very little for more than a couple of minutes. It is very important to realize that most people cannot work for very long at even 90% of their maximal aerobic capacity. This is because everyone has a threshold at which the balance between aerobic and anaerobic energy systems begins to favor the anaerobic; your muscles cannot extract enough oxygen to produce the required energy. This is called your **anaerobic threshold;** the turning point can be monitored by the accumulation of lactate in your blood. Of course, your body will know when there is too much lactate, because once lactate goes above a certain value, it starts to accumulate and unless you decrease your work rate, you will become too tired to continue working.

This anaerobic threshold, or "break point" varies among individuals, but ranges between 60% and 100% of your VO_{2max}; all SEALs should be able to work at 70% of their VO_{2max} for an extended period and should have a break point above 70%. Conditioning programs for SEALs should strive to raise the anaerobic threshold or break point to as high as possible, because that means you can work at a higher rate for a longer period of time.

Interval workouts stress the anaerobic energy systems and will increase your anaerobic threshold and power.

Interval and fartlek workouts for running and swimming are described in their respective chapters, and such workouts for other forms of exercise are described later in this chapter.

Determination of Work Rate

One common denominator across all types of cardiorespiratory conditioning programs is exercise intensity and work rate. The term exercise intensity typically refers to how hard you are working as a percent of your maximal aerobic capacity. For example, you could work at an intensity equivalent to 50% (easy), 70% (moderate), or 90% (strenuous) of your maximal aerobic capacity or maximal heart rate. You will learn how to estimate your maximal aerobic capacity below, but on average, a maximal capacity of 45 to 55 ml of oxygen/kg/min and a maximal heart rate of 200 beats per min would be typical for a 20 to 29 year old SEAL. Table 3-1 presents the relation between exercise intensity, oxygen uptake, and heart rate for a 20 year old SEAL with a maximal heart rate of 200 and a maximal oxygen uptake of 55 ml of oxygen/kg/min. Easy exercise would use 25 to 30 ml of oxygen/kg/min or a heart rate of about 130 bpm, whereas strenuous exercise would require a heart rate of around 180 bpm. However, you must know your maximal capacity or your maximal heart rate to actually quantify your exercise intensity in this way.

Table 3-1. Example of the Relation Between Exercise Intensity, Aerobic Capacity, and Heart Rate

Exercise Intensity (% of Maximal)	Oxygen Uptake (ml/kg/m in)	Heart Rate (bpm)
100% - Maximal	55	200
90% - Strenuous	50	187
70% - Moderate	39	160
50% - Easy	28	131

Factors Affecting the Training Response

The terms duration, frequency, and intensity are commonly used when talking about training for fitness or health. All training programs, whether running, biking, swimming, or climbing, strive to vary in duration, frequency, and intensity so as to optimize conditioning and minimize injuries. Five major factors determine the extent of your maximal aerobic capacity and the magnitude of your response to training. These include:

◆ Initial level of aerobic fitness
◆ Duration of exercise
◆ Frequency of exercise
◆ Intensity of exercise
◆ Genetics/heredity

General principles apply to all types of physical activities. Take the following general principles and apply them to your individual program.

◆ The degree of aerobic training is closely tied to intensity and total work, not to frequency of training. However, a minimum of 3 days per week is recommended.
◆ A greater training improvement (up to a point) will be noted if you exercise above 85% of VO_{2max} or 90% of your maximal heart rate once a week or every other week: interval training.
◆ Aerobic capacity will improve if exercise increases your heart rate to at least 70% of your maximum heart rate.
◆ A lower exercise intensity can be offset by exercise of longer duration.
◆ Maximal heart rate for swimming and other upper body exercise is lower than maximal heart rate for leg or whole body exercise. Thus, training heart rate (THR) can be 13 to 15 bpm lower for swimming/upper body exercise than when running, biking, or other whole body exercises.
◆ A threshold duration per workout has not been identified to maximize aerobic capacity.

Active Recovery

Throughout this guide, we will continually stress the importance of warming up, cooling down, and stretching. These are integral parts of any workout, regardless of the activity. The cool down, or recovery period, is very important because it will determine how you feel several hours after your workout. There are two types of recovery: active and passive. Passive recovery, in other words, just resting, was recommended many years ago, and is still recommended when you exercise below 50% of maximal capacity. Active recovery is now preferred for exercise exceeding 60% of maximal capacity to accelerate removal of lactate. This may help prevent muscle cramps, stiffness, and preserve performance during subsequent strenuous exercise.

Active recovery involves exercising at 30% to 50% of maximal capacity for 5 to 10 minutes after a strenuous workout.

Blood lactate removal after strenuous exercise is accelerated by active recovery: mild aerobic exercise.

How to Estimate Your Maximal Aerobic Capacity

Exercise testing is often conducted for assessment of cardiorespiratory fitness. Types of protocols currently used to assess cardiorespiratory fitness or aerobic capacity are **incremental work rate tests**, where the exercise work rate is increased by a uniform amount at predetermined time intervals, and **constant work rate tests**, where the subject works at a submaximal constant work rate for a specified time period. Your heart rate at the specific work rates are used to estimate maximal oxygen uptake. Although the most accurate test is conducted on a treadmill, a bicycle will give a good estimate. If you have access to a stationary bicycle, you can test yourself by using the incremental test protocol described. Although it is best to use a heart rate monitor, you can manually take your pulse at various times during the test.

Bicycle Exercise Test Instructions

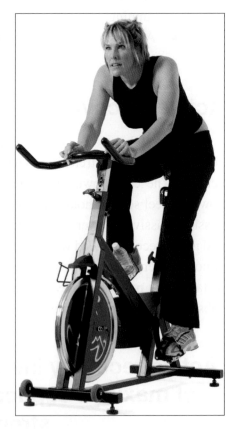

This test is an incremental submaximal test with four stages; each stage lasts two minutes. If desired, you can continue to increase the work rate and exercise for five to six stages. If you use a bike that monito ^) revolutions per min (RPM), your RPM must be maintained at 60. This seems like a slow pace, since you would usually bike at 70 RPM, but in order to achieve the desired work rate, 60 RPM pace is critical. Whatever type of bike you use, you must check to determine how to regulate kcal/hr.

Test Procedures

Adjust height of seat and handle bars to fit you, then if available, hook up a heart rate monitor and then start pedaling at a comfortable workload (See Table 3-2). If the bicycle permits, key in your body weight. This will make the test more accurate. After a couple minutes of warm-up, begin to exercise at level 1 or around 450 kcal/ hr (± 25 kcal/min); record heart rate after two minutes

---

(end of stage one). Increase the workload to level 2 or approximately 550 kcal/hr and continue for two more minutes. Remember that all stages are 2 minutes, so proceed to levels 3 (650 kcal/hr) and 4 (750 kcal/hr) at the appropriate time. The test should take no longer than 8 minutes, after warming-up. Record your heart rate at the end of each stage (Table 3-3).

DO NOT STOP Pedaling While Recording Your Heart Rate.

Table 3-2. Stages and Work Rates for Cycle Ergometer Exercise Testing

Stage	Work Rates
0	Warm-up
1	450 kcal/hr
2	550 kcal/hr
3	650 kcal/hr
4	750 kcal/hr

Table 3-3. Cycle Ergometer Test Form

Name:_____ Age:_____

Weight in kg*:_____ Estimated Max HR **:_____

Stage	Kcal/hr	Heart Rate
1	450	
2	550	
3	650	
4	750	

* To convert your weight from pounds to kg, divide by 2.2. ** Estimate your maximal heart rate as 220—your age.

Estimating Maximal Aerobic Capacity

Look at the example in the figure on the following page. Heart rate has been plotted against each energy expenditure. Estimate your maximal heart rate as 220—YOUR AGE. Plot your heart rate values at each kcal/hr and draw the line of best fit through your points as in the following figure (This should be a fairly straight line). Extend the line so you can also plot your estimated maximal heart rate on the line. Estimate your maximal aerobic capacity (in L/min), and then normalize for body weight: divide your VO_{2max} by your weight in kg. For example if your maximal oxygen uptake was 4.2 L of oxygen/min (4,200 ml) as in the examples below, and you weigh 85 kg, your normalized maximal oxygen uptake would be 4.2 L or 4,200 ml/85 = 49 ml/kg/min. To convert your weight in lb to kg divide by 2.205. Normalizing for body weight allows you to determine how you rate relative to other persons of your age (Consult Table 3-4).

Example of How to Estimate Maximal Oxygen Uptake for an 85 kg, 24 year old SEAL

Table 3-4. Cardiorespiratory Fitness Classification: Maximal Oxygen Uptake (ml/kg/min)

Age	Low	Fair	Average	Good	High
20-29	<25	25-33	34-42	43-52	53+
30-39	<23	23-30	31-38	39-48	49+
40-49	<20	20-26	27-35	36-44	45+
50-59	<18	18-24	25-33	34-42	43+

Figure 3-1. Plot Your Heart Rate to Estimate Maximal Oxygen Uptake

Kcal/hr	300	400	500	600	700	800	900	1000	1100	1200	1300	1400	1500	1600	1700	1800	1900	2000	2100
O₂ (L/min)	1.0	1.3	1.7	2.0	2.3	2.7	3.0	3.3	3.7	4.0	4.3	4.7	5.0	5.3	5.7	6.0	6.3	6.7	7.0

Estimated VO₂max _____ (ml/min) or _____ (ml/kg/min)

Types of Aerobic Activities and Basic Workouts

Outdoor Activities

Aerobic activities, other than running and swimming, are briefly described below. More extensive discussions are provided in the section on indoor activities, since equipment used indoors typically has information about work rate and intensity. However, Table 3-5 presents the amount of energy expended per hour (kcal/hr) in these activities as a function of work rate. The values are for a 70 kg male. To get a more accurate estimate for yourself, multiple the number by your weight in kg and divide by 70.

Table 3-5. Typical Energy Requirements for Various Outdoor Activities

Activity	Work Rate	Energy Expenditure (kcal/hr)
Bicycling	6 mph	270
	10 mph	420
	20 mph	720
Cross-Country Skiing	Moderate	504
	Strenuous, Uphill	1140
Jumping Rope	70 Jumps/minute	690
	145 Jumps/minute	840

Bicycling

Bicycle riding, or biking, is an excellent activity for improving overall cardiorespiratory fitness. Importantly, indoor bicycle ergometers have been used for many years to study the responses of the body to exercise. The work rate you maintain while biking varies according to the terrain and your motivation. As such, biking outside offers many challenges. It is also a very efficient means of locomotion: the energy cost of biking is only 20% of walking, but you can travel almost five times faster on a bicycle. The quadricep muscle in the front part of

---

the thigh is the primary muscle for high rates of power output, and seat height can markedly affect overall muscle involvement. Although pedaling rates vary from 40 to 100 RPM, a rate of 70 appears to be the most comfortable.

A high pedaling rate offers advantages in terms of a high power output.

All in all, biking is a great alternative to running and should be considered as a suitable activity for maintaining fitness, even if it is not part of a SEAL's mission. Biking complements other activities and is often used in rehabilitation from other musculoskeletal injuries. More details with respect to biking will be provided under the section on stationary cycles.

Cross-Country Skiing

Although cross country skiing is discussed in detail under winter warfare below, it should be noted that this is an excellent method of training for cardiorespiratory fitness. It engages almost all of the major muscle groups and thus, the overall energy expenditure may be as high or higher than when moving the body over the same distance on foot. Importantly, the intensity of the effort varies greatly as a function of the terrain: climbing uphill requires tremendous effort whereas going downhill represents a light load. High caliber cross-country skiers have some of the highest maximal oxygen uptakes ever recorded (see Chapter 2). However, the appropriate equipment and environment are necessary for cross-country skiing.

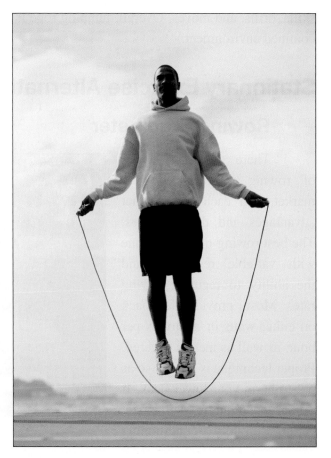

Jumping Rope

Jumping rope is a great way to maintain fitness on board a ship or in confined spaces. It can provide a high intensity, cardioresnprvtory workout if done long enough and fast enough. If the pace is fast, it is equivalent to running in terms of energy expenditure.

Jumping rope does not have to be boring, especially if you use different types of jumps. Table 3-6 provides the names and an explanation for alternatives to the basic jump.

Table 3-6. Different Types of Jumps for Jumping Rope

Type of Jump	Description
Boxer's Dance	With both feet together, shift weight from right to left with each jump.
Run	Jump to the left while lifting left knee, then switch.
Shuffle	Start with right foot forward and left foot back, then switch each jump landing on both feet at same time.
Knee-Toe	Tap right toe on the floor, then jump from your left foot to your right; at the same time lifting left knee as high as possible. Switch legs.
Double Rotation	Twirl the rope around twice between each jump.
Jumping Jack	Jump two times with feet together, then do a jumping jack every third time.

In terms of gear, many different types of rope are available, and rope jumping can be limited by the quality of the rope. Most experts recommend lightweight leather ropes. Believe it or not, many books have been written about jumping rope, with basic to advanced skills, drills, and moves. Overall, jumping rope is a great activity, especially if you are in a confined environment.

Stationary Exercise Alternatives

Rowing Ergometer

There are many types of rowing machines on the market, and each has distinct advantages and disadvantages. The best rowing machine is one with variable resistance and the ability to regulate rowing rate. Most provide feedback on either watts or kcalories per hour, as well as meters covered. Proper technique is critical so as not to harm your lower back. If proper technique is maintained, cardiorespiratory conditioning

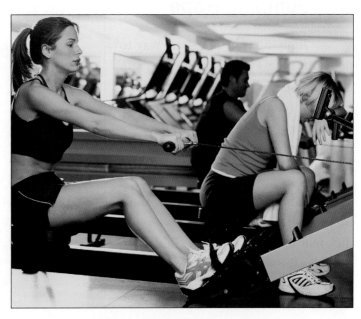

can easily be achieved. In fact, both the upper and lower body are exercised, and it promotes flexibility by emphasizing maximum joint range of motion, so it is a total body workout. It is also impact-free so it is a great alternative to running! Some key points to remember are:

- ◆ The motion of the entire stroke should be fluid.
- ◆ A stroke rate between 24 and 30 per minute should be the goal.
- ◆ Your grip should be loose and comfortable with wrists level.
- ◆ The rule of thumb should be a longer not a harder workout.

Just plain rowing can become a bit boring, but there are many ways to make it fun and varied. Table 3-7 presents descriptions of various workouts for a rowing ergometer.

Table 3-7. Various Workouts for a Rowing Machine

Workout	Description
Steady State	20 to 40 minutes at a pace which barely allows you to chat with a partner
Intervals	3 to 5 sets of 300 to 500 meters at a fast pace with 2 minutes of rest between each set
Fartleks	Alternate 1 minute hard and 1 minute easy for 20 minutes
Long and Slow	6,000 meters at an easy pace
Time Trial	2,000 meters at a record pace
Pyramids	1 min hard, 1 min rest, 3 min hard, 2 min rest, 5 min hard, 3 min rest, 7 min hard, 5 min rest, 5 min hard, 3 min rest, 3 min hard, 2 min rest, 1 min hard

How do you know if the workout is hard or light? Your body is the best judge, but knowing the kcal/hr will also help. A pace of 500 meters/4 minutes would be a light workout whereas a pace of 500/2 minutes would be strenuous. These paces equate to 385 and 970 kcal/hour for a 70 kg man.

Bicycle Ergometers

Cycle ergometers have been around a long time and are still the mainstay in exercise/fitness testing. Monitors on the bicycles available today typically display kcal per hour. Table 3-8 presents kcal/hour values for stationary bicycle workouts at various intensities. These values can be used to gauge your work rate during indoor biking.

Table 3-8. Energy Expenditure (kcal/hr) for Stationary Cycling at Various Intensities and Body Weights

Body Weight (lbs)	Intensity			
	Light	Moderate	Vigorous	Strenuous
155	320	450	600	770
175	360	520	680	880
200	400	590	760	990
220	450	650	850	1100

Treadmills

Despite the fact that it is much nicer to run outside than inside, the treadmill is an extremely efficient way to maintain and/or improve cardiorespiratory conditioning. Unlike the cycle and rowing ergometer, jogging or running on a treadmill is weight dependent: the energy expended is determined by your body weight. In addition, it is an impact sport and should not be the only form of conditioning so joints are protected and injuries minimized. However, if you are on a ship or in another type of confined space, a treadmill could maintain your fitness!

What kind of workouts should you do on a treadmill? Three days per week is more than enough if you do other types of exercise on off days. On a treadmill, you can mix up your pace and/or change the resistance by changing the incline. The incline and speed will determine the intensity of the workout. Remember, a strenuous workout is over 750 kcal/hr and a moderate workout would be 450 to 600 kcal/hr. Table 3-9 presents kcal/hr values for treadmill workouts. These values can be used to determine the speeds and grades for indoor running.

Table 3-9. Approximate Energy Requirements (kcal/ hr) for Horizontal and Uphill Running on a Treadmill

% Grade	Speed (mph)				
	4	5	6	7	8
0	425	515	610	700	800
2.5	470	570	670	775	880
5.0	510	620	740	850	970
7.5	550	670	800	920	1045
10.0	600	720	850	990	1125

Ski Machines

The simulated skiing machine provides an excellent mode of exercise for whole body conditioning. It uses both the upper and lower body and offers a range of settings so your workout can be light, moderate, vigorous, or exhausting. Maintaining a comfortable rhythm is most important during a moderate workout and is essential for progressing to a strenuous workout. Importantly, unlike running outside or on a treadmill, minimal stress is placed on the joints. Most models have various settings for modulating leg resistance, and typically the resistance ranges from 4 to 32 lbs. Once you have determined your desired resistance, the intensity of your workout will be determined by your average speed. Numerous tables are available which allow you to determine the number of calories expended per minute at various resistance settings and speeds. However, they are far too detailed to include here. Table 3-10 presents the kcal/hr expenditures for various settings and speeds for a 70 kg (155 lb) man. These values can be used as to estimate your actual work rate.

Table 3-10. Energy Expenditure (kcal/hr) on a Ski Machine at Various Settings and Speeds

Setting	Speed (kilometers per hour)					
	5	6	7	8	9	10
3	485	530	575	620	670	710
4	550	600	645	690	735	780
5	620	660	710	755	800	850
6	680	730	775	820	865	910
7	750	800	840	885	930	975
8	815	860	905	950	1000	1045

Some indoor skiing machines also have multiple settings for arm resistance and adjustments to these settings should be made to ensure a moderate to vigorous workout. However, kcal/hr expenditure for arm settings becomes quite complicated and will not be presented here. All in all, ski machines provide great exercise and would be extremely beneficial for SEALs involved in winter warfare training.

Stair Steppers

Stair steppers provide an excellent alternative to running, biking, and other forms of aerobic exercise. Although stair-stepping is a weight-bearing exercise, the impact is much less than with running. However, to get the full effect, instructions must be followed. Most people hang on to the handles and this diminishes the conditioning effect. An equally good workout could be gained by actually climbing real stairs for the same period of time; many people climb stairs without holding the handles, and thus carry their full weight up the steps. By hanging on, you allow your arms to support a portion of your body weight and the energy demands are less.

Most stair steppers have a variety of computerized, pre-designed programs to meet the needs of devoted users. There are interval training programs, climbing programs, manual programs, and many other creative exercise programs to vary the intensity of the exercise. Although each manufacturer has its own energy cost equations, the way to determine work intensity is to determine the number of steps per minute; one step is typically 8 inches of vertical climb. A low intensity exercise would be a step rate of less than 35 steps/minute, whereas a high intensity workout would require a step rate in excess of 95. This is not an easy exercise routine. Table 3-11 presents the approximate energy expenditure in kcal/hr for a 155 lb SEAL at various stepping rates.

Table 3-11. Energy Expended (kcal/hr) during Stair Stepping at Various Step Rates

Step Rate in Steps/minute	35	60	95	120	140
Approximate kcal/hr	250	390	580	730	820

Climbers

Workouts on a climber will build upper body strength and provide excellent cardiovascular conditioning. Different types of climbers are available, and each has specific characteristics. Regardless of which variety is used, climbers have common features: weight dependent exercise that conditions primarily the upper body.

Energy expenditure on a climber depends on your speed of climbing and your body weight. Some authorities would say that climbing results in a greater energy expenditure than most other activities, but this depends on your strength and how hard you work. Table 3-12 provides kcal/hr at selected weights and ascent rates.

Table 3-12. Energy Expended (kcal/hr) on a Climber at Designated Weights and Feet per Minute

Weight in lbs	Feet Climbed Per Minute					
	40	60	80	100	120	140
140	360	480	600	690	810	930
160	420	520	670	800	930	1050
180	460	600	750	900	1050	1200
200	510	670	840	1020	1170	1320
220	570	750	930	1100	1270	1450

Basic Workouts

The most important issue with respect to workouts is recovery. Rest is an exceedingly important factor in recovery from strenuous workouts, so back-to-back high intensity workouts are not encouraged. Experts recommend a hard day followed by an easy day and at least one day of rest over a seven day period. This can be an excellent plan, but you should also let your body be your guide. Some days when you go to workout and feel great, this day can and should be a hard workout day. On other days when it is an effort to even get your workout clothes on, this should either be a rest day or an easy day.

Easy days could be a run, bike, or swim at a very comfortable pace for 60 minutes or more, an easy short workout, or a short hump with a light load. A hard day may be intervals, fartleks, a fast pace for a specified period of time, a long hump with a heavy load, or a competition among team members. The key is to make it fun, challenging, and interesting.

Other Terms for Work Rate

Other terms are frequently used to describe exercise intensity and work rate. These include:

◆ Work
◆ Power
◆ METS
◆ Watts

If these terms and concepts are learned, they will apply to almost all exercise equipment and conditioning programs. The terms work and power are often used incorrectly.

Because these terms can be expressed in a variety of ways, it is useful to understand or at least be familiar with the basic units of measurement.

Work and Power

Work = Force x Distance and is measured in kcal

Power = Rate of Doing Work and is measured in watts

METs and Watts

The term MET, which was used in the national recommendations for exercise, is often used to estimate energy expenditure and work rate.

A MET is defined as a multiple of resting metabolic rate or energy expenditure.

One MET is between 0.200 to 0.250 liters (of oxygen)/min, or approximately one kcal/min, depending on the weight and body type of the person. Two METS would be two times resting metabolic rate or approximately 0.5 liters (2 X 0.200 to 0.250) of oxygen/min, or 2 kcal/min. Likewise, 3 METS would be 0.75 liters (3 X 0.200 to 0.250) of oxygen/min, or around 3 kcal/min.

Watts, as stated above, are units used to quantify the rate of doing work, or work/ time. Most new exercise equipment express work rate in terms of watts, although many use METS instead of or as well as watts. Table 313 presents the relationship between various terms denoting exercise intensity. These can be used to monitor exercise intensity.

Table 3-13. Workload Conversion Sheet

Watts	Oxygen Uptake (L/min)	Work Rate	Energy Output (kcal/hr)	METS
50	0.9	Easy	270	4.0
100	1.5	Fairly Easy	450	6.7
150	2.1	Moderate	630	9.3

Cardiorespiratory Conditioning

200	2.8	Moderately Hard	840	12.4
250	3.5	Very Hard	1050	15.5
300	4.2	Very, Very Hard	1260	18.7

Summary

No doubt new modes of exercise will be appearing in the future. What you choose to use will depend on many factors. The important issue is whether you are able to achieve the desired work rate and conditioning level. A recent study of indoor exercise machines examined energy expenditure at given ratings of perceived exertion. They compared a treadmill, a rowing ergometer, a combination cycle/arm ergometer, a cycle ergometer, a stairstepper and a cross-country skiing simulator. Surprisingly they found that rates of energy expenditure varied by as much as 261 kcal/hour for the exercise machines when subjects exercised at self-selected work rates corresponding to fairly light, somewhat hard, and hard. The treadmill came out with the greatest energy expenditures, followed by the rowing and stairstepping ergometers; the cycle and combination cycle/arm ergometers came out with the lowest values. If exercise intensity is established by perceived effort, treadmill running/walking will result in greater energy expenditure and a stronger cardiorespiratory training stimulus for a given duration of exercise as compared to other modalities.

Chapter 4

Running for Fitness

Running is a fundamental part of your physical training program and provides an excellent aerobic workout. Moreover, it is not expensive; most of the cost of running involves buying a pair of "good" running shoes. If you train intelligently and have the right gear, you can continue to enjoy the fitness and general sense of well-being that accompanies running while avoiding running injuries. In this chapter, basic information is provided for maintaining a sound, middle distance running (20 to 40 miles/week) program; this is adequate for running 10K and half marathon races. Some of you may consider running

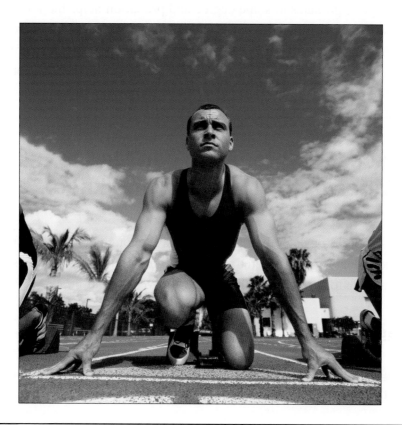

a marathon in the future; at such a time you may want to get training tips from experienced marathoners, trainers at a running club, or running magazines.

Running Gear

Running Shoes

A good pair of running shoes will provide shock absorption, cushioning, motion control, and durability and ultimately help prevent injuries. Under no circumstance should you buy shoes if they do not fit correctly. Running magazines usually have a yearly review of various running shoes, newest models of shoes, and the type of runner the shoes are most suited to. You can also obtain current information from "Running Sites/Pages" on the worldwide web. It is wise to try on several different shoes at a sporting goods store to determine which one might be best for you. This is also important if you are planning to buy shoes from a catalog.

Pronation

It is important to understand this term because the type of running shoe you buy depends on whether you are a normal, over-, or under-pronator. While running, the outside of the heel strikes the ground first. Next, the foot rotates inward and downwards: this process is called pronation. Everyone pronates to some degree and pronation helps the foot absorb the shock of impact. However, some runners over-pronate: their feet roll too far inward. Put your running shoes together and look at their heels/backs; if they lean inward, you are probably over-pronating. Another way to check pronation is to have a friend run behind you and have them watch the back of your heel as it makes contact with the ground: the greater the inward roll of your heel, the more you pronate.

Excessive pronation can lead to injuries of the lower leg and knee.

Other runners under-pronate or their feet do not have enough inward roll after striking the surface. Such individuals are considered to have "rigid" feet or feet that absorb shock poorly. Shoes are available to correct for either under- or over-pronation.

Shoe Terminology

When buying running shoes, it is helpful to be familiar with some common terms. Figure 4-1 presents the various parts of a running shoe.

Figure 4-1. Parts of a Running Shoe

Some General Terms

◆ **Outsole** is the material on the bottom of the shoe that comes in direct contract with the running surface.

◆ **Midsole** is the layer of cushioning that is placed between the upper and outsoles.

◆ **Lateral** is the outer-edge of the shoe.

◆ **Medial** is the inner or arch side of the shoe.

◆ **Upper** is the part of the sole that is above the midsole.

◆ **Achilles notch** is the U- or V-shaped cut at the top of the heel collar which prevents irritation of the achilles tendon.

◆ **Heel counter** is a firm cup usually made of plastic that is encased in the upper and surrounds the heel to control excessive rear foot motion.

◆ **External heel counter** is a rigid plastic collar that wraps around the heel of the shoe to provide support and control excess pronation.

◆ **Motion control designs** or devices control the inward rolling or pronation of the foot. Some amount of pronation is normal: corrective measures are necessary only if there is excessive rolling or under-pronation.

Terms Related to Cushioning

◆ **Cushioning** is provided by midsoles and is needed for shock absorption.

◆ **Cantilever** is a concave outsole design in which the outer edges flare out during foot strike to provide better shock absorption.

◆ **EVA** is a foam-like material which is used in midsoles to provide cushioning.

◆ **Polyurethane (PU)** is a synthetic rubber that is used with EVA. in midsoles. It is more durable than EVA. but provides less cushioning. PU is used in the rear foot for firmness and EVA in the forefoot for flexibility and lightness in many shoe models.

◆ **Metatarsal pad** is a soft wedge of EVA that is placed under the ball of the foot to increase cushioning and shock absorption for runners who are fore-foot strikers.

Terms Related to Shape

◆ **Last** is a foot shaped piece of wood, plastic or metal which is used as a frame for building a shoe. Lasts can be straight or curved as shown in Figure 4-2.

◆ **Straight-lasted shoes** are relatively straight shaped on the inner or medial side and provide support and stability and are recommended for runners who over-pronate.

◆ **Curve-lasted shoes** are shaped to curve inwards (see figure). This shape allows greater foot motion and such shoes can be worn by runners with normal pronation and arches.

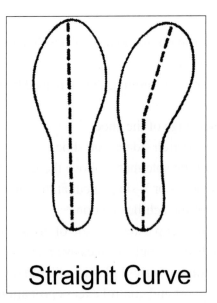

Straight Curve

Figure 4-2. Types of Lasts Used for Running Shoes

Terms Related to Shoe Construction

◆ **Board lasting** increases stability and is good for orthotics. A board-lasted shoe is made by gluing the upper to fiber board before it is attached to the midsole.

◆ **Slip lasting** is the most flexible shoe construction wherein the shoe upper is stitched together like a moccasin before it is glued to the midsole.

◆ **Combination lasting** as the term suggests is partly board and partly slip lasting. Such shoes are board lasted in the rear foot for stability and slip lasted in the fore-foot for greater flexibility. If you removed the sockliner you would see stitching in front and a fiber-board in the rear foot.

Figure 4-3. Shoe Construction: Lasting

Slip   Board Combination

Pointers for Buying Running Shoes

◆ **Maximum emphasis on shock-absorbing characteristics.**
◆ **Know your foot type.**
◆ **Look for shoes that come in widths.**

Do you have normal arches, high arches, or are you flat footed? You can assess your foot type by what is known as the "wet test": simply wet your feet and briefly stand on a piece of paper or on a dark, bare floor; look at the imprint left by your feet. Compare them to the impressions shown in Figure 4-4 to determine your foot type.

If you have high arches you will need a shoe with more cushioning for shock absorption whereas if you are flat footed you will need a shoe with more support and heel control (see Table 4-1).

Flat   Normal High

Figure 4-4. Types of Arches

◆ **Know whether you over- or under-pronate.**

If you over-pronate you need shoes that provide stability, whereas, if you under-pronate you need shoes that provide shock absorption and cushioning.

◆ **Know if you are prone to running injuries.**

See a sports medicine doctor if you are predisposed to training/overuse injuries to determine if your injuries are related to biomechanics. Biomechanical conditions, such as being an over- or under-pronator, or having one leg shorter than the other, often result in running injuries. In some cases, you may benefit from using orthotics (see section on orthotics) in your running shoes. Also, take your running shoes with you when you go to see your doctor.

◆ **Try on shoes towards the end of the day.**

Feet are smallest first thing in the morning and swell slightly as the day progresses. Also, wear running or sports socks while trying on shoes since they are generally thicker than regular socks. Walk around the store in the shoes to check the fit, cushioning, and stability of the shoe. If you use orthotics, lifts, or other inserts, bring them with you when you try on shoes.

◆ **Do not buy shoes based on their brand name.**

Buy shoes that suit your biomechanical needs and work for your foot type, not shoes that a friend highly recommended or shoes you have seen a "good" runner wear. Consider going to a specialty shoe store where a knowledgeable salesperson can evaluate your running style and biomechanical needs and recommend a shoe.

◆ **Replace worn out shoes in a timely manner.**

Wearing worn out shoes can eventually lead to injuries and cause knee or hip pain. It is a good idea to replace running shoes every 400 to 500 miles, or sooner, if your shoes wear down quickly. One way to keep track of your running mileage is to establish a running log. A running log will not only help in keeping track of your running distance, but it will also help in tracking factors such as sudden increases in mileage or the onset of injury.

Table 4-1. The Right Shoe for Your Foot Type

Shoe Features	Flat Feet	Normal Feet	High-Arched Feet
Last - Shape	Straight	Semi-curved	Curved
Last - Construction	Combination	Combination	Slip
Midsole	Firm	Soft or firm	Soft
Motion Control	Yes	No	No
Orthotic Sole	May be needed to correct for over-pronation	No	No
External Heel Counter	Yes	No	Yes
Recommended Shoe Type	Motion control or stability shoes with firm midsoles	Stability shoes with moderate control features such as two-density mid-sole	Cushioned shoes to provide lots of flexibility and promote foot motion
Avoid	Highly cushioned and curve-lasted shoes		Motion control or stability shoes

Orthotics

Individuals with biomechanical conditions that result in pain and injury may benefit from using orthotics in their running shoes. Orthotics are shoe inserts that are customized to an individual's biomechanics and foot type to provide good foot support and motion control. First, a plaster mold of the foot is made and then inserts are developed to correct the biomechanical problem(s). These inserts are usually made of cork soles covered by flexible leather or hard plastic. Orthotics should be gradually broken in; first wear them while walking and then progress to running. If not properly fitted, orthotics may worsen the problem. A podiatrist or sports medicine specialist is required to have them custom-made.

Sometimes low cost, over-the-counter, commercial orthotic inserts can work as well as customized inserts. For example, if the amount of pronation is not too much, over-the-counter inserts may correct the problem. Commercial inserts are sold by shoe size. If you find that the pain lessens, but does not go away or that the pain returns when you increase your mileage, you may need custom-made orthotics.

Cleats for Cold Weather Running

By putting on rubber cleats over a pair of running shoes you will be able to run outdoors under icy conditions. Personnel in the Arctic Warrior Brigade in Alaska use cleats when training in frigid weather. To obtain information about ordering these cleats, call Ft. Wainright (DSN 317-353-6048).

Clothes

Unlike many sports, running is not seasonal and with the right clothes, it is possible to continue to train outdoors on very hot or very cold days (see Chapter 11: Special Considerations for Training to review training under adverse environmental conditions). When weather conditions are extreme, as in ice storms, blizzards, or a major heat wave, outdoor training can be substituted with running on a treadmill in the gym. Thus, running clothes can range from a simple pair of running shorts and a singlet to running tights and gortex jackets, depending on environmental temperatures. Cold weather running requires dressing in layers. Always keep your head and extremities warm in cold weather. Experience will teach you what to wear when running in the cold. If you wear too much, you may get hot after warming up, i.e., within the first mile or so.

Running socks tend to cost a bit more, but they are thicker and provide more cushioning than average sports socks. In most cases, sports socks are recommended as they provide adequate cushioning.

Other Gear Items

Heart Rate Monitors

You may have seen these advertised in running and fitness magazines. Some athletes use these for monitoring their training intensities. Such monitors consist of a wrist watch and a chest strap: the chest strap has an electrode which picks up your heart beat and transmits it to the watch which in turn displays your heart rate in beats per minute. If you know your target training zone (see Chapter 1) you can check and maintain your heart rate within that zone. Heart rate monitors are not a training necessity and can be expensive.

Reflectors

Putting reflectors on your shoes and running clothes is a great idea if you routinely run late in the evening, at night, or very early in the morning when visibility is particularly poor. This is especially important in urban areas where motorists may not be paying particular attention to runners. Note that you should also run against the traffic.

Fluid Containers that Strap onto Belts

As you already know, it is very important to maintain fluid balance and prevent dehydration. Thus, if your long runs include running for more than 90 minutes, especially in hot weather, it is advisable to strap on a fluid container and drink fluid (8 oz.) at 30 minute intervals (refer to *The Navy SEAL Nutrition Guide*). If your running route provides access to water fountains then you need not carry your own fluid supply.

Portable Radio/Cassette Player/Walkman

Running with headphones can really help during long runs. However, it is not advisable to wear headphones and run on city streets as it may reduce your awareness of your surroundings. Running with headphones on base may be prohibited.

Running Surfaces

The ideal running surface is flat, firm, smooth and, provides some shock absorption. Surfaces in the order of most to least desirable are listed in Table 4-2.

Table 4-2. Running Surfaces: From Best to Worst

Surface	Comment	Rating
Soft, smooth cinder track, unbanked	Least likely of all to aggravate biomechanical injuries. Change direction frequently on any track to reduce mechanical problems.	1-Best

Table 4-2. Running Surfaces: From Best to Worst

Surface	Comment	Rating
Artificially surfaced track, unbanked	Provides less shock absorption than the cinder track.	2
Soft, smooth dirt trail	Provides reasonable cushioning and holes and ruts are clearly visible.	3
Flat, smooth grass	Grassy areas including golf courses make relatively poor running surfaces since they hide uneven areas.	4
Asphalt street or path	Poor surfaces since typically sloped to facilitate rain water run-off. Surface slant causes one foot to pronate more and other to supinate more. Biomechanical problems are aggravated especially if runner tends to run in the same direction each time. Changing directions is highly recommended.	5
Hard, dirt track or trail	Watch out for ruts, holes, loose stones.	6
Concrete sidewalk or road	A very hard surface: wear good shock absorbing shoes.	7
Banked or cambered surface	Severe incline puts stress on the knees.	8
Hard-sand or soft sand beach	Beaches are slanted and can aggravate biomechanical problems. Do not run barefoot.	9
Rough, pot-holed, dirt trail or grass	A particularly hazardous surface. An unexpected hole or rut can result in ankle sprains.	10 - Worst

Source: Running *Injury-Free* by Joe Ellis with Joe Henderson, Rodale Press, 1994

Other running surfaces include treadmills and water. Treadmills are very popular at fitness centers and may also be available to you when deployed aboard a ship. Most treadmills are state of the art in terms of cushioning and you can control the speed and intensity of your work out. Perhaps the biggest problem when working out on a treadmill is the boredom that is often associated with the monotony of the unchanging environment and the consistent pace. A portable cassette player or radio may be helpful, particularly during longer runs.

Deep water or aqua running is mainly used for rehabilitating injured athletes as it takes the pressure off of injured muscles and joints while providing cardiovascular benefits similar to those obtained with running on surface. This type of running is becoming popular at various swim centers.

Warm-Up

A warm-up to lengthen short, tight muscles before running is crucial for preventing injuries that may result if muscles are "cold." A longer muscle is less likely to get injured than a short, tight muscle because it can exert more force with less effort than a short muscle. Another benefit of warming up is that it protects tendons. Warm up by slow jogging or walking for 5 to 10 minutes before you run. **After you warm up you need to stretch your hamstrings, quadriceps, hip flexors, groin, calves, achilles, and the iliotibial band.** Exercises to accomplish these stretches are provided in the chapters on "Flexibility" and "Calisthenics" and are included in your recommended PT (Chapter 15).

Cool-Down and Stretching

After completing your run, walk for a few minutes to cool-down. It is not a good idea to sprint at the end of your run and then come to a complete stop; this practice may result in an injury. Cooling down helps to shift the blood flow from the muscles to the heart and other vital organs. A cool down lets your heart rate slow down and your body gradually return to its preexercise physiological state. **Cooling down properly and stretching (see Chapter 7: Flexibility) after your run will go a long way towards preventing injuries.**

Running Gait or Form

Different runners may have different running styles. Running is a function of footstrike, forward stride, body angle, and arm drive. The key is:

Run naturally and remain relaxed.

Footstrike

For most runners, other than sprinters or very fast runners, the heel-ball footstrike method works well: (1) the outside of the heel strikes the surface; (2) the foot rolls inwards to the ball of the foot while the knee is slightly bent; and (3) the foot lifts off from propulsion provided by the big toe. This method provides good shock absorption.

Forward Stride

The point of foot contact should occur in line with the knee which should be slightly flexed. As you improve and get faster, the length and frequency of your strides will increase and you will begin lifting your knees higher. Do not overstride such that your foot hits the ground ahead of the knee flex (i.e. leg should not be straight at point of impact). Overstriding is hard on the knees, back, and the hips and can cause injuries. Short, choppy strides, which usually result from tight or inflexible muscles, require more energy and are inefficient. Run with a relaxed stride and do not exaggerate the knee-lift or back kick.

Body Angle

Keep your back as straight as naturally possible, your head up and look ahead. Of course, depending on the terrain you may have to look down to avoid tripping or landing in a hole or rut. Lean forward only when going uphill or sprinting as this motion will put stress on leg muscles and may cause back pain and shin splints. Leaning back is not recommended as this puts tremendous pressure on the back and legs and has a "braking effect." The key is to run "tall" and remain relaxed; allow your shoulders to hang in a relaxed manner and let your arms drop from time to time.

Arm Drive

While running relax your shoulders, elbows, wrists, and fists and occasionally let your arms hang down at your sides and loosely shake them out. Whereas vigorous pumping of the arms helps sprinters, it is unnecessary during distance running.

Building Your Mileage

Increasing mileage too quickly can cause training injuries. Your running mileage should be gradually increased and not by more than 10% to 20% from one week to the next. For example, if you can comfortably run four miles, increase your distance by a mile and maintain this new mileage for at least one to two weeks or until this distance is consistently easy for you. Also, remember consistency is more important than speed.

A good rule of thumb: increase your mileage by no more than 20% a week.

When you can continuously run for 40 minutes, begin thinking about your running mileage or distance. Most of you, unless coming back from an injury or returning from a deployment, are already running 30 to 40 minutes as part of your fitness routine. However, if you have been unable to run for some time due to reasons mentioned above or other reasons, start out slowly; this will prevent you from getting injured and benefit you in the long run.

Running Frequency

Run at least three to four times per week or every other day. It is a good idea to build in one or two rest days in your weekly running schedule. These rest days do not necessarily mean no exercise, but rather an alternate type of exercise, such as biking or swimming. This allows your "running muscles" time for rest and recovery and helps prevent overuse training injuries.

Running Speed and Intensity

When running for exercise and not competition, you should run at an even pace that allows you to talk comfortably. If you run too fast and get breathless, you may not be able to go the distance. Also, speed work tends to tighten muscles and must be properly stretched afterwards. Failure to stretch may lead to an injury. One way to estimate your training intensity is to check your heart rate and see if it falls within your target training zone

(See Chapter 1). As previously mentioned, speed is not as important as being able to go the distance consistently. Figure 4-5 presents tips on how to increase your running speed.

Figure 4-5. Ways to Increase Running Speed

Increase length of stride: do not overstride

Increase frequency of stride

Increase length and frequency of stride

Do not increase speed and distance simultaneously.

Increasing both at the same time may cause an injury. Hold one constant while you gradually increase the other. After you have been running 30 minutes continuously 3-5 times per week, you can begin increasing your running distance. Running 20 to 30 miles per week is a good training distance for an intermediate runner. If you would like to further increase your weekly mileage, remember to increase it by no more than 20% per week. Table 4-3 provides a nine week program for running up to 40 miles per week.

Table 4-3. A Program to Run 40 Miles per Week

Week	Mon	Tues	Wed	Thur	Fri	Sat	Sun	Total
One	4	CT*	5	3	CT	3	5	20
Three	5	CT	5	5	CT	5	5	25
Five	5	CT	6	6	CT	6	6	29
Seven	7	CT	7	8	CT	5	8	35
Nine	6	CT	8	8	CT	8	10	40

*CT=Cross train on these days.

The program in Table 4-3 provides a basic template for you. Based on your own routine, you could modify this program to fit your schedule and requirements. Another way to vary your workout is to have one long slow run and one fast run per week. Remember if you feel over tired, cut back your mileage or take a day off from running. With a running base of 40 miles per week you can easily run a half marathon.

Training for a Marathon

If you have been running 35 to 40 miles per week for 1 to 2 months, you have a good endurance base for running a marathon after 3 additional months (12 weeks) of training (Table 4-4). To run a marathon, you must complete some long training runs in the weeks leading up to the marathon. The week that you run the marathon, however, should include only a few short runs. Your goal for your first marathon should be to complete it.

Table 4-4. A 12 Week Marathon Training Program Starting at 40 Miles/Week

Week	Mon	Tues	Wed	Thur	Fri	Sat	Sun	Total
One	-	5	8	5	5	4	15	42
Two	-	8	5	10	5	5	12	45
Three	-	6	8	6	6	4	15	45
Four	-	8	8	10	5	5	14	50
Five	-	6	8	8	6	4	18	50
Six	-	6	10	12	5	8	14	55
Seven	-	5	10	10	6	4	20	55
Eight	-	8	10	10	10	8	14	60
Nine	-	8	10	10	6	6	20	60
Ten	-	8	4	10	10	8	15	55
Eleven	-	5	10	10	5	4	18	52
Twelve	-	8	6	4	-	2	Marathon	

Other Points to Consider

 ◆ Make sure you eat enough carbohydrates and are well hydrated before the marathon. Refer to The Navy SEAL Nutrition Guide for information about high carbohydrate diets and fluid replacement beverages.
 ◆ Start out slowly and pace yourself.

- Walk for a while if you get cramps or feel fatigued.
- Consider the environmental temperature; if it is a hot and humid day, it is especially important to pay attention to your fluid and electrolyte needs (Refer to Chapter 11 and to *The Navy SEAL Nutrition Guide*).
- After you finish, stretch and walk around. Take a hot bath.
- Slowly return to running.

Interval Training

Various interval training techniques can be used for building speed. Ideally, speed work would be done on a measured track. Sample interval training workouts are provided in Figure 4-6. Two important points are:

- Rest periods between reps for intervals to train the anaerobic energy systems should be equal or slightly less than time to cover distance (quarter mile: 60 seconds; rest: 60 seconds)
- Rest periods to train aerobic system should be less than one-half time to cover distance (half-mile: 2:50; rest: 60 seconds)

Figure 4-6. Sample Sprint and Distance Running Interval Workouts

---

Sprint

One mile warm-up, slow pace

10 minutes lower body stretching

Quarter mile sprint w/ 60 to 90 second jogs: Repeat five times

Half mile sprints/ 2 to 3 minutes jogs: Repeat three times

One mile cool-down, easy pace

Whole body stretching

Distance

One mile warm-up, slow pace

10 minutes lower body stretching

One mile sprints/ 1 to 2 minute/s jogs: Repeat four times

Two mile cool-down, easy pace

Whole body stretching

These are not the only interval workouts, so you may modify them to suit your requirements. For example, you could do pyramids: you would start with a quarter mile, followed by a half mile, 3/4 mile, and mile, then go back down in reverse. Between each speed set, it is best to jog one quarter to one half the distance to accelerate recovery.

Interval workouts are a great way to improve performance.

Varying Your Workouts

It is good idea to vary your daily running mileage so you have some "light" days in between heavy training. Avoid running long distances on two consecutive days, unless you are training for a marathon, to give your body time to recover. Listen to your body and pace yourself accordingly.

Most importantly, it is good to cross-train.

Consider biking, swimming, stair-climbing, or other activities that will provide a good aerobic workout while mainly using muscles other than those used during running. A major benefit of cross training is that it prevents the onset of over-use injuries while maintaining fitness. For information about cross-training see Chapter 3: Cardiorespiratory Conditioning. Strength training, especially upper body strength workouts, have become an important part of a "runners'" overall workout. It is recommended that you strength train two to three times a week (see Chapter 6).

Common Running Injuries or Problems

Most running injuries are due to "over use" from running too much, i.e. too fast, too far, or too often. See Chapter 12: Training and Sports Related Injuries for more information about injuries. The following table shows the incidence of various running injuries that were reported by male runners

---

in a recent survey (Adapted from *Running Injury-Free* By Joe Ellis with Joe Henderson, Rodale Press, 1994).

Table 4-5. Frequency of Running Injuries Reported by a Sample of Male Runners

Injury	Frequency (%)
Knee	23
Achilles Tendon/Calf	16
Metatarsal	11
Hip/Groin/Toenails/Blisters	9
Plantar Fascia/Heel	8
Ankle Sprain	7
Shin Splints	6
Nerve/Quadriceps/Hamstring/Back	2

If you train sensibly there is no reason why you should not be able run injury-free. Should you get injured, information on how to go about seeking treatment for training related injuries is provided in Chapter 12. Keep in mind the three principles of a good running form as shown in Table 4-6.

Table 4-6. Three "Principles" of Good Running Form

Run Tall
Run Relaxed
Run Naturally

Resources

- ◆ Joe Ellis with Joe Henderson, *Running Injury-Free*, Rodale Press, 1994.
- ◆ Bob Glover and Jack Shepard, *The Runner's Handbook,* Penguin Books, 1985.

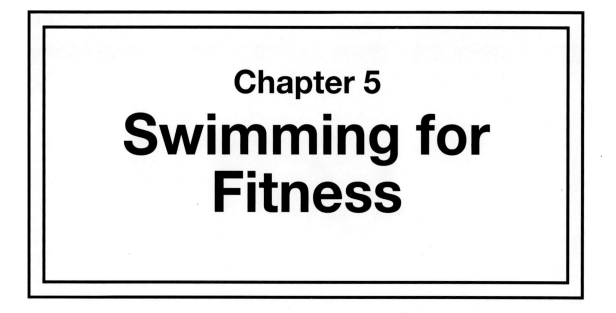

Chapter 5

Swimming for Fitness

As a SEAL you are required to be a swimmer. Swimming is an excellent exercise for overall fitness; aerobic endurance, power, strength, and flexibility are all enhanced by swim training. It is generally gentle on the joints and provides excellent cross training for running and other gravity-intensive forms of exercise by providing load-bearing joint rest. However, training must be specific for the anticipated operational environment, including cold water acclimatization. This section will give you the tools to improve your swimming skills, thus enhancing your fitness for combat swimmer missions.

You must primarily train for endurance while preserving the significant power and strength required by other phases of SEAL operations. This section includes information on competitive swimming strokes and pool training, but it is important to emphasize that most training for SEAL combat swimmer operations should consist of open water swims with fins. Open water training is essential for SEALs as a part of a comprehensive training program under the general principle of "specificity of training." Surf and high sea state swimming provides specific training for potential operational situations by increasing your sense of timing and confidence.

Swim training should focus primarily on open water swims with fins.

Swim training is best accomplished with others for a variety of safety reasons. There should always be a guard or buddy available to you, even if you swim in a pool. You certainly should not train alone in open water.

Open Water Gear

In the pure sense the only gear required is a set of trunks. Look at the gear list for the UDT swimmers at Omaha Beach in 1944. It did not even include fins and masks. However, today there are some significant gear issues. Goggles are necessary for any real swim training. Operational and open water swimming requires more gear. There are specific training aids that help develop strength and technique in pool training. Swimming is still an inexpensive sport with respect to gear; a complete set of the most expensive training gear for pool training will not cost over $100.

Wet Suits

Open water swimming may require thermal protection for safety. Males in particular may be susceptible to hypothermia and the first symptom in an open water swimmer may be unconsciousness from cardiac arrhythmia. Thermal protection in swimmers means a wet suit worn over an anti-chafing shirt.

Wet suits designed for open water swimming are generally of a Farmer John design with the arms free for stroking. In all but the coldest water, a 1/8" wet suit is best for surface swimming. Unlike diving, there is no need to factor in the loss of insulation due to compression of the neoprene with depth. However, this is not true for the combat swimmer operations that may entail prolonged periods in the water.

Anti-chafing shirts are generally made of nylon without elastic properties. Worn under the wet suit, the nylon shirt allows arm strokes and head rotation without getting chafing from the wet suit. If you don't use anti-chafe shirts, then this would not matter.

Hood, Gloves and Booties

◆ Good open water swimming hoods allow the head to be turned with minimal chafing. Thermal protection is not as good with the neck exposed. A good hood preserves a great deal of the swimmer's heat.

◆ Gloves may have webbed fingers to allow sidestroke pulling to be more efficient. They work great for freestyle, too. Neoprene web gloves are popular and work like paddles.

◆ Thin 1/8" booties without soles maximize the power delivered by the swimmer's legs to the fins.

Fins and Fin Selection

There are three factors to keep in mind when you are selecting a fin; the specific design characteristics of the fin, the physical attributes particular to your body, and operational constraints. Fins, by increasing the surface area of the foot, serve to magnify the thrust delivered by the legs. Kicking with fins involves a forward stroke and a backward stroke. Several examples will illustrate how the three factors interact to influence the SEAL's fin selection.

◆ SDV operations require an operator to sit with fins on for a long period of time. The operator may require thermal protection and he may have a flexible ankle. Space is limited, so a shorter fin is necessary. For this situation, the operator should select a short, wide fin with a strap that can be adjusted for varying amounts of thermal wear.

◆ Surface swimming with gear will involve a sidestroke flutterkick. In the sidestroke, forward is toward the front of the swimmer's body and backward is toward the swimmer's back. Applied force is typically much greater during the forward stroke, and fins are often designed with this fact in mind. When power is needed for both forward and backward kick, like in sidestroke, a straight symmetrical fin may be more efficient for you.

◆ Underwater swimming involves a face down position, where the forward stroke is down and the backward stroke is up towards the surface of the water. In this position, gravity assists with the downstroke and produces a less symmetrical type of thrust than seen with sidestroke kick. You should select a high-tech diving fin with moderate flexibility and an integral type footbox. The fin should have an offset design to allow a more efficient transfer of propulsion force.

◆ For body surfing, use short surf fins.

The main principle of fins is to increase the surface area of the foot.

Table 5-1. Recommended Fin Types

Type of Swimming	Type of Fin
SDV Operation	Short fin (Beware of compromised propulsion power. Rocket fin is wide and may provide extra safety factor.)
Underwater Swimming	Offset fin
Surface Swimming	Straight fin

Figure 5-1. Examples of Traditional Short and Long Fins (Left) and Newer Long Blade Fins with Innovative Buckles (Right)

Specific Design Characteristics of Fins:

◆ Size or surface area of fin blade
◆ Stiffness of fin blade
◆ Configuration or shape of fin blade—length and width
◆ Integral footbox versus strap-type fin
◆ "Offset" or angle of pitch between footbox and fin blade
◆ Buoyancy of fin

Physical Attributes Influencing Fin Selection:

◆ If your ankle range of motion is inherently limited, long fins will assist in transmitting lower extremity forces to the water.

◆ If your ankles are inherently flexible, short fins may be more efficient as well as less stressful on relaxed ankle joints.

◆ Your natural kick frequency will also influence your choice of fin stiffness and size. Larger sizes and stiffness produces a slower rate of kicking, while short flexible fins allow a higher kick rate.

Operational Constraints:

◆ Face down versus sidestroke position

◆ Surface versus submerged

◆ Space limitations (SDV)

◆ Thermal protection

The fit of the fin is critical.

If the fin is too tight, the finbox may make your foot cramp up and more susceptible to cold. If it is too loose, energy is lost in the slop between foot and footbox; slop also translates into foot chafe! Booties provide grip for the foot within the footbox and the neoprene acts to even out areas where stress is concentrated.

Other Fin Selection Considerations

Fins vary slightly in buoyancy; about half of sport fin models float and the remainder sink. This may be an operational consideration. In the April 1996 Rodale's Scuba Diving fin test, fins testing as "outstanding" in the area of power included the expensive Scubapro Gorilla, Mares/Plana Avanti, Ocean Edge Spectra, and the U.S. Divers Blades. However, so did the IDI Frog Foot and Power Fin models, which have been the standard fins in the Teams for many years.

The authors of the article reveal honestly that, "In spite of extensive research and a multiplicity of designs applied to modern fins, there are still tried and true fins that perform as well as many of the top newer models." The older, buckle-style strap fasteners have the advantage of being reversible and are far less likely to foul in fishing line or seaweed than fasteners on newer models, many of which have quick-release buckles. The simple straps on older models have no plastic to break, are easy and inexpensive to replace, and can be found in almost any dive store. These fins are also not as slippery on deck as newer designs.

As a SEAL, you will need to evaluate individual fin performance carefully. You should not only consider characteristics of the fin, but know your own physical attributes and any particular operational constraints in making your decision.

When buying fins consider:

◆   Size, stiffness, weight, buoyancy, buckles, and releases.

◆   Getting the best possible fit; try on
    fins with booties or other foot gear
    that you'll be using with the fins.

Face Masks

A face-mask is required for swimming as prolonged exposure to salt water and/or stinging marine organisms may cause eye irritation or injury.

For open water swimming, you should use your face mask.

Open Water Training

There is no substitute for ocean or lake swimming. Training in open water will force you to swim straight and develop a cycle of breathing that allows you to look forward in order to navigate. This is an essential skill for operational swimming. Group swims in open water are an excellent way to maintain fitness and should be used extensively in SEAL training programs. Open water training will maximize the training effect of using fins.

For operational open water swimming, the sidestroke with a flutterkick is superior to freestyle.

In rough open water and under operational circumstances you may want to combine a scissor kick with a sidestroke pulling technique to maximize your navigational ability and watch for breaking waves. However, sculling is as important in the sidestroke as it is in freestyle. Both arms should be used to incorporate sculling motions and to stabilize the swimmer's trunk while the kick provides the main thrust. There are stroke efficiency issues with the sidestroke just as there are in other swimming strokes. Stroke coaching is invaluable in developing good technique.

Water Temperature Issues

Cold water is an issue to be addressed by SEALs training in open water. Although the work of swimming generates heat, there is heat loss created by movement of the swimmer into new "unheated" cold water. Thus, open water swimming may require various combinations of passive thermal protective gear, in particular, wet suits. The three determinants for passive thermal protection are:

◆ Temperature

◆ Length of the swim

◆ Effort level

It is important to remember that wet suits operate by allowing the body heat to be transferred to a layer of water caught between the body and the neoprene material of the suit. Convective heat loss from the swimmer's body is greatly reduced by this mechanism and as a result, swimming at a high effort while wearing a wet suit allows the swimmer to generate and retain heat. Guidelines have been developed for training and are presented in this section.

Research has established some known "bench mark" facts about operating in a cold water environment. In very cold water (below 40° F), the unprotected swimmer loses heat faster than an immobile person immersed in the same cold water. Heat generation simply does not keep up with losses. The immobile person warms the cold water immediately around his body thereby limiting total heat loss. However, in moderately cold water (around 68° F), an elite class swimmer may stay active, and the heat generated by swimming keeps pace with overall losses (although the swimmer may develop cold feet and hands). In this situation, the active swimmer outperforms the immobile person with respect to maintenance of core body temperature. Currently we do not know the crossover temperature point or the water temperature at which it is better to remain stationary than active in the water for thermal balance.

Passive thermal protection modifies this balance by reducing the convective component of heat loss. As a result, a swimmer may extend training durations beyond those possible without passive thermal protection. Diving medicine specialists at BUDS have developed guidelines for use of passive thermal protection during training in cold water environments. Note that Table 5-2 is limited to high energy swims at a set distance of 2 miles.

Table 5-2. Distance, Temperature, and Protection Requirements

Swim	Water Temperature (°F)	Protection
	>64°	None
	63 - 64°	Hood Only
Swim of 2 miles	60 - 62°	Wet-Suit Top/Hood
	50 - 60°	Full Wet Suit/Hood

Special Open Water Training Issues

It is easy to have chafing from the wet suit around the arms and also for the fins to chafe. Get thin booties without soles for fin use and consider using some vaseline or aquaphor ointment for other chafe points.

If you swim regularly in cold water, your body will undergo some adaptive changes. This will increase your tolerance to some extent. You will also begin to actually crave fatty foods, an instinctual tendency of cold water swimmers to want extra body fat to protect them! This is a natural adaptation, but this may be undesirable for your running and overall fitness.

Surf training is great for honing your aquatic skills and for developing confidence in big water. For body-surfing, use a medium fin, like short surfing fins, that permits quick acceleration but is small enough not to get caught in moving parts of the wave. Use velcro-elastic "keepers" for your fins unless you are sponsored by a fin manufacturer!

Keep your head down and always surf with an arm extended up over your head.

It is far better if you get folded by a big chopping wave to have your shoulder dislocated than for you to become quadriplegic from a cervical spine injury. Avoid shorebreaks; the waves are unpredictable and going over the falls may yield a screaming descent straight onto the beach sand. Instead try to find a good "grab and release" break where the wave stands up nicely and then breaks back into deeper water.

Another open water issue you may be faced with is that of sharks. They commonly attack solitary swimmers, particularly freestylers: the solitary, beefy organism making arm slaps against the surface of the water. Avoid swimming in places where you may resemble part of the food chain, but even then there appears to be protection in numbers. A good example is La Jolla Cove near San Diego. Here triathletes swim and Great White sharks eat small mammals all in the same day. Avoid swimming in the evening and get out of the ocean if you get bloodied too much in the surf.

Sharks virtually never attack swimmers in groups.

Swimming Pool Gear

Goggles

The most important gear for pool training is a good set of goggles. Get goggles that can be adjusted across the bridge of the nose. The fog-free goggles work better than they used to, but they do lose this quality relatively quickly under hard use and are much more expensive.

Kickboard

A kickboard is essential. They come in a wide variety of sizes and shapes, but all do basically the same thing.

Pullbuoy

A cheap, but essential, piece of training gear, the pullbuoy fits between the swimmer's legs for specific types of swim drills.

Hand Paddles

These are useful to develop the feel of sculling during freestyle pulling.

Zoomers

A unique and expensive short fin, the Zoomer is helpful but not essential. This special fin is designed to allow the swimmer to use flip turns during pool training sessions with minimal interference with technique. Other short fins may be substituted, notably the short, surf fins.

Nose Clips

Many individuals develop low grade nasal reaction to pool water. Use of a nose clip will allow a swimmer to complete some of the backstroke drills presented in this chapter much more comfortably.

Pool Training: Building Strength and Endurance

The major reason to use a pool is the quality of training. Swim sessions may be closely monitored and are safe. Controlled interval workouts used in pool training sessions provide good feedback; the pace clock doesn't lie. Pool sessions allow you to design workouts that vary in intensity and emphasis, which is not possible in open water. Pool training and acquisition of improved stroke skills are elective elements of a SEAL's training program. Pool training will increase your comfort level in open water, thus enabling you to significantly improve your operational capabilities.

Swimming is not an intuitive activity like running.

Warming Up

Warming-up should consist of at least 400 meters of swimming, along with some kicking and pulling drills. Warming-up is essential for swimming to avoid developing problems of the shoulder joint and upper back.

Target heart rate during warm-up should be about 60% of maximal.

During your warm-up, work on efficient stroke "stealth" swimming! Warming-up is an appropriate time to include stroke drills. This serves the purpose of providing stroke patterning along with the warm-up.

Basic Principles of Interval Training

SEALs need to concentrate on swim training that will enhance endurance: interval swim training will allow this to happen. Interval training sets (for both strength and endurance) are generally comprised of repeated swims lasting 45 seconds to 4 minutes. Basics of interval training include the following:

- ◆ Swim at a slow to moderate pace for five to ten minutes to warm-up muscles and cardiorespiratory system.

- ◆ For anaerobic training, sets should be performed until repeat times can no longer be held. There is no magical number of repetitions for a set, but the distance is typically 50 to 100 meters, or a time of about 45 seconds.

- ◆ Swimming at a prescribed intensity pace for as long as possible is most important. When desired pace can no longer be sustained, the set should be terminated.

- Work:recovery ratios play an important part in the type of adaptation that occurs. A 1:1 work:recovery ratio would be to swim 45 seconds and rest 45 seconds, whereas a 1:2 ratio would be to swim 45 seconds and rest 90 seconds.

- To stimulate endurance adaptations, recovery intervals between repetitions should be less than 30 seconds. For maximum benefit, it is best to keep the interval less than 15 seconds.

- For anaerobic adaptations to occur, recovery intervals should be in excess of one minute and up to at least twice the duration of the repetition swim. These effects occur independent of the repetition distance or pace.

- The longer the rest interval, irrespective of the distance being repeated, the greater the use of the anaerobic system. With long rests, it takes considerably longer for the aerobic energy system to be reactivated. Short rest intervals keep the aerobic system functioning, particularly during initial recovery.

Interval training is the backbone of a swimming workout.

Figure 5-2 illustrates how the different energy systems can be trained in an interval workout. Swim 1 is a hard effort, short distance and a lot of rest; this type of effort builds the anaerobic (CP) and transitional (Lactate-CP) energy systems. The second swim consists of fewer sets at a longer distance and with shorter rest intervals; this swim would challenge the aerobic system.

Figure 5-2. Energy Systems Used During Interval Sets

Lactate-CP System

Swim 1: 10 X 100 m with 45 sec. rest
10 = Repetitions (Sets)
100 m = Distance in Meters

Aerobic System

Swim 2: 5 X 200 m with 5 sec. rest
5 = Repetitions (Sets)
200 m = Distance in Meters

A swimming pace clock is the best way to time intervals: a diving watch works fine.

Interval Sets - Endurance

Freestyle Swim: 10 x 50 m with only 5 sec. rest

- ◆ Rest 5 seconds between each swim.
- ◆ Start with efficient "stealth" stroke, work into distance race pace. Don't overkick.
- ◆ Try to match your 1000 meter pace with this set.

Freestyle Swim: 50-50-100 m with 5 sec. rest

- ◆ Swim 2 x 50 meters with 5 seconds rest, then swim 100 meters: Repeat 3X.
- ◆ This set builds into a 100 meter swim where the swimmer tries to match the pace set in the 50 meters.
- ◆ Back off of the 50 meters a little to save up for the 100 meters.
- ◆ If you want, add an extra 15 seconds of rest between each 50-50-100 to keep the quality up.
- ◆ A "buildup" set like this will do great things for your endurance and sense of pace.

Freestyle Swim: 10 x 100 m with 10 sec. rest

- ◆ Rest 10 seconds between each 100 meter swim.
- ◆ Swim smoothly and efficiently. This is the set where you may exceed your long, slow swimming 1000 meter time!

Breaststroke Swim: 50-50-100 m - 5 sec. rest

- ◆ Done like the freestyle 50-50-100 set outlined above.
- ◆ Concentrate on keeping effort level up.

Interval Sets - Strength and Power

Freestyle Swim: 10 x 50 m with 30 sec. rest

- ◆ Begin at a strong pace. Build to race pace with a strong turn and an extra strong finish. Try to be within 5 seconds of your race 50 meters pace, usually equal to your race 200 meter pace.
- ◆ At first, try just 5 x 50 meters with 30 second rest.
- ◆ This is the most power-oriented freestyle set. It will also allow you to discover your true maximal heart rate. If you start to die off at the end, increase your rest a little to keep your pace.
- ◆ If you are particularly strong and want to build more speed, do this set with zoomers.

Freestyle Swim: 10 x 100 m with 45 sec. rest

◆ Same pace approach as the 50 meter interval set. This is for advanced swimmers with a refined stroke. It will build power, but this set should be used no more than once every two weeks.

◆ The rest interval should be 45 seconds for this length of swim; adjust your interval accordingly.

Breaststroke Swim: 10 x 50 m with 30 sec. rest

◆ Like backstroke, work on hard swimming with about 30 seconds of rest. Breaststroke is very taxing when done hard but like bicycling it is easy to throttle back and have the appearance without the substance.

Integrated Workouts

For pool training it is necessary to integrate your sets into a comprehensive workout. At first you will want to limit your hard sets, but as your fitness improves, hard drills can be extended. It's also worthwhile alternating between anaerobic and aerobic workouts. In this way your performance for combat swimmer operations should be optimized.

Figure 5-3. Sample Anaerobic and Aerobic/ Endurance Swim Interval Workouts

Anaerobic

600 m warm-up

5 x 50 m with 15 sec rest between each

5 x 50 m with 30 sec rest

5 x 50 m freestyle swim with 45 sec rest

200 m easy swim

5 x 100 m freestyle, 45 sec rest

5 x 100 m freestyle with 90 sec rest

500 m easy swim

Aerobic

400 m warm-up

5 x 200 m freestyle with 30 sec rest

10 x 100 m freestyle, keep distance pace, 10 sec rest

200 m easy swim

5 x 200 m freestyle with 5 sec rest

10 x 100 m freestyle, keep distance pace, 5 sec rest

400 m cool down

Underwater Training

Swimming underwater requires breathholding. While this is an activity that is not endorsed by the diving manual, it may be something you will need to do as a SEAL. Given this fact, specific training will enhance your performance and extend your operational capabilities. The following rules apply to underwater swim training:

◆ DO NOT hyperventilate prior to your underwater swim.

◆ Use a buddy to observe during pool drills.

Varying Your Workout

Swimming workouts should be varied between easy days and hard days. For competitive speed, it is good to swim at least four days a week; this will help keep stroke efficiency. Swimming days provide good relief for tight muscles generated by running and weight training.

Swimming has some specialized weight training techniques. The primary issue is that swimmers have full range of motion of their arms during exertion. Muscle contraction is fairly constant over the entire arm motion requiring balanced power throughout. Weight training must complement this fact, or muscle tightness develops that actually works against the swimmer (see Chapter 6).

Pulley pulls are excellent weight training techniques for a swimmer. The classic is the lat pull-down station present in virtually all weight rooms and multi-station machines.

A better arrangement is for weights and pulley setups to be individualized for each hand. Pulley pulls are "isotonic" and mimic the constant resistance of water. Weights should be kept on the low side, permitting high speed weightlifting of between 1-1.5 seconds per repetition. Hold slightly at the end of each lift to prevent banging weights and getting thrown out of the weight room.

Swimmers use high reps, never less than 10.

Many dedicated swimmers own an Exergenie, which is a truly simple piece of equipment that permits a realistic workout in freestyle or backstroke. It is a nylon line rigged up through a little cylinder that twists the line and provides resistance. This workout is possible even within the confines of a cramped 688 class (40 - 50 reps) can be done daily because the motion is so much like swimming. Thus, it is a portable weight room for swimmers.

Cross training includes canoeing, rowing, kayaking, and cross country skiing.

All of these involve repetitive arm use in a pattern that is generally complementary to a swimmer's stroke. These sports will impart strength to the shoulder and chest muscles that will help your swimming.

Developing Stroke Skills

Basic stroke mechanics will prohibit you from increasing your respiratory rate (except during backstroke). Because you can't pant, you will quickly become limited by not getting enough oxygen or not getting rid of carbon dioxide before it starts building up. This is different than in running and is the reason for the universal use of interval training in swim training programs. Runners often go out for long steady runs, but a swimmer who trains this way becomes a slow and inefficient swimmer. While operational SEAL swimming is a long, slow activity, it is best for you to acquire a broad base of swimming skills. This will increase your efficiency during SEAL operational swimming.

This section will discuss three main swimming strokes; crawl stroke (usually called freestyle or "free"), breaststroke, and sidestroke. These particular strokes are the most useful to you as a SEAL. Most swimmers use a variety of strokes in a workout to provide cross training and avoid overuse injuries. Skills must be developed over a long period of time in order for the swimmer to become proficient. Good stroke mechanics are not only necessary to develop speed; injury may occur in swimmers from poor technique. A proper stroke may only be developed by getting feedback from others. This factor makes a buddy system or partner coaching an essential component of your training program. Obtain periodic stroke coaching from a qualified instructor—no matter how good you are.

General Stroke Principles

Water causes a large amount of drag on the swimmer's body, thus streamlining becomes extremely important. The key to swimming fast is reducing drag as much as possible while maximizing propulsive forces. One specific technique includes rolling from side to side to clear high resistance parts of the swimmer's body for arm recovery. Swimming in salt water is faster than swimming in fresh water because of the increased buoyancy of the swimmer, reducing resistance. There are many other subtle ways to reduce water drag in swimming, and learning them is one of the benefits of getting coaching from a qualified instructor or swimming coach.

The Strokes

Freestyle

For beginning freestyle swimmers, a pullbuoy will help the swimmer concentrate on proper arm stroke, and additionally help keep the hips positioned high in the water which minimizes drag. Approximately 90% of the work with the freestyle is due to the arm stroke.

The correct arm pull incorporates several elements of sculling. In overall terms, the arm of the swimmer resembles a turning propeller. The diagrams in Figure 5-4, Figure 5-5, and Figure 5-6 outline the hand motion relative to the water and present front, side, below the water views of the free-style arm stroke of Mark Spitz, as analyzed by swimming physiologist, James Counsilman. Notice the circular motion of the swimmer's arm.

In Figure 5-5 you can see the "catch" that a championship swimmer develops as he sculls downward at first and then sweeps his hand quickly back toward his body.

As shown in Figure 5-6, you can see how the hand is used to seek out still water from below the swimmer. The swimmer initially sculls outward, then he directs his hand inward at the same time he is "catching" back upward toward his body. The freestyle stroke is then completed with an outward scull.

Figure 5-4. Comparing the Free-Style Stroke to the Blades Turning on a Propeller

---

Figure 5-5. The Free-Style Stroke of Mark Spitz

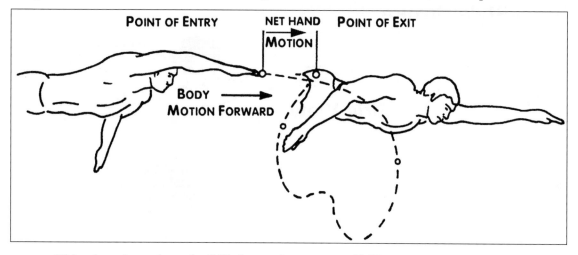

POINT OF ENTRY   NET HAND   POINT OF EXIT
                  MOTION

BODY →
MOTION FORWARD

This view shows best the "S" shape of a proper pull. Keep in mind that the "S" occurs in both the horizontal and vertical planes—a very complex motion indeed! You can appreciate how necessary coaching is in developing a proper arm stroke.

Several of the drills are designed to break this down for you. One arm freestyle allows you to concentrate on the arm's motion. Catchup freestyle slows everything down so that you can coordinate body roll with arm pulls. Using hand paddles will help you feel the water and the sculling sensation is also greatly accentuated.

Using hand paddles will help you develop a strong sculling motion.

Other views (Figure 5-7) show how the arms move during the freestyle stroke. From the front, the hand roughly describes a loop. Finally, you can see again from a side view of Mark Spitz that there is an aggressive "catch" action in the arm pull as he sculls back toward his body.

Breaststroke

The key to breaststroke is the kick. Propulsion is provided by drawing the feet up towards your body in the direction of motion, and then sweeping both feet backward in a circular

Figure 5-6. Below the Swimmer View of Mark Spitz's Free-Style Stroke

Figure 5-7. Side and Front Views of Mark Spitz's Free-Style Stroke

motion, pushing motionless water backward with the inside and bottom portions of the swimmer's feet. Coaching is essential to develop good technique as the kick is very subtle.

Pulling is done by a sweeping sculling motion. A good stroke drill to work on for a strong sculling motion is to use only your arms and not your legs, in other words, "pull breaststroke." This drill develops a feel for the water that is needed for all three strokes.

Sidestroke

Sidestroke is extremely important for you to master. SEALs are required to swim in open water under challenging conditions. Arm pulling and kicking should be coordinated to maximize thrust and conserve energy over a long swim. It is necessary to learn sidestroke using either side in order to be able to face away from heavy ocean chop and swells. You can't afford to have a favorite side.

Sidestroke is a "stealth" stroke, unlike freestyle. SEALs can stay in contact with each other over a long swim distance. The sculling motions that have been diagrammed in this chapter for freestyle, also apply to sidestroke. Use a sweeping action with your hand and visualize that your upper hand is like a helicopter blade grabbing still water out in front of you while your bottom hand grabs water ahead and below you.

The power of fins can be used with your flutterkick, not broaching on the surface of the water. Sidestroke is efficient, conserving your energy over a long swim. With fins, the majority of thrust comes from the legs and arm stroke is less important.

Swimming Drills

Fin Drills

Kicking with fins is fantastic training. Be careful of using a kickboard too much while training with fins; this may cause back pain. Sidestroke is good but you will need lane lines and flags to prevent careening off course and acquiring a nice scalp laceration. The mainstay of kicking strokes is still prone flutterkick.

Fin kicking drills are essential to building leg strength and specific training for SEAL combat swimmer duties. These drills are effective when imbedded within a pool workout where there are swimming sets that accentuate arm and chest muscle training. This is because the swimmer's legs will be warmed up but relatively fresh and ready for a strenuous workout with fins. Use high numbers of repeats in sets, 10-12, with relatively short rest intervals of 10-15 seconds. A total set length of around 10 minutes is optimal; any longer and the set begins to degrade into a long, slow distance set which is best done in open water.

- ◆ **Fin Sprints:** Sprinting 25 meters with fins will allow you to feel flaws in your arm strokes. This drill will consume an extraordinary amount of oxygen and provide a good anaerobic and strength workout for your legs. It also feels great to go fast.

- ◆ **Fin Fartlek:** Do this set without a kickboard. Kick one length with an easy flutter kick, then flutterkick the next length on your right side with both hands out of the water—effort level high—then back to face down for a length of easy flutter kick, then back at it over a hard length, this time on your left side, again hands out of the water. Repeat several times. This drill is particularly effective in a long pool (45m).

- ◆ **Fin Repeats:** Do with a kickboard. Kick flutterkick hard for 50m, rest 10 seconds, repeat for 10 repetitions.

Other Specific Freestyle Drills

- ◆ **One Arm Freestyle:** May be done with or without a pull-buoy. Emphasizes body rolling without corkscrewing. This drill will allow the swimmer to concentrate on proper pulling technique.

- ◆ **Catch-Up Freestyle:** Hold arm out in front while pulling with the other arm. Recover the pulling arm and then touch hands out in front before initiating the pull with the other arm. This drill will help timing of pull.

- ◆ **Fist Freestyle:** Swim with fists. This will make the swimmer concentrate on forearm sculling. Do this drill without the pull-buoy.

- ◆ **Finger Drag Freestyle:** Recover arm with fingers skimming the water. This provides the swimmer with feedback regarding arm and hand position during arm recovery.

Common Problems

Swimmers often develop hypersensitivities and allergies with pool swimming. The source of the problem is the inhalation of chlorinated organic material (guess where this comes from in a public pool). These hypersensitivity reactions may include lung conditions that are quite disabling. Prevention is the key. Ways to minimize your chances of such problems include:

- ◆ Wearing goggles.

- ◆ Using a nose clip.

- ◆ Avoiding any situation where you might breathe a mist or spray that is generated from pool water

Chapter 6
Strength Training

Muscular strength and endurance training enhance agility, speed, strength, and endurance, all of which are essential to the SEAL operator. This chapter will help to establish an understanding of the principles of muscle strength and endurance training and their application in the use of weight equipment. The focus of strength training should be its functional use for specific missions. Pure strength alone will not improve mission performance, but conversion of strength to muscle endurance should. The main objective of your strength training program should be to increase your applied strength—an increase in applied strength will enhance your performance on physical tasks required during missions. As such, this chapter introduces concepts and practical information for achieving optimal muscle strength and endurance for job performance and prevention of injuries.

Weight Training Gear and Equipment

Weight training requires minimal personal gear. Other than the weights themselves, equipment such as a pair of supportive shoes, fitted lifting gloves, and standard PT attire is all that is needed. A weight lifting belt should be used for back protection.

Technology has allowed the development of exercise equipment that efficiently adapts to the changing needs of a body in motion. Consider the choice of free weights, machines, or a combination of both for development of strength and balance when starting a weight training regimen. Table 6-1 presents a comparison of free weights and machines.

Table 6-1. Free Weight and Exercise Machine Comparison

Issue	Free Weights	Exercise Machines
User Friendliness	Usually available; Require minimal space; Require spotters for some evolutions	Must have access to sophisticated equipment; Doesn't require spotters
Skill	Require more skill than machines	Require less skill than free weights; Easy to use
Type of Movement	Dynamic	Limited range of motion
Variety in Workout	Allow for a variety of exercises; Useful for correcting strength imbalances between muscles on both sides of the body	Provide variable resistance; Availability of equipment may limit variety
Application	Primary muscles plus peripheral muscles	Tend to isolate muscles

Strength Training Guidelines and Terms

Performing operational tasks requires all muscles of the upper and lower body to be developed in a balanced way. *Circuit weight training* or *Split-routine workouts* are the most common ways to maintain a musculoskeletal balance. Circuit weight training consists of a progression from one station to the next such that over the course of the training period, both the upper and lower body are exercised. For split-routine training, different body areas are exercised on alternate days. For example, on Monday and Thursday, the upper body would be exercised whereas on Tuesday and Friday the lower body would be exercised. By having a well designed strength program, you can expect to maintain a high level of fitness while reducing your risk of injury and fatigue.

Repetition Maximum or RM

One term routinely used in strength training is that of repetition maximum. **A repetition maximum or RM is the maximum amount of weight you can lift for a given number of repetitions.** For example, your 1RM would be the amount of weight you could lift for only 1 repetition. Your 5RM would be the amount of weight you could lift for 5 repetitions. For example: if a SEAL can do 5 repetitions of an exercise with 50 lbs., he has a 5RM of 50 lbs.

Your 1RM would be the amount of weight you can lift for only 1 repetition

FITT: Frequency, Intensity, Time, Type

In order for the SEAL operator to perform mission-related tasks, strength training is a key aspect that must not be overlooked. Understanding the concepts of **Frequency, Intensity, Time,** and **Type (FITT** principle) will help you understand and maximize your training.

The **FREQUENCY** of training should be determined by the amount of time one has to spend on strength training. As SEAL operators, your weight training time is limited due to busy schedules, so keep this in mind when your start a program. For example, total body circuit training only needs to be performed twice a week, along with other training modes for optimal results. If two days of training cannot be achieved, one session will be better than none. Split-routine training should be performed a minimum of two sessions per muscle group weekly to ensure total muscular balance, and thus consumes a greater amount of time than circuit training.

Circuit weight training optimizes the time available for SEAL operators.

Training **INTENSITY** is considered to be the most critical aspect of strength and conditioning. Intensity of weight training can be referred to as load, which is the amount of weight per repetition. It is defined as the percentage of the RM that is being used to perform

---

an exercise. Various intensities are recommended for optimal results. The program phase focusing on muscular endurance would involve training at 30% to 50% of your 1RM with 20 to 60 repetitions per set, whereas the phase focusing on strength with 20 to 60 repetitions per set, whereas, the phase focusing on strength development would require training at 65% to 90% of your 1RM, with 1 to 12 repetitions per set, depending on the week of training (Table 6-1). SEAL training should focus on both strength and muscular endurance and cycle between 30 and 90% of maximal strength. This approach will yield maximum results and increase your performance as a SEAL operator.

The **TIME** you spend on weight training might vary depending on the program chosen. Generally, 30-60 minutes is sufficient, whether a circuit or split routine is implemented.

The **TYPE** of exercise will vary throughout your strength program and can include free weights or machines. For platoon evolutions, circuit training is more adaptable, while split routines may be used for individual strength programs. Figure 6-1 provides an example of the FITT principle.

Strength training, along with various other mission-related practices (such as obstacle courses, swims, runs, jumps, and climbs) will develop an overall well-conditioned SEAL operator.

Figure 6-1. Applying the FITT Principle to Total Body Circuit Weight Training

Muscle Balance and Exercise Selection List

Total Body Circuit

F: 2 times weekly

I: 30% to 90% of 1RM

T: 30 to 60 minutes

T: Circuit weights

It is extremely important to consider muscle balance when designing your workouts. Building strength in the triceps should be balanced by strengthening the biceps, and strengthening the quadriceps should be balanced by strengthening the hamstrings. **Without proper balancing of opposing muscle groups, you become vulnerable to injury.**

The main goal of a weight training regimen is to produce a gain in overall strength for operational tasks.

Many exercises can be incorporated into your strength training program. **Table 6-2 presents a list of exercises by specific body parts, all of which are demonstrated in Appendix A.** This translates into a complete body workout from the calves to the neck.

Table 6-2. Exercise Selection List by Body Part

Body Part	Exercises	
Legs:	Squats Leg Press 3/4 Squat Standing Calf Raises	Leg Extensions Leg Curls Leg Press
Back:	Curl Grip Lat Pulldown Reverse Barbell Row	One Arm Dumbbell Row Hyperextensions
Chest:	Bench Press	Incline Dumbbell Press
Shoulders:	Behind-the-Neck Press	Upright Row
Arms:	Triceps Pressdowns	Curls

Determining Repetition Maximums

The purpose of knowing your RM is to allow you to adjust the exercise intensity. As a safety measure, it is best to start out by determining your 5RM. To do this, you should have not had any strenuous activity on the day of the test, and you should be properly warmed up. A spotter should always be available when conducting this test. Free weights are the recommended form of weight for this test.

- ◆ Select a weight you know is light enough for 10 repetitions.
- ◆ Perform 10-15 repetitions with that weight.
- ◆ Rest for two minutes.
- ◆ Increase weight 2%-10%, depending on difficulty of previous set.
- ◆ Perform 6-8 repetitions.
- ◆ Rest for two minutes.
- ◆ Increase weight 2%-10%, depending on difficulty of previous set.

- Rest for three minutes.
- Perform 5 repetitions—this should be close to your 5RM.

Perform sets with increasing weights and decreasing repetitions until a weight that can be comfortably handled for 5 reps is reached.

Table 6-3 provides an example of how you might determine your 5RM for the bench press, starting with a weight of 110 lbs. Typically, your 5RM is 87% of your 1RM, and your 10RM is 75% of your 1RM. Thus, if your 5RM is 160, your 1RM would be approximately 184 lbs, and your 10 RM would be about 138 lbs. After determining your 5RM, it will be easy to establish your 1RM and loads for workouts (See Figure 6-2). See Table 6-4 for intensity as a percent of maximum strength, repetitions, energy systems, and rest intervals. Remember, the three energy systems are:

- ATP-PC System for speed work activities, such as sprinting.
- Lactic Acid and ATP-PC System for all-out exercise that continues beyond 30 seconds, but lasts less than 3 minutes.
- Oxygen system for aerobic energy to support long-term steady state exercise, such as long distance running or swimming.

Multiply your 5RM times 1.15 to establish your 1RM.

Figure 6-2. Determining Your 1RM from 5RM

5RM = 75
1RM = 75 X 1.15 = 86
5RM = 136
1RM = 136 X 1.15 = 156

Table 6-3. How to Determine Your 5RM for a Bench Press

Set	Repetitions	Weight	Rest Intervals Between
10 Minute Warm-Up			
1	15-Dec	110 lbs	2 minutes
2	12-Oct	120 lbs	2 minutes
3	8-Jun	135 lbs	3 minutes
4	5	160 lbs	Completed

Table 6-4. Intensity Levels Relative to a 1RM*

% of 1 RM	Number of Repetitions	Rest Intervals Between Sets (minutes)	Energy System
>95	1	3-5	ATP/CP
80-95	2-5	3-5	ATP/CP
65-80	6-10	2-4	ATP/CP/LA
50-70	8-15	2-4	ATP/CP/LA
30-50	15-60	1-2	LA/Aerobic

*Adapted with permission from *Strength Training for Sports;* Applied FuturisticsSM, Inc.

Periodization

Periodization of training is a technique that involves altering training variables (such as the number of repetitions per set, the exercises performed, training intensity, and the amount of rest between sets) to achieve well-defined gains in muscular strength, endurance, and overall performance. For example, if you were working towards a particular mission or athletic competition, you would want to peak at that moment and not earlier. Your training schedule would be adapted to achieve that goal.

There are several phases to periodization and weight training in general. The first phase is one of activation, or getting the body ready for a new activity. It would typically last four weeks. Most of you are already weight training and thus have completed the true activation phase, but it is okay to start anew. The second phase is for strength development, and it would last about 4 to 7 weeks, depending on how long you have been weight training. The next phase is the muscular endurance phase, and lasts 8 to 12 weeks, depending on your schedule. Table 6-5 presents a one year plan for training, with three seven week periods of strength development followed by 12 weeks of conversion to muscular endurance. Note that this schedule can be modified and is presented here to emphasize the concept of periodization.

The goal of the muscular endurance phase is to take strength gains and convert them into applied strength for operations.

Table 6-5. An Annual Plan for Activation, Strength Development, and Muscular Endurance*

Sept	Oct	Nov	Dec	Jan	Feb	Mar	April	May	June	July	August
Develop Strength		Muscle Endurance			Develop Strength		Muscle Endurance			Cross-Training/ Active Rest	Develop Strength

*Adapted with permission from *Strength Training for Sports*; Applied FuturisticsSM, Inc.

Training intensities should be varied weekly, depending on whether you are in the strength or muscular endurance phase. Table 6-6 and Table 6-7 present the percent of maximum (%1RM) and number of sets for the strength and muscular endurance phases, respectively. These templates can serve as guidelines for creating your own periodized program. Remember, this program should be followed two times per week.

30°

Table 6-6. Strength Development Phase: 2-Day Circuit Weight Training Routine

Week	Set 1	Set 2	Set 3	Set 4	Set 5
Perform a 5RM test to start Week 1					
1	50% X 12	70% X 8	70% X 8	80% X 6	80% X 6
2	50% X 12	70% X 8	80% X 4-6	80% X 4-6	85% X 3-5
3	50% X 12	75% X 8	85% X 3-5	85% X 3-5	90% X 3-5
4	45% X 15	75% X 6-8	75% X 6-8	80% X 4-6	80% X 4-6
5	55% X 12	75% X 8	85% X 3-5	85% X 3-5	85% X 3-5
6	55% X 10	75% X 8	85% X 3-5	90% X 1-3	90% X 1-3
7	55% X 12	75% X 6-8	75% X 6-8	80% X 4-6	80% X 4-6

Table 6-7. Muscle Endurance Phase: A 2-Day Circuit Weight Training Routine

Week	Set 1	Set 2
	Perform a 5RM test at Week 1	
	Start at 30%: Reps are more important than%	
1	30-50% X 20	30-50% X 20
2	30-50% X 30	30-50% X 30
3	30-50% X 40	30-50% X 40
4	30-50% X 35	30-50% X 35
5	30-50% X 45	30-50% X 45
6	30-50% X 50	30-50% X 50
7	30-50% X 40	30-50% X 40
8	30-50% X 55	30-50% X 55
9	30-50% X 60	30-50% X 60
10	30-50% X 50	30-50% X 50
11	30-50% X 40	30-50% X 40
12	30-50% X 30	30-50% X 30

Although it may seem a bit foreign to you to see up to 60 reps per set in Table 6-7, this is the best way to convert your strength gains to applied strength, or functional strength. You will be amazed at your muscular endurance and ability to perform mission-related tasks and other strenuous physical tasks if you truly stick with a program such as this

Weight Lifting Techniques

Correct lifting techniques are critical for achieving maximum benefits and preventing injury. Lifting form, speed, and breathing techniques are all important for weight training. The lift should be performed as a controlled movement with proper form. Do not compromise your form as it will not help but rather increase your chance of injury. The appropriate speed of lifting needs to be applied to all exercise movements. When performing exercises, such as the bench press, squat, biceps curl, lat pull-down, etc., the weight should be moved at a rate of 1-2 seconds in each direction. This will ensure your safety and optimize strength training.

Controlling the rate of movement affects the muscle you intend to strengthen.

Always make use of a spotter if you are using free weights. Refer to Appendix A for form illustrations and instructions so you can change your technique if you are not following the proper directions.

Exhale when moving a weight against gravity.

Proper breathing techniques must be used during weight training. Exhale during positive weight movement (moving the weight against gravity). This helps prevent the valsalva maneuver (an increase in internal pressure caused by holding your breath during lifting exercises) which can result in damage to the cardiovascular system. Never hold your breath while performing any exercise task.

Types of Workouts

A *Circuit Routine Training* for the first week of the strength development phase and muscular endurance phase is presented in Table 6-8 and Table 6-9, respectively. Workouts for the other weeks can be obtained by reviewing Table 6-6 and Table 6-7. Remember, periodization is the key to improving overall muscle strength and endurance.

Table 6-8. Week 1: Circuit Training Strength Development Phase

Exercises	Sets (% of 1 RM and Reps)				
	1 (%/Reps)	2 (%/Reps)	3 (%/Reps)	4 (%/Reps)	5 (%/Reps)
Squats or Leg Press	50/12	70/8	70/8	80/6	80/6
Curl Grip Pulldowns	50/12	70/8	70/8	80/6	80/6
Leg Curls	50/12	70/8	70/8	80/6	80/6
Bench Press	50/12	70/8	70/8	80/6	80/6
Standing Calf Raises	50/12	70/8	70/8	80/6	80/6
Behind-the-Neck Press or Upright Row	50/12	70/8	70/8	80/6	80/6
Tricep Pressdown	50/12	70/8	70/8	80/6	80/6
BB Curls	50/12	70/8	70/8	80/6	80/6

DB = Dumbbell; BB = Barbell; See Appendix A for pictorial representation.

Table 6-9. Week 1: Circuit Training Muscle Endurance Phase

Exercises	Set 1 (%RM/Reps)	Set 2 (%RM/Reps)
Squats or Leg Press	30-50/20	30-50/20
Curl Grip Pulldowns	30-50/20	30-50/20
Leg Curls	30-50/20	30-50/20
Bench Press	30-50/20	30-50/20
Standing Calf Raises	30-50/20	30-50/20
Behind-the-Neck Press or Upright Row	30-50/20	30-50/20
Tricep Pressdown	30-50/20	30-50/20
BB Curls	30-50/20	30-50/20

DB = Dumbbell; BB = Barbell; See Appendix A for pictorial representation.

Warming Up

It is imperative to warm-up prior to a strength training workout. An active and dynamic warm-up will elevate the body temperature so that the muscles respond better to the training. An increase in circulation to the joints and tissues allow more elasticity and may decrease the risk of injury. The warm-up should last long enough to break a sweat then stretching should be initiated. Thus, the major component of a warm-up session for weight training is a cardiovascular workout, or a general warm-up designed to increase your circulation and direct blood flow to the muscles for the upcoming workout. This should be low intensity exercise for 10 to 20 minutes.

- ◆ Biking
- ◆ Stairclimber
- ◆ Treadmill/Jogging
- ◆ Jumping Rope
- ◆ Rowing Ergometer
- ◆ Jumping Jacks/Calisthenics
- ◆ One or Two Exercises with Light Weights

Cooling Down and Stretching

Upon the completion of a training routine, cooling down and stretching should not be overlooked. The cool-down should be gradual to normalize body temperature, prevent pooling of blood in the muscles and return metabolic rates to pre-exercise levels. It also speeds the removal of waste products which tend to increase muscle soreness and prolong recovery. Stretching after weight training maintains joint and muscle flexibility while minimizing muscle spasms and weight training injuries. In brief, the components of a cool down include:

◆ Low intensity cycling or walking
◆ Complete body stretching
◆ Relaxation

Common Problems

You need to listen to your body and be able to recognize the signs of problematic conditions associated with weight training.

◆ **Injuries -** Lack of warm-up and improper lifting techniques (form) can cause muscle damage.
◆ **Overuse Syndrome -** Occurs when you engage in frequent repetitive exercises to a specific area or use an improper technique during an exercise. The knee, elbow, and shoulder are most susceptible to these injuries.
◆ **Delayed Onset Muscle Soreness (DOMS) -** Potentially severe pain experienced 24 to 48 hours after the activity.

In order to allow the body to heal, the improper routine and/or techniques must be altered. Proper technique, progression, variation, rest, and recovery will minimize training related injuries. More information can be found in the training related injuries chapter.

Conclusions

Strength training with weights is an important component to the complete PT program of the SEAL operator. Training with weights 2-3 times per week can help optimize preparations for mission-related tasks. It is important to understand that one should focus on the SEAL mission when developing a weight training regimen. A proper weight training routine will help prevent injuries and accelerate recovery from an injury to the musculoskeletal system. Following the principles and examples in this chapter will help you develop a well balanced lifting routine. Optimal conditioning can be obtained without injury to the body if weight training is included in your overall PT program.

Resource

◆ Fred Koch, *Strength Training for Sports;* Applied FuturisticsSM, 1994.

Acknowledgment

The editors thank Mr. Fred Koch for sharing his expertise and experience in strength training. His comments and suggestions were invaluable to the development of this chapter.

Chapter 7
Flexibility

Most trainers, exercise physiologists, and health care professionals agree that flexibility training, although often overlooked, is an important component of a physical fitness program. Stretching becomes even more important as athletes and/or SEALs achieve advanced levels of muscle strength and endurance. If optimum performance is the goal, then adherence to a consistent flexibility program is required.

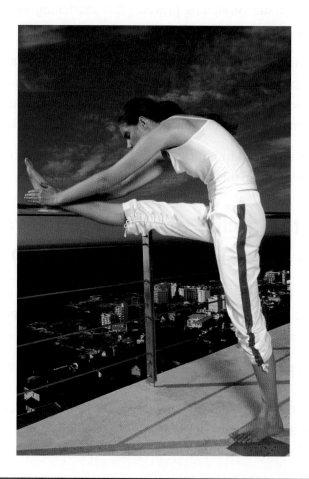

Flexibility Benefits

Proper use of stretching increases flexibility and provides the following benefits:

- Improved performance
- Reduced potential for injury (i.e., muscle strain or sprain)
- Reduced muscle soreness
- Decreased risk and severity of low-back pain
- Increased agility
- Increased blood flow to the joints

Proper physical conditioning is necessary for successful mission performance. Flexibility is an integral part of a conditioning program and enhances performance by extending the range of motion in which one can optimally perform. SEALs are at high risk for musculoskeletal injuries. Joint stability and consequent protection against injury are best achieved through a balanced physical conditioning program designed to improve both muscle strength and flexibility. Strength and flexibility training should be considered interdependent since both are involved in the degree and quality of movement across a joint.

Muscles that are strengthened should be stretched, and vice versa. An intense strength workout can cause microtrauma to the muscles, and the process of recovery can shorten the muscles and connective tissue. Stretching prevents this shortening which could contribute to muscle strains or other overuse injuries (e.g., tendonitis, fasciitis).

Flexibility training, without concurrent strength training, weakens the muscles and connective tissue and places the joints and muscles at risk for sprains, partial and complete dislocations, and muscle strains. Strengthening the muscles surrounding a stretched joint helps stabilize the joint and improve muscular function, thus decreasing the likelihood of injury.

Overstretching may lead to injury; however, as long as a flexibility program is well balanced with strength training, this possibility is negligible.

Flexibility is the ability of a limb to move freely about a joint through a full range of motion.

In the case of Special Warfare Operators, flexibility refers to the optimum range of motion surrounding a particular joint that is necessary for peak performance. Range of motion is specific to each joint and dependent upon:

- Joint surfaces and capsule and the degree of movement required for the joint to function
- Muscles, tendons, ligaments, and connective tissue associated with limb movement around a joint (for definitions see Chapter 1)
- Strength of the musculature surrounding the joint

There are two types of flexibility: dynamic and static.

Dynamic or active flexibility refers to the speed attained within a range of motion at the joint during physical performance. This type of flexibility involves the intrinsic musculature surrounding the joint and its ability to overcome resistance to motion. An example would be the flexibility required to throw a baseball, punch a boxing opponent, or perform a martial arts kick. Static or passive flexibility refers to the maximal range of motion of a joint during passive movement induced by an external source (e.g., a partner, equipment, gravity). The range of static flexibility is always greater than that of dynamic flexibility.

The Stretch Reflex and the Lengthening Reaction

The stretch reflex and the lengthening reaction are joint-protective mechanisms in which sensory organs, located in the muscles and tendons surrounding a joint, are activated when muscles are stretched. As seen in Figure 7-1, the two sensory organs involved in monitoring muscle tightness are the muscle spindle cells and golgi tendon organs (GTOs).

Figure 7-1. Graphical Representations of Muscle Spindles and Golgi Tendon Organs

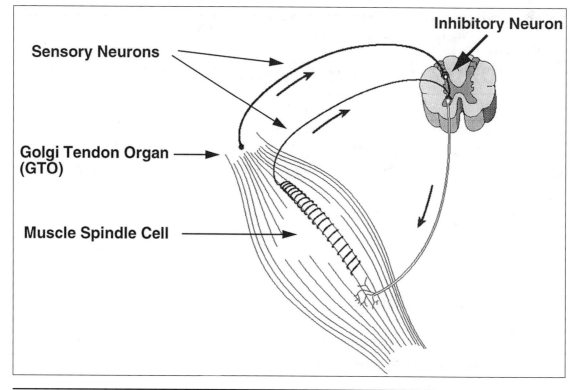

The stretch reflex involves muscle spindles which lie parallel to the muscle fiber. These spindles are very sensitive to changes in muscle length. When the muscle stretches, muscle spindles send signals to the spinal cord, which in turn, sends signals to the muscle telling it to contract in order to protect the muscle from potential tissue damage. The classic example of the stretch reflex occurs when a physician taps a patient just below the kneecap. The quadriceps muscle is quickly stretched, and the muscle spindles react by contracting the quadriceps muscle causing the knee-jerk response. The greater or more rapid the stretch, the greater the response of the muscle spindles and the resultant muscle contraction. Signals are high in frequency at the beginning of a stretch, but then slow down as they adapt to the new length.

The lengthening reaction engages GTOs, which are located in the muscle-tendon junctions, and activates them when the tension in a tendon is increased as a result of either muscular contraction, stretching the muscle beyond its resting length, or a combination of the two. When muscular tension increases, the GTOs respond by sending inhibitory signals to the muscle; this causes the muscles to relax and protects the muscles and tendons from tearing due to tension overload. Knowledge of the stretch reflex and the lengthening reaction is useful for effective stretching.

The most effective stretches are performed slowly and held for 15-30 seconds.

Performing the stretch slowly avoids excessive activation of the muscle spindles and resultant muscular contraction. Holding the stretch allows time for the muscle spindles to adapt to the new muscle length, and eventually, to achieve greater lengths. The length and duration of the stretch should also be sufficient to activate the GTOs so that they override the muscle spindles and induce muscular relaxation.

Flexibility Training Methods

There are several training methods used to develop flexibility; however, most fall under the following general categories:

- ◆ Dynamic
- ◆ Static
- ◆ Ballistic
- ◆ Proprioceptive neuromuscular facilitation (PNF)

Dynamic Stretching

Dynamic stretching (sometimes referred to as active stretching) consists of controlled movements which increase in range and/or speed so that you gradually reach your full range and speed of movement (e.g., slow, controlled leg swings or kicks, controlled arm swings, back bends). This type of stretching often mimics the activity that is to be performed and prepares the muscles for that activity.

There is some controversy surrounding the effectiveness of dynamic stretching and its role in the development of flexibility. Some experts believe that the short, intermittent movements involved in this type of stretching activate the stretch reflex and cause the stretched muscle to contract. Others maintain that dynamic stretching is beneficial for quick, explosive activities like gymnastics or martial arts. However, in general, dynamic stretching should not be used to develop static flexibility or long-standing changes in range of motion. If used at all, dynamic stretching functions best before exercise to enhance performance. This type of stretch is often performed after a warm up and prior to an exercise session in anticipation of a particular activity. Dynamic stretches should mimic the activity that is to be performed.

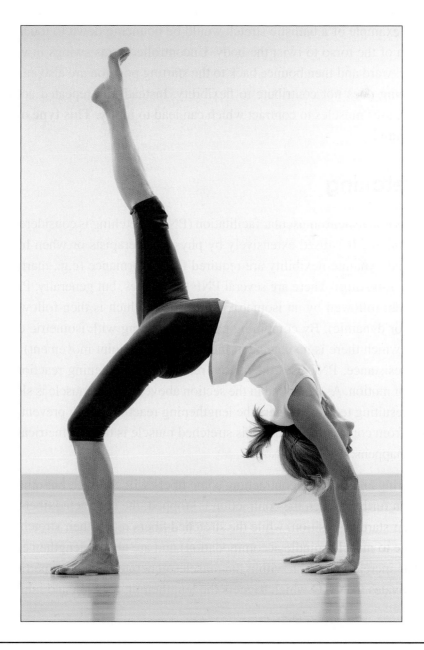

Static Stretching

Static stretching (sometimes referred to as passive stretching) develops static flexibility and uses slow, controlled movements through a full range of motion. This type of stretch is performed by holding a position using a part of the body, the assistance of a partner, or some other apparatus such as a pole or the floor (e.g., lifting one leg up and holding it with the hand, the splits). Slow, static stretching helps relieve muscle spasms due to exercise, and is used for cooling down after a workout to reduce muscle fatigue and soreness.

Ballistic Stretching

Ballistic stretching uses the momentum of the body or a limb to force a stretch past the normal range of motion and then return to the starting position. Ballistic stretching incorporates bouncing or jerky movements and should not be confused with dynamic stretching. An example of a ballistic stretch would be bouncing down to touch toes or using the momentum of the torso to twist the body. Uncontrolled arms swings in which the arms are thrown backward and then bounce back to the starting position are also an example. This type of stretching does not contribute to flexibility. Instead, the repeated activation of the stretch reflex causes muscles to contract which can lead to injury. **This type of stretching is not recommended.**

PNF Stretching

Proprioceptive neuromuscular facilitation (PNF) stretching is considered an advanced stretching technique. It is used extensively by physical therapists or when high degrees of both passive and dynamic flexibility are required for performance (e.g., martial arts, ballet, gymnastics, kick-boxing). There are several PNF techniques, but generally, PNF consists of a passive stretch, followed by an isometric contraction, which is then followed by another stretch (static or dynamic). By combining passive stretching with isometric contractions (a contraction in which there is no change in muscle length or joint movement) with a partner or object for resistance, PNF uses the stretch reflex and lengthening reaction to achieve a greater range of motion. As described in the section above, when a muscle is slowly stretched and held, the resulting tension triggers the lengthening reaction which prevents the stretched muscle fibers from contracting. When this stretched muscle is then isometrically contracted, the following happens:

◆ During an isometric contraction, some fibers will contract, but others will stretch even further. When the contraction is stopped, the contracted fibers return to their starting position, while the stretched fibers retain their stretched position (due to muscle spindle accommodation) and are able to lengthen even further.
◆ The increased tension within the muscles generated by an isometric contraction activates the GTO which triggers the lengthening reaction and inhibits further

contraction. When the isometric contraction is stopped, the muscle is still inhibited from further contraction and able to lengthen further.

The final stretch, which follows isometric contraction, takes advantage of the muscle's ability to elongate further, and allows the muscle, tendon, and sense organs to adapt to greater lengths.

It is best to have a partner help when using PNF techniques.

A common PNF technique is referred to as the **"contract-relax method."** Instructions for and a pictorial representation of this method are provided in Figure 7-2. This technique uses passive stretch and isometric contractions, followed by muscle relaxation and passive stretching to the new range of motion. For example, if you are stretching your hamstrings, you first passively take the stretch to the point of tightness and hold. Then you isometrically contract the hamstrings by using this muscle to apply force against an object or partner (See Figure 7-2). Following the contraction, the muscle is allowed to relax and the muscle is then passively stretched and held. Current recommendations suggest performing this technique with one to five repetitions, but like weight training, it needs to be done no more than three to five times a week.

Figure 7-2. Contract-Relax PNF Technique

1. Passive stretch for 15 sec

2. Isometric contraction for 7 - 15 sec

3. Passive stretch to new end ROM for 15 sec

Repeat 1 - 5 times

It is interesting to note that many stretches (including some of those illustrated in this chapter) can be performed statically, dynamically, or using PNF, depending on the goals of a stretching program.

Warming-Up and Stretching

Stretching is not the same as a warm-up.

Many individuals stretch in a misguided attempt to warm-up; however, stretching and warm-up should be considered distinctly different activities. A warm-up prepares the body for the activity that is to follow. The two types of warm-up are general and activity-specific. Physiologic changes that occur during warm-up include increases in muscle temperature, blood flow, oxygen delivery to the muscles, and skeletal muscle metabolism. Warm-up benefits include injury prevention and an improvement in performance.

A warm-up should always precede any physical activity whether it be stretching, exercise, sports, or mission-related training.

Cold muscles don't stretch, and there is a high chance of injury when stretching is performed without first warming up. Stretching (especially dynamic stretching) may be part of (or follow) a warm-up, but should not exclusively comprise the warm-up.

Stretch only after an adequate warm-up has been performed.

General Warm-Up

General (or unrelated) warm-up involves movements (e.g., running in place, jumping jacks, and other calisthenics) that are different from, or unrelated to, the specific activity that is to follow. This type of warm-up should be performed prior to high-intensity activities (e.g., O-Course, power-lifting, "burn-out PT," gymnastics, etc.) when immediate participation in the actual activity is likely to result in joint or muscle injuries.

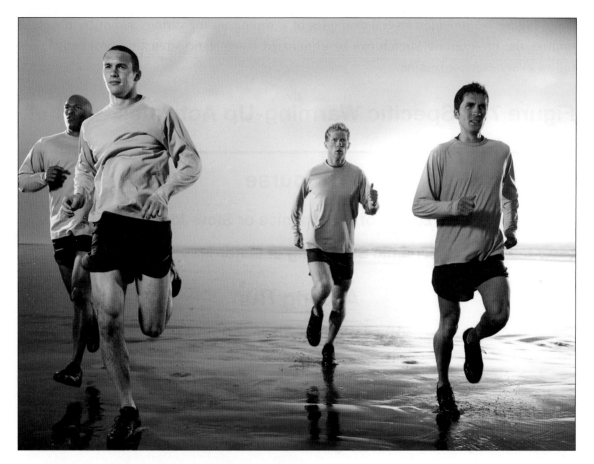

Activity-Specific Warm-Up

Activity-specific (or related) warm-up occurs with a low-intensity version of the activity that is to follow. Examples of activity-specific warm-up include a slow jog prior to a long run; slow cycling in preparation for a cycling event; or slow karate moves prior to practice. A related warm-up starts out slowly and progresses to more intense activity. Depending on the intensity of exercise to be performed, a warm-up of anywhere between 10-30 minutes may be required—the greater the intensity of the workout, the longer the warm-up.

All warm-ups should be of sufficient intensity to elevate body temperature; sweating is a good indication that you are ready to move on to the next phase of your workout.

Both general and activity-specific warm-ups may incorporate some type of stretching, especially if the activity to be performed is one of high intensity and imposes a good chance of acute injury. After a short period of warming-up, some pre-exercise stretching should be done. Figure 7-3 provides several examples of warming-up for various activities. If time is limited, the pre-exercise stretch can be eliminated but a static stretching program should follow every exercise session.

Figure 7-3. Specific Warming-Up Activities

O'Course

10 - 20 min of Calisthenics or Slow Jogging

Dynamic Stretching of Major Muscles

A Long Run

10 - 15 min of Slow Jogging

PT

Jumping Jacks, Slow Jog or Other In-Place Activity for 10 - 20 min

Dynamic Stretching of Muscles to be Used in PT

Exercise should not be ended abruptly, but gradually slowed, to avoid pooling of blood in the skeletal muscles and to facilitate the removal of metabolic end products. Exercise should be followed by a cool-down and stretching session.

Since most of the benefits from stretching occur post-exercise, a 10-15 minute stretching program should follow every exercise session and should be incorporated as part of the warm-down while the muscles are still warm. Stretches should be slow and static, held for 15-30 seconds, and taken to the point of tightness, not pain. Static stretching provides a good warm-down after a workout, reduces post-workout muscle fatigue and soreness, and is useful for relieving muscle spasms that occur as a result of exercise. Once muscles have been stretched, standing in cool/cold water, or running cool water over the legs or muscles used during the exercise, can also reduce soreness, and seems to speed recovery between exercise bouts. Figure 7-4 represents the ideal recommended exercise sequence.

Figure 7-4. Recommended Exercise Sequence

Recommended Stretches

Dynamic Stretching

Dynamic stretches of the muscle groups to be exercised during PT should be performed following a warm-up. Dynamic stretches should not be jerky movements. In fact, any slow, controlled movement that simulates the activity to be performed, executed for approximately 2 seconds, is sufficient. Some suggested dynamic exercises are provided in Table 7-1.

Table 7-1. Dynamic Stretch Exercises to be Used in Physical Training

Name	Description	Muscle Group(s)
Neck Rolls	No count exercise: From a standing position, slowly roll the head to the side, toward the back, to other side, etc.	Neck muscles
Hi Jack, Hi Jill	4-count exercise: Begin from a standing position with one arm elevated above the head and other arm down and slightly away from body. On count 1 both arms are pulled backward stretching chest muscles and released. Count 2 repeats first movement. On count 3, arms exchange positions and again pull toward back and release. Repeat this movement on count 4.	Chest and anterior shoulder muscles
Up-Back-and Over	3-count exercise: Begin from standing position, arms at sides. On count 1, bring both arms forward and upward. On count 2, bring both arms down and back. On count 3, bring both arms forward, up, back, and around to complete a full circle.	Shoulders, chest, and back

Flexibility

Table 7-1. (Continued)

Name	Description	Muscle Group(s)
Press-Press-Fling	3-count exercise: Begin from a standing position with arms bent, fists midline at chest level, and elbows out to the side. On count 1, pull elbows backwards towards the midline of the back, stretching the chest muscles and release. Repeat the same movement on count 2. On count 3, extend the arms out and back- wards, stretching the chest muscles.	Chest and anterior shoulder
Standing Toe Pointers	No count exercise: Start from a standing position with body weight over the heels. Flex and extend the feet and toes. Stretch Standing Toe should be felt in both the calf muscles (gastrocnemius) and muscles in front of the shins (anterior tibialis). As an alternative, walk on the heels with toes pointed upward.	Gastrocnemius and anterior tibialis muscle. (A good pre-running stretch.)
Four-Way Leg Swings	No count exercise: Standing upright, slowly swing 1 leg to front and to back and to side and across front or Four-Way Leg back of body. Swing should be a slow, controlled movement. Pointing the toes up or forward will stretch different muscles in leg.	Hip and lower leg muscles

Table 7-1. (Continued)

Name	Description	Muscle Group(s)
Four-Way Lunges	No-count exercise: Begin from a standing position. Extend 1 leg forward into a lunge so that body weight is distributed on both legs. When lunging forward, the knee should not extend beyond the toe of that leg. Use the forward leg to push off and return to starting position. Repeat this movement, using the same leg to the side. Then, perform exercise with the opposite leg.	Leg muscles
Trunk Rotations	4-count exercise: begin in a standing position with legs shoulder-width apart, knees slightly bent. On count 1, bend forward at the waist flexing torso. On count 2, bend torso laterally. On count 3, extend torso backward, and on count 4, bend torso laterally to remaining side. When bending backward, keep legs slightly bent to avoid hyperextending back.	Abdominal muscles, including obliques and hip flexors

Table 7-1. (Continued)

Name	Description	Muscle Group(s)
Trunk Twisters	No count exercise: Starting from a seated position with hands behind the head, twist the upper / torso to one side, and then to the other.	Abdominal muscles, including obliques
Trunk Bending Fore/Aft	No count exercise: Standing straight, knees slightly bent, bend the trunk forward and then back.	Hip flexors

Static Stretching

Most of the benefits derived from flexibility training are obtained with a consistent, post-exercise, static stretching program. The stretching that is performed following exercise on one day helps to prepare the muscles for the next day's exercise session.

The following exercises (Table 7-2) can be incorporated into a postexercise stretching program by selecting 1-3 stretches for each anatomical location listed below. Remember to balance the front of the body with the back (e.g., hip extensors with hip flexors, hamstrings with quadriceps). Select more stretches for those body areas exercised (e.g., legs after a run, shoulders after a swim). Perform 2-5 repetitions per stretch, hold for 15-30 seconds, then relax for 10-15 seconds. Note: these stretches are all no count exercises.

Table 7-2. Static Stretch Exercises to be Used in Physical Training

Name	Description	Muscle Group(s)
	Neck	
Lateral and Forward Neck Stretch	In a standing position, clasp hands behind back, with left hand grasping right wrist. Bend head to left bringing left ear toward left shoulder while slowly pulling down on right arm with left hand for added stretch (do not shrug shoulder up to ear). Stretch should be felt on right side of neck and shoulders. Perform stretch on left side by grasping left wrist with right hand. Bring right ear toward right shoulder while pulling down on left arm with right hand. Return to upright position and flex head forward and down using either hand to hold stretch. Return head to upright position.	Neck muscles
	Shoulders, Chest, and Arms	
Chest Stretch	Begin from a standing position with arms extended to side at shoulder level. While keeping thumbs pointed up, extend arms backward. Either have another person hold stretch or use a pole for resistance.	Anterior shoulder and chest muscles
Swimmer's Stretch	Perform seated. Clasp hands together behind lower back, palms up, thumbs pointed down. While bending over from waist, slowly pull arms up and toward head.	Chest and anterior shoulder muscles

Table 7-2. (Continued)

Name	Description	Muscle Group(s)
Upper Back Stretch	While standing or seated, extend and clasp arms together in front of body turning palms outward and pressing forward until shoulders and back are rounded.	Posterior shoulders, upper back, and triceps muscles
Posterior Shoulder Stretch	Bring arm that is to be stretched across chest. Use opposite arm to pull arm being stretched toward chest until stretch is felt in posterior shoulder.	Posterior Shoulder muscles
Forearm/ Wrist Stretch	Begin with knees and hands on deck, wrists turned so fingertips are pointing toward knees, thumbs to outside. Keep palms flat, and lean back, stretching front part of forearm.	Forearm and wrist muscles
Triceps Stretch	Standing erect, bring arm to be stretched up and back so that elbow is pointing toward sky and hand rests between shoulder blades. Gently pull arm toward midline behind head to stretch triceps muscle. NOTE: To extend stretch down side of body, bend to opposite side of arm being stretched.	Triceps muscles

Table 7-2. (Continued)

Name	Description	Muscle Group(s)

Torso: Abdominals and Back

Name	Description	Muscle Group(s)
Supine Back Stretch	While lying on back (supine), bring both knees up and toward chest. Place hands behind knees and gently pull both legs toward chest, stretching back muscles. Excellent stretch for lower back. Can help relieve muscle spasm and reduce risk of injury (muscle strain) to back muscles. When performing stretch, one may initially feel increased tightness or pain. HOLD stretch until you can feel muscles relax and tightness subside. May hold stretch for as long as a minute.	Back extensor muscles
Overhead Trunk Side Stretch	This exercise may be performed from a standing position or while lying on deck. From a standing position with arms above head, grasp wrist of arm on side that is to be stretched and slowly bend torso to opposite side that is to be stretched. Return to starting position and repeat on other side. While lying on side, slowly lift torso off deck and hold.	Abdominal muscles
Torso Prone Stretch (Press-Ups, Lizard)	Begin lying on stomach (prone) with hands flat on deck as for a push-up. Extend arms so that upper torso lifts off deck.	Abdominal muscles

Hips

Name	Description	Muscle Group(s)
Hip Cross-Over	Begin from a lying position (on back) with legs extended. Bring one knee toward chest at a 90° angle. Using opposite hand, pull leg over other leg and toward floor. Stretch should be felt in lower back and side of hip.	Iliotibial band and hip abductor muscles

Table 7-2. (Continued)

Name	Description	Muscle Group(s)
Iliopsoas Stretch	This exercise is essentially a standing lunge with a pelvic tilt. Begin from a standing position. Step forward with one leg, placing one foot in front of the other. Keep both legs slightly bent. Weight should be distributed toward the front foot. Flatten the back and tuck the hips under, stretching the iliopsoas muscle on the front of the back leg. For added stretch, either lean slightly back with the upper torso or bend further at the knees.	Iliopsoas
Hip Stretch	Begin by lying on back, knees bent, and feet flat on the deck. Cross one leg so that the ankle is resting on the knee of the other leg. Slowly lift the one leg off the deck and move it toward the chest. The stretch should be felt in the hip of the crossed leg. NOTE: May also be performed seated using arms to pull leg, as one unit, toward body.	Hip extensors
Kneeling Lunge with Pelvic Tilt	Begin kneeling on deck with toes pointed straight back. Move one leg forward until knee of forward leg is directly over ankle of forward foot. Without changing position of either leg, lower front of hip downward until a stretch is felt in front of back leg. Then, perform stretch on other side. NOTE: Placing front leg slightly to the side will also stretch leg adductors.	Iliopsoas

Table 7-2. (Continued)

Name	Description	Muscle Group(s)
Butterflies	Begin by sitting with legs bent and bottoms of feet together. Grasp ankles and push legs to floor using elbows while bending upper torso toward feet keeping back flat. NOTE: Leaning upper body over one knee instead of straight ahead engages hip abductors. Bend from hips and not the back.	Hip/thigh Adductors
Groin Stretchers	Begin standing erect, with legs far enough apart to allow for sufficient stretch, and toes pointed slightly outward. Shift body weight to one side while bending the leg on the same side. The knee of the bent leg should always be aligned over the toe to avoid stress in the ligaments and menisci of the knee joint.	Hip/leg adductors

Legs

Name	Description	Muscle Group(s)
Standing or Prone Quad Stretch	While standing, bend one leg back toward buttocks, stretching front of bent leg. Use hand on same side as bent leg to hold stretch. Tilting pelvis forward will engage hip flexor. Knees should be kept parallel, underneath hips. This exercise may also be performed while lying face down (prone) on deck.	Leg extensors and hip flexors
Shin/Quad Stretch	Begin kneeling on deck, toes pointed straight back, palms on deck. Slowly lower hips toward heels until tightness is felt in quads and shins. If unable to rest hips on heels, place hands on outside of legs and support body weight with arms. If more stretch is needed, place hands behind feet and lean slightly back, supporting body weight with arms.	Shins, ankles, and quadriceps

Table 7-2. (Continued)

Name	Description	Muscle Group(s)
Hurdlers Stretch (Quadriceps)	Sit with one leg bent and tucked under hips so that heel lies just outside hip; the other leg may be bent or straight. Foot should be extended straight back (not flared out to one side). Slowly, lean back until stretch is felt in top of bent leg. NOTE: To stretch upper thigh and hip flexors, tighten buttocks and lift hips on side of leg that is tucked under while performing this stretch. Bending front leg can provide a further stretch.	Quadriceps
3 Way Hurdlers Stretch - (Hamstring)	From a sitting position, extend one leg out while tucking other in front of hips with knee pointing outward. Bend torso forward toward deck keeping back straight, stretching muscles of inner thigh. Hold stretch and return to starting position. Next, turn torso toward knee of extended leg and bend over from waist. Keeping back straight, bring chest toward knee while stretching muscles in back of leg. Return to starting position. Using arm opposite extended leg reach up and over while bending body to side. Keeping back straight, bring shoulder toward knee while reaching with opposite arm toward foot of extended leg. Stretch should be felt on side of torso and hamstrings.	Leg flexors, leg adductors, and side of body
Seated Head to Knee (Sitting Hamstring)	From a sitting position, extend the legs forward and bend the torso toward the knees, stretching the back of the legs. Keep knees slightly bent and the back flat throughout.	Leg flexors

Table 7-2. (Continued)

Name	Description	Muscle Group(s)
Supine or Sitting Hamstring	Begin by lying with back flat on deck (supine), legs extended. Bring one leg toward chest grasping ankle with 1 hand and outside of knee with other hand. Pull leg toward chest until a stretch is felt in back of leg. This exercise may also be performed sitting. Keeping back straight, bring knee of one leg toward chest. Grasping ankle with one and outside of knee with other, extend leg until a stretch is felt in hamstrings.	Leg flexor
Achilles Stretch	Kneel on deck, toes pointed straight back, palms on deck. Bring hips back toward heels supporting body weight with arms if necessary. Bring one foot forward until toes are parallel to knee of other leg. Let bent heel come off the ground an inch or so. Lower heel of forward leg toward ground while pushing forward on thigh with chest and shoulder. Perform stretch on other leg. Goal is not to flatten heel on deck, but rather to use forward pressure of chest and shoulders on thigh to slightly stretch Achilles tendon.	Achilles tendon
Soleus Stretch	Standing on a tilt board, on edge of a stair, or curb, flex foot, stretching calf muscles. Bending knee of leg being stretched will engage soleus.Note: soleus and gastrocnemius comprise the calf musculature.)	Soleus

Table 7-2. (Continued)

Name	Description	Muscle Group(s)
Gastroc Stretch	Standing on a tilt board, on edge of a stair, or curb, flex foot, stretching the calf aV| muscles. Keep leg of stretched muscle straight.	Gastrocnemius
BUD/S Knee (ITB Stretch)	Perform while seated, with one leg extended, and other leg crossed over extended leg at knee. Turn upper torso toward bent leg, stretching iliotibial band (ITB) of that leg. Use elbow on side of straight leg to hold stretch.	Trunk and iliotibial band

A Post-Exercise Total Body Stretching Program

A suggested post-exercise total-body stretching program is outlined in Figure 7-5. Stretches are grouped by the position in which they are performed. To make the most efficient use of time, perform stretches in the sequence provided. The outlined program takes ten minutes if stretches are held for 15 seconds and performed once on each side of the body. Ideally, stretches should be performed twice on each side of the body.

Figure 7-5. Total Body Post-Exercise Stretching Program

1. Standing

Lateral/Forward Neck Flexion

Upper Back Stretch

Posterior Shoulder Stretch

Overhead Side Stretch

Triceps Stretch (and side bend)

2. Sitting

Swimmers Stretch

ITB Stretch

Butterflies

3-Way Hurdler's Stretch

Seated Head to Knee Stretch

3. On Back

Supine Back Stretch

Hip Stretch

Hip Cross-Overs

4. On Stomach

Prone Quad

Torso Prone Stretch

5. Kneeling

Shin-Quad Stretch

Achilles Stretch

Forearm-Wrist Stretch

Kneeling Lunge with Pelvic Tilt

6. Standing

Iliopsoas Stretch

Gastrocnemius Stretch

Soleus Stretch

Resources

◆ Alter, MJ. *Sport Stretch.* Champaign, IL: Leisure Press, 1990.

◆ Anderson, B. *Stretching.* Bolinas, CA: Shelter, 1980.

◆ Appleton, B. *Stretching and Flexibility: Everything You Never Wanted to Know,* 1995. Available: Chesapeake http://www.ntf.ca/ NTF/papers/rma/stretching_toc. html.

◆ Tritschler, T. *Stretching and Strengthening Exercises.* New York: Thieme, 1991.

◆ Sudy, Mitchell (Ed.). *Personal Trainer Manual: The Resource for Fitness Instructors.* Boston: Reebok University Press, 1993.

◆ Cantu, RC and Micheli, LJ. (Eds.). *ACSM's Guidelines for the Team Physician.* Philadelphia: Lea & Febiger, 1991.

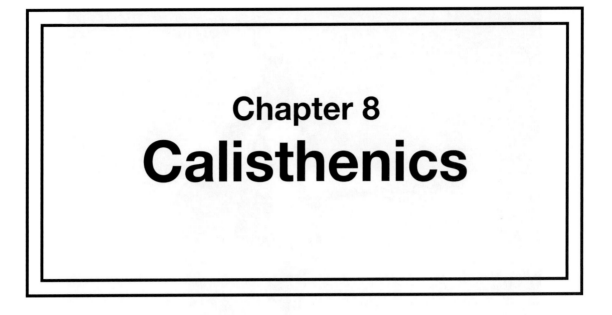

Chapter 8
Calisthenics

Calisthenics are a traditional and integral part of the SEAL's training program because they require minimal equipment and can be performed in almost any location. Calisthenic exercises, depending on how they are performed, can be used to develop flexibility, muscle strength, muscle endurance, and/or muscle power. These terms have been previously defined in Chapter 1. In this chapter we will discuss the benefits and proper use of calisthenics within the Special Warfare training environment.

The Muscle Strength-Endurance Continuum

Muscle strength and muscle endurance exist on a continuum. Given that muscle strength is the amount of force generated by one repetition and muscle endurance is the ability to exert force repeatedly over time, improving muscle strength will improve muscle endurance. If your one repetition maximum weight is increased, your submaximum multiple repetitions can be performed with more weight (resistance).

Muscle strength is developed by performing low-repetition (6-12), high-resistance exercises. When more than 12 repetitions can be performed, the resistance should be increased, and the repetitions decreased. Muscle endurance is developed by high-repetition (>12), low-resistance exercises.

A set for an exercise is the number of repetitions performed per unit weight.

Increasing the number of repetitions per set develops endurance. For example, if an individual can perform only 10-12 sit-ups using proper technique, the exercise will develop muscle strength. Once an individual can perform over 15 repetitions per set, muscle endurance is being developed. Table 8-1 outlines the strength-endurance continuum and illustrates the training schedules used to develop various degrees of endurance. Note that strength and short-term efforts have no effect on aerobic capacity because the aerobic/endurance system is not recruited with maximal or heavy loads. In contrast, sustained efforts with a light load recruit the aerobic system and have minimal effect on strength. Generally, activities of longer duration require more muscle endurance. SEALs should modify their training programs according to the principles of strength and endurance specific to mission requirements.

Table 8-1. The Strength-Endurance Continuum

	STRENGTH	SHORT-TERM EFFORT	INTERMEDIATE EFFORT	SUSTAINED EFFORT
Goal	Maximum force 3 sets 3 times/week	Endurance with heavy load 3 sets 3 times/week	Endurance with intermediate load 2 sets 3 times/week	Endurance with light load 1 set 3 times/week

	STRENGTH	SHORT-TERM EFFORT	INTERMEDIATE EFFORT	SUSTAINED EFFORT
Recommendation	6-10 RM*	6-12 RM	12-50 RM	Over 100 RM
Enhances Strength	Muscle contractile proteins; actin and myosin; connective tissue	Some strength; anaerobic metabolism	Some aerobic and anaerobic metabolism; slight strength improvement	Aerobic enzymes; fat utilization
Does Not Alter	Aerobic Capacity	Aerobic Capacity		Strength

*RM = Repetitions Maximum Effort
Modified from Sharkey, BJ: *Physiology of Fitness,* 3rd Ed. Champaign, IL: Human Kinetics, 1990, p 91.

In general, calisthenics develop muscle endurance. There are two occasions, however, when calisthenics develop muscle strength. The first occasion depends on individual fitness level and how many repetitions can be performed. Individuals who can only perform a low number of repetitions of a calisthenic exercise (less than 10-12) will develop muscle strength. Those who can perform a higher number (more than 10-12) will develop muscle endurance. For example, when you first start doing pull-ups you may only be able to perform 9 repetitions. At this point, you are developing muscle strength. As your performance improves, and you are able to perform over 12 repetitions, you begin to develop muscle endurance.

The second occasion occurs when calisthenics are modified to overload the muscles so that they contribute to strength development. This can be achieved by any of the following:

- ◆ Adding weight (e.g., pull-ups or push-ups while wearing a weighted pack)
- ◆ Using a buddy for resistance (e.g., having a buddy sit on your hips while doing bent over calf raises; buddy-assisted leg extensions)
- ◆ Exercising on one side of the body only (e.g., one-legged squats or calf raises)
- ◆ Modifying the exercise (e.g., elevating the legs during push-ups)
- ◆ Super sets/pyramids

These modifications can be particularly helpful if weight training facilities are not available and a strength workout is required.

Calisthenics in Naval Special Warfare

Muscle strength and endurance are both essential for operational performance. Muscular strength is also required for many Special Warfare missions. Muscular endurance is needed when work is required over longer periods of time (e.g., patrolling with a heavy load, climbing with equipment, swimming, or carrying a buddy).

The goal of a physical training (PT) program for the SEAL should be to develop complete muscular fitness (i.e., strength, endurance, and power). Muscle strength provides the foundation for muscle endurance and power. An adequate strength base not only improves performance, but also decreases the likelihood of injury. For this reason it is recommended that at least two strength workouts (low-repetition [10-12 reps], high resistance exercises per muscle group per week), as described in Chapter 6, be part of the SEAL's physical fitness program. Traditional calisthenic exercises performed two to three times a week will develop and maintain muscle endurance. A plyometric program (See Chapter 9) when necessary, can also be used to develop muscle power.

Mission-related training schedules, lack of exercise equipment, and inadequate nutrition can keep operators from maintaining required fitness levels in the field. Calisthenics, however, are practical for field situations because they can be performed anywhere with minimal equipment. Moreover, calisthenics can also be modified to provide a strength workout.

A unit's PT schedule should be flexible enough to accommodate different training needs

It may take one to four weeks for an operator or platoon returning from the field to completely regain levels of aerobic and muscular fitness comparable to those when exercising regularly in a basic unit PT program. Allowing time to gradually increase fitness will improve performance, prevent overtraining, and decrease the likelihood of overuse injury or reinjury. Those returning to PT following surgery and/or rehabilitation need to return to basic PT gradually. When performing calisthenics, **more is not necessarily better,** and in fact, can be harmful. Too many repetitions can cause an overuse injury or worsen an existing injury.

The goal of a PT program should be to develop aerobic capacity, muscular strength, endurance, power, and flexibility, NOT TO OUT PERFORM OTHERS

Competitive exercise situations, such as "Burn Out" PT and pyramid sets, can be challenging, but if not handled correctly, can cause injury. SEALs should train like elite athletes and avoid situations that could contribute to injury.

Calisthenic sessions occasionally include holding an exercise in the halfway position for 2-10 seconds. This technique is often applied to pull-ups, dips, or push-ups in an attempt to make the exercise more difficult or alleviate boredom. For example, when performing a pull-up, the operator will maintain the position halfway between the starting position and the bar, while the chin is over the bar, and again halfway down the bar. This technique is NOT recommended.

Holding a mid-exercise contraction stresses the joints, tendons, and ligaments and can cause an injury or worsen an existing injury.

Slowing the cadence throughout the entire exercise (i.e., 10 seconds up to the bar, 10 seconds back to the starting position), is recommended for added strength gains, alleviation of boredom, or to increase the difficulty.

Balancing Abs and Hip Flexors and Extensors

Many calisthenics performed to strengthen the abdominal (Abs) muscles, are actually exercises for the hip flexors (muscles that move the hips and legs toward the chest). This causes over-development of the hip flexors and under-development of the abdominals. Although both hip flexor and abdominal strength is necessary for operational performance, overdeveloped hip flexors play a significant role in the development of lower back problems. Overdeveloped hip flexors not only change the curvature of the spine, but also stress the front portion of the vertebral discs. **Many experts contend that much of the low-back pain in the SEAL community is due to an overabundance of hip flexor calisthenics.** Hip flexor strength is necessary, but it should be balanced with equally developed strength and flexibility in the hip extensors (muscles which move the legs away from the chest) and abdominals.

A balanced workout incorporates abdominals, hip flexors, and hip extensors.

Therefore, it is important to identify which exercises are appropriate for each muscle group (i.e., abs, hip flexors, hip extensors) and include all three in a PT program. A calisthenic program should also incorporate a flexibility program in order to prevent the exercised muscles from becoming too tight (see Chapter 7: Flexibility).

Exercises that anchor or elevate the legs and feet off of the deck (e.g., Hello Darlings, Flutter Kicks, Leg Levers, Inboard Outboards) are actually working the hip flexors. When performing these types of exercises, the torso and upper abdominals act to stabilize the pelvis during the movement. For this reason it is suggested that **hip flexor exercises be performed first.** Exercising the abdominals first causes them to become fatigued and therefore unable to stabilize the pelvis. The following recommendations will strengthen the abdominals:

- Identify exercises which are true abdominal exercises versus those which work the hip flexors.
- Decrease the number of hip flexor exercises performed to two sessions per week with fewer repetitions per session.
- Increase the number of true abdominal exercises (e.g.,Crunches, Elbow to Knee/ Cross Overs, Hip Rollers, Side Flex).
- Abdominal exercises can be performed daily or as limited by muscle soreness.
- Add hip extensor exercises (e.g., Prone Back Extension, The Superman, Donkey Kicks).
- Incorporate a total body flexibility program into Special Warfare training and include stretches for the hip flexors, abdominals, and hamstrings.
- Focus on proper technique as presented below.

Proper technique is important when performing all calisthenics.

If the muscles are not strong enough to perform an exercise properly, other muscles will come into play. The result: the wrong muscles get developed and can lead to injury. For example, exercises that are too difficult for the lower abdominals will rely on the hip flexors. Hip flexors which are relatively stronger than the abdominals, result in the stomach protruding. This may lead to injury and low-back pain. Proper technique is essential.

The following suggestions should decrease mechanical stress on the low back during hip flexor exercises:

- Keeping one foot on the deck minimizes the stress placed on the lower back and spine. Many exercises that require both legs to be off the deck simultaneously can be modified so that one foot is constantly on the deck supporting the low back (Figure 8-1 and Figure 8-2).
- Placing a fist under the lower part of the buttocks helps to keep the spine in a neutral position.
- Lifting the head and slightly rolling the shoulders helps maintain the position of the spine.
- Performing hip flexor exercises prior to abdominal exercises.

Figure 8-1. Modified Flutterkick: Keeping One Foot on the Deck Protects the Lower Back

Figure 8-2. Modified "Knee Bender": Keeping One Foot on the Deck Protects the Lower Back

Another change that should be incorporated in an abdominal workout is the addition of a 2 inch thick towel or an "Ab Mat" beneath the lower spine. The anatomical range of motion for the abdominals is from 30' extension to approximately 75-90° flexion (Figure 8-3). When performing abdominal exercises on a flat surface (i.e., the deck) you are limiting your exercise to only half the normal abdominal range of motion. In other words, when abdominal exercises are performed on a floor, deck, or mat, only half the work necessary to develop abdominal strength is being done. Abdominal strength is best developed by exercises performed within the full anatomical range of motion, with some curve in the lumbar spine (i.e., towel or Ab Mat) as opposed to a flat back. By placing a towel or the Ab mat beneath your lower spine you can achieve the right form for these exercises (see Figure 8-4).

Figure 8-3. Range of Motion for Flexion and Extension of the Upper Body Based on Anatomy

Flexion (75° TO 90°)

Neutral (0°)

Extension (30°)

Figure 8-4. Placing a Towel Beneath the Lower Spine Can Help Achieve the Right Form for Abdominal Exercises

Towel

Because of limited flexibility, it is better to start abdominal exercises at approximately 15° of extension and eventually work toward 30° of extension. A towel is particularly useful because you can adjust it to provide inclines of 15° and 30°

Recommendations for Sit-Ups

In recent years, the sit-up technique has undergone many modifications. Because sit-ups compose a large portion of the SEAL training program, some specific comments regarding their proper use are crucial.

When performing sit-ups, the preferred technique is to bend the legs at the hips (at 45°) with the feet flat on the deck shoulder width apart. Legs should be slightly abducted (turned outward). If hands are placed behind the head, care should be taken not to force the neck into flexion. The fingertips of the hands should just barely touch the back of the head. Elbows should remain back at all times. Concentration on using the abdominals (not the head) to pull through the movement is essential. Keeping the eyes focused on the ceiling helps prevent neck strain and isolate the abdominals. Lifting the torso until the shoulder blades come off the floor engages the majority of the abdominal musculature. Lifting the torso further off the deck will safely engage the internal obliques and the hip flexors, if that is the goal (see Figure 8-5).

Figure 8-5. Proper Technique for Sit-Ups: Legs Slightly Turned Outward and Elbows Behind Neck at All Times

When first performing the sit-up from an extension position, you may not be able to perform as many repetitions. This should not be surprising since essentially, you have been performing only half a sit-up in the past.

The focus should be on the quality, not the quantity, of sit-ups.

The same principles that govern the muscle strength-endurance continuum apply to the abdominal musculature. The muscular fitness component you will develop (i.e., strength vs. endurance) is determined by the number of sit-ups performed using a towel or "Ab Mat" beginning with 15° of extension. If muscle strength is the goal, you may want to move to 30° extension. Once you are performing over 15 reps per set at 30° extension, you can increase the difficulty of the exercise by changing the position of the arms, adding weight, or performing sit-ups on a decline. Variations in arm positioning, from the easiest to the most difficult, are shown in Figure 8-6:

- ◆ At the side of the body
- ◆ Across the chest
- ◆ Behind the head
- ◆ Clasped together above the head; weight can be added for more resistance

Figure 8-6. Variations on Sit-Up Routines

Arms at Sides   **Arms across Chest**

Arms behind Head   **Arms above Head**

If the goal is to develop muscle strength, enough resistance should be added to keep the repetitions per set below 15. Once there is a sufficient foundation of muscle strength, muscle endurance can be developed. As with calisthenics, when muscle endurance is the goal, enough weight should be added to keep the repetitions between 15-50 per set. These principles apply to all other types of sit-ups as well (i.e., Crunchers, Vee-Ups, Cross Overs).

Recommendations for Calisthenics

Two evolutions per week on nonconsecutive days are recommended for calisthenic (muscle endurance) training. Additionally, weekly PT sessions using the calisthenic modifications for muscle strength are recommended. Calisthenics may be performed in conjunction with plyometrics, strength training, or aerobic training. Static stretches for specific body areas may be performed (filler stretches) once the workout for that area of the body is complete; however, a significant drop in exercise tempo should be avoided in order to keep exercising muscles warm.

For a 30-minute workout, choose one to three exercises from each of the following categories in Table 8-2. For a 60-minute workout, choose three to six exercises from each of the categories. Remember to balance the front of the body with the back (e.g., hip flexors/abdominals with hip extensors, quadriceps with hamstrings, hip adductors with hip abductors). The resting period between exercises may vary depending on individual or group fitness level.

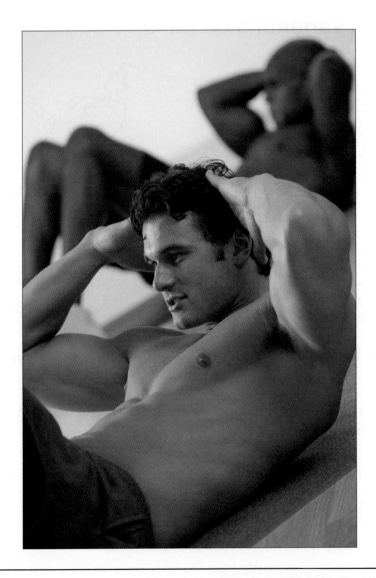

Calisthenics

Calisthenic Exercises

Table 8-2. Recommended Calisthenics for Physical Training

Name of Exercise	Description of Exercise	Muscle Group(s)
	Overall Exercise	
Jumping Jacks	A 2-count exercise from a standing position with feet together and hands at sides. Count 1: jump up while bringing hands together over head and landing with feet shoulder width apart. Count 2: jump back to starting position	Aerobic: A good warm-up exercise
Eight-Count Body Builders	An 8-count exercise from a standing position. Count 1: bend legs and place hands on deck. Count 2: extend both legs backward supporting body weight with extended arms (starting position for a push-up). Count 3: bend elbows, lowering chest toward deck (a push-up). Count 4: extend arms. Count 5: separate legs while keeping arms extended. Count 6: bring legs back together as on count 4. Count 7: flex legs and bring them back to count 1 position. Count 8: stand and return to starting position.	Chest and leg muscles

Table 8-2. (Continued)

Name of Exercise	Description of Exercise	Muscle Group(s)
	Neck Exercises	
Neck Rotations	A 4-count exercise. Begin lying on back. Count 1: lift head up and over to side. Count 2: lift head straight up. Count 3: bring head to other side. Count 4: head returns to starting position. Can also be performed on stomach facing deck in order to condition neck extensors.	Neck flexors and extensors
	Chest, Shoulders, and Arms	
Triceps Push-Ups	A 2-count exercise. Begin by lying on stomach with feet and hands on deck, fingers spread, thumb and index fingers on both hands almost touching each other, elbows extended, and body straight. Count 1: bend elbows at least 90° using arms to support body weight. Count 2: return to starting position.	Triceps and muscle groups used in regular push-ups
Push-Ups Wide, Standard, and Narrow	A 2-count exercise. Begin lying on stomach with hands and feet on deck, arms extended, and head facing forward. Count 1: bend elbows to at least a 90° angle, lowering chest toward deck. Count 2: extend arms back to starting position. Should be performed first with hands placed wider apart than shoulder-width (Wide Push- Ups), then, gradually move hands closer together so that smaller muscles (i.e., triceps) are worked last. Starting wide minimizes problem of fatiguing triceps before pectorals.	Chest, anterior shoulder, triceps, and abdominal muscles

Table 8-2. (Continued)

Name of Exercise	Description of Exercise	Muscle Group(s)
Dive Bomber Push-Ups	A 2-count exercise. Start by assuming a leaning rest position with feet spread 3 ft. apart, palms on deck, elbows fully extended, and hips slightly lifted. Count 1: upper torso sweeps down toward deck between and through hands while bending elbows. Resting position is same as down position of basic push-up. Count 2: upper torso sweeps back and up while elbows extend to return to starting position.	Chest, forearms, triceps, and anterior deltoids
Finger-Tip Push-Ups	A 2-count exercise: Perform same as a regular push-up, but support weight on fingertips.	Forearm and muscle groups used in regular push-ups. Good for forearm and grip strength

Back

Training Tip: Putting tape around pull-up bar or using wider pull-up bars will develop more grip strength. Many athletes have difficulty transferring strength gains achieved during exercise into actual performance gains because many of the movements performed during sports are done with a more open-handed grip. This is particularly relevant to the SEAL community where many of the movements necessary for operational performance require a more open-handed grip (i.e., lifting yourself up and over a barrier). Adding a piece of athletic tape to pull up bars with each successive workout (i.e., gradually increasing the thickness of the bar) steadily develops open-handed grip strength.

Dips	A 2-count exercise which requires use of parallel bars. Flex and extend arms while supporting body weight.	Triceps, back, and to some extent, chest and shoulder muscles

Table 8-2. (Continued)

Name of Exercise	Description of Exercise	Muscle Group(s)
Chin-Ups	A 2-count exercise beginning at a dead hang (i.e., full extension) from a horizontal bar with arms shoulder-width part and palms facing inward. Pull body upward on count 1 until chin touches top of bar. Return to starting position on count 2. No kicking or kip-up allowed.	Back and bicep muscles
Pull-Ups (Wide, Standard, Narrow, Behind the Neck, Interlocking)*	A 2-count exercise beginning at a dead hang from a horizontal bar with arms shoulder width apart and palms facing outward. Pull body up on count 1 until chin touches top of bar. Return to starting position on count 2. No kicking or kip-up allowed.	All muscles of back and forearm (Especially good for grip strength)
Incline Pull-Ups	A 2-count exercise. Requires a low bar (i.e., a dip bar). While lying or sitting on ground (depending on how low bar is), grab bar with both hands and pull upper body toward bar at a 45° angle. Emphasis: pulling shoulder blades together during movement.	Posterior shoulder muscles and triceps (Need to balance extensive # of pushups in SEAL training.)

Table 8-2. (Continued)

Name of Exercise	Description of Exercise	Muscle Group(s)
	Abdominals	
	These exercises will help develop abdominal strength	
Vee-Ups	A 2-count exercise. Lie on back with arms behind head, legs vertical. Lift arms and upper torso toward feet. Only upper torso should elevate off deck. Variations: Keep upper body on deck with arms to sides and legs vertical. Lift only hips off ground a few inches as if pushing feet toward ceiling. This movement, although small, burns after only a few reps.	Abdominals
Crunches	A 2-count exercise. Start by lying on back with legs bent and elevated off deck and placing hands behind head. Lift upper torso 10 to 12 inches off ground, then return to starting position. Variations: legs may be bent with feet on deck, bent with knees toward chest and feet elevated, or extended vertically (as in VeeUps). Arms may be placed in several positions (easy to most difficult): alongside body, across chest, hands behind head, or hands clasped above head. Adding a pelvic tilt at peak of abdominal contraction engages lower abdominals.	Abdominals
Sit-Ups	A 2-count exercise. Described in detail above. Ideally, should be performed within full range of motion (30° extension to 75°-90° flexion), but may be performed so that upper or entire torso is lifted off floor. Lifting only upper torso will engage most abdominals; lifting entire torso will engage internal obliques and hip flexors.	Abdominals

Table 8-2. (Continued)

Name of Exercise	Description of Exercise	Muscle Group(s)
Elbow to Knee/ Cross Overs	A 2-count exercise. Lie on back with hands clasped behind head. Legs can be bent at knees (feet on deck), with one leg crossed over knee of opposite leg or bent with knees toward chest (feet elevated from deck). Slowly lift and twist torso bringing one shoulder toward knee of opposite leg. Engaging obliques requires rotation to start immediately at beginning of exercise, not at top. Return to starting position. Perform exercise by turning torso to both left and right knees.	Abdominals and obliques
Hip Rollers	A 2-count exercise. Lie on back with legs bent and elevated off deck, slowly bring both knees down together on one side until low back begins to lift off deck. Bring knees back to starting position, then repeat on other side.	Abdominals

Abdominals and Hip Flexors

Note: These exercises should be limited to twice per week to prevent over-development of hip flexors. Proper technique is essential; performing these exercises improperly can contribute to or worsen low-back pain.

Name of Exercise	Description of Exercise	Muscle Group(s)
Good Morning Darlings	A 2-count exercise. Lie on back with palms on deck and hands under hips, legs extended, and feet together, 6" above deck. Count 1: spread legs 2-3 feet apart. Count 2: bring legs back together.	Abdominals and hip flexors

Calisthenics

Table 8-2. (Continued)

Name of Exercise	Description of Exercise	Muscle Group(s)
Flutter Kicks	A 4-count exercise. Lie on back with hands under hips, legs extended, and feet together 6"above deck. Count 1: lift right leg 1 1/2 feet, keeping leg straight. Count 2: lift left leg to same position while returning right leg to starting position. Count 3: bring right leg back up and return left leg to starting position. Count 4: repeat.	Abdominals and hip flexors
Sitting Flutter Kicks	A 4-count exercise. Flutter Kick performed from a seated position.	Abdominals and hip flexors
Knee Benders (Supine and Seated)	A 2-count exercise. Lie on back with arms at sides. Bring both legs 6" off deck, bend at knees, bringing legs toward chest. Straighten knees and lower legs down again. Variation 1: Perform same leg movements from a seated position. Variation 2: Begin with hands clasped behind head, one leg bent with foot on deck, and other leg extended. Bend extended leg, keeping foot off deck, and bring it toward chest while lifting shoulders off deck. Return to starting position.	Abdominals and hip flexors

Variation 1

Variation 2

Table 8-2. (Continued)

Name of Exercise	Description of Exercise	Muscle Group(s)
Inboard/ Outboards	A 2-count exercise. Lie on back, hands under hips, feet 3 feet apart and 2 feet above deck. Make small circles by bringing feet out, around, up, in, and down: inboard circles. Change directions for outboards.	Abdominals and hip flexors

Back and Hip Extensors

The Superman (Prone and Kneeling)	A no count exercise. Either lie on stomach or on hands and knees. Opposite arm and leg (i.e., right arm, left leg) should be lifted and held for 3 to 5 seconds, then slowly lowered. Same movements should then be made with other arm and opposite leg. Superman can be made more difficult by adding weights to arms and legs. To avoid hyperextension of back, leg should not be raised higher than hip when in kneeling position.	Back muscles and hip extensors (Helps develop balanced strength between hip flexors and hip extensors. Very safe, but can burn after a while.)
Donkey Kicks	A 2-count exercise. On hands and knees, extend one leg out and behind, then bring it back. Repeat this movement using the same leg until a burn is felt in the hips and lower back. Then exercise the opposite leg. To avoid hyperextension of back, the leg should not be raised above hip.	Hip extensors

Table 8-2. (Continued)

Name of Exercise	Description of Exercise	Muscle Group(s)
Prone Flutter Kicks	A 2-count exercise. Flutter Kick performed lying on stomach. Avoid hyperextension of back.	Back and hip extensors (Highly recommended; helps balance hip flexor conditioning.)
Prone Back Extension	A no count exercise. Lie face down on deck, hands clasped behind back, lift Prone Back upper torso off Extension deck, hold, and return to starting position. Avoid hyperextension of back. Placement of hands alters difficulty; behind back is easiest, behind head is more difficult, straight out in front is most difficult.	Back and hip extensors

Hip/Leg Abductors and Adductors

Note: It is highly recommended that exercises for both leg abductors (i.e., muscles that carry leg away from body) and leg adductors (i.e. muscles that bring leg toward body) be added to the special operations PT program. No exercises that effectively exercise these muscle groups are currently used in team PT sessions.

Leg Lifts	Lie on side: bend legs at a 90° angle from torso. Lift and lower top leg. Knee and ankle should always be in the same plane. Weights can be added to legs if more resistance is needed. Variation 1: 4-count exercise: on count 1 lift leg; on count 2 extend leg while elevated. Count 3: bend leg and return to count 1 position. Count 4: return leg to starting position	Hip and thigh abductors

Table 8-2. (Continued)

Name of Exercise	Description of Exercise	Muscle Group(s)
Burt Reynolds	A 2-count exercise. Lie on side with head supported by hand. Bend top leg and place it in front of the knee of opposite leg. Raise and lower straight leg approximately 8" off deck until fatigued. Should be felt in inner thigh and balances hip abductor exercises.	Hip adductors. Beneficial for rock climbing
Other Leg Lift	Variation2: On count 4 do not return leg to starting position, but keep leg elevated while extending then flexing leg until a burn is felt in hip. Lift and lower top leg. Variation 3: Keep bottom leg at 90° angle while keeping top leg straight. Top leg should remain aligned along bottom leg. Other Variations: Use foot to draw circles in the air; keep leg elevated, and move foot toward head and back; make an arch in air so big toe touches ground above knee then below.	Hip and thigh abductors

Leg Muscles: Extensors and Flexors

Hand to Knee Squats	A 2-count exercise. Feet flat on deck, shoulder width apart with arms relaxed at sides. Keep back straight and feet flat, bend at knees until your fingertips pass knees, then return to starting position.	Hip and leg thigh muscles

Table 8-2. (Continued)

Name of Exercise	Description of Exercise	Muscle Group(s)
One-Legged Squat	A no count exercise. Use one leg to support body weight: bend leg until thigh is almost parallel to ground and return to starting position. Repeat using other leg. Squat should not pass position where upper portion of legs are parallel with ground. Going lower places excessive stress on knee.	Hip and thigh muscles (Useful when equipment and/or weights are not available)

Lower Leg Muscles

Name of Exercise	Description of Exercise	Muscle Group(s)
Calf Raises	A 2-count exercise. Standing on deck or surface (e.g., a curb) which allows heels to hang over side. Raise and lower body weight by raising and lowering heels no more than 3 inches. Perform exercise with toes pointed inward, straight, and turned outward.	Calf muscles

Modified Calisthenic Exercises

Calisthenic exercises can be modified to provide a strength workout by increasing resistance, using a buddy, or some other source of added weight. Many experts recommend buddy-assisted exercises for the following reasons:

◆ Can be performed in any location with no equipment.
◆ Help to maintain strength base in the field.
◆ Teach reliance on another operator.

Most buddy-assisted exercises are designed to develop strength, depending on the amount of resistance one's partner applies. As with regular calisthenics, the muscle strength-endurance continuum applies. If you can only perform 4-10 reps per set, you are building strength. If you can perform over 10 reps per set you are beginning to build muscle endurance. Depending on the fitness goal, the partner can apply as much resistance as necessary to control the number of repetitions. For maximum benefit, perform these exercises slowly. Table 8-3 provides suggestions to aid in developing a buddy-assisted exercise program.

Table 8-3. Tips for Developing a Buddy-Assisted Exercise Program

---

A 5-10 minute warm-up should precede each exercise session followed by stretching for the part of the body to be exercised.

Perform 6-10 reps per set. Each partner should perform 1-3 sets per exercise.

Completion of exercises for a muscle group should be followed by stretches for body area exercised.

Partners should be of similar height and weight.

Some examples of buddy assisted exercises are provided in Table 8-4. Additional exercises and illustrations can be found in Gain W., Hartmann J. *Strong Together! Developing Strength with a Partner,* 1990.

Table 8-4. Buddy Exercise

Exercise	Description	Muscle Group(s)
	Chest, Shoulders, Arms	
Front Push-Up	Lead partner in leaning-rest position. Support partner grabs ankles and lifts to hip level. Lead partner performs push-ups from this position. Body straight.	Chest, triceps, anterior shoulder, and abdominal muscles
Push-Up Walk (Wheelbarrow)	Lead partner in leaning-rest position. Support partner grabs ankles and lifts to hip level. Lead partner walks on hands. May also be performed with arms bent.	Shoulder, chest, triceps, and abdominal muscles
Back or Side Push-Ups	Lead partner is in back or side push-up position. Support partner grabs ankles and lifts them to thigh/hip level. Lead partner performs a backward push-up with both arms or side push-up with one arm. Keep body straight throughout movement.	Back Push-Ups: back, triceps, shoulders, and muscles. Side Push-Ups: triceps, shoulders, upper back, and chest muscles
Backward Push-Up Walk	Lead partner is in Back Push-Up position. Support partner grabs ankles and lifts them to thigh/hip level. Lead partner walks backward with hands.	Shoulders, back, and abdominal muscles
Handstand Push-Ups	Lead partner performs a handstand. Support partner grabs ankles to balance lead partner. Lead partner then bends and straightens arms. Do not touch head to deck.	Shoulders, chest, and triceps muscles
Resistance Exercises-Arms	Lead partner lies on back. Support partner applies resistance against movement of arms up and toward head, down and toward hips, and straight out from body. Resistance can be applied in both directions. For example, resistance can be Shoulder, chest and back applied against arms while they are extended outward pushing toward floor or muscles while arms are extended outward pulling to midline.This exercise can also be performed with lead partner lying on stomach.	Shoulders, chest, and back muscles

Table 8-4. (Continued)

Exercise	Description	Muscle Group(s)
	Back	
Trunk Drops from Bench	Lead partner kneels with hands behind head while support partner holds ankles of lead partner. Lead partner lowers trunk until forehead touches ground and then returns to starting position.	Back extensors
Arm Raises from Bench Position	Lead partner kneels with hands extended above head while support partner holds lead partner's ankles. Lead partner then brings hands to the side and back to starting position.	Back extensors
	Abdomen	
Trunk Lifts	Lead partner lies on back with hands behind head. Feet are held by support partner at hip level. Lead partner then raises and lowers head and trunk.	Abdominals
Trunk Twisters and Trunk Side Bends	Starting position is fireman's carry with lead partner carrying support partner on shoulders. With feet shoulder-width apart, lead partner twists to right and then to left. Lead partner may also bend from waist to right and to left. Be careful not to use momentum of support partner's weight to carry movement beyond a controllable range.	Obliques
	Hips, Legs, and Calves	
Two-Man Squat	Partners stand with backs to each other leaning into each other's weight. Simultaneously, both partners squat until thighs are parallel to floor. Both partners return to starting position keeping backs together for support.	Hips quard and hamstrings

Table 8-4. (Continued)

Exercise	Description	Muscle Group(s)
One-Legged Squat	Start from standing position. Support partner holds leg and opposite arm of lead partner. Lead partner performs a squat until thigh of bent leg is parallel to ground using support partner for balance. Lead partner returns to starting position.	Hips, quads and hamstrings
Fireman Squats and Lunges (Cartilage Crunchers)	Lead partner holds support partner in fireman's carry. Using support partner's weight for resistance, lead partner performs a squat until thighs are parallel to floor and then returns to standing position. Lead partner may also perform forward and side lunges using support partner's body weight for resistance.	Hips, quads and hamstrings
Resistance Exercises—Legs	Lead partner lies with back on deck or stands. Support partner applies resistance as lead partner moves bent leg down toward floor or up toward chest.	Hip flexors and extensors
Fireman Toe Raisers	Lead partner holds support partner in fireman's carry. Using support partner's weight for resistance, lead partner raises up on toes, and then lowers himself. Should be performed with toes straight, pointed outward, and turned in.	Gastrocnemius
Push-Up/Squat	Partner 1 in leaning rest with feet resting on shoulders of Partner 2. Lead partner bends arms to a push-up position while Partner 2 bends legs to a squat position. Return to starting position at same time.	Partner 1: Chest, triceps, anterior shoulder, and abdominals Partner 2: Hips, quads, and hamstrings

Resources

◆ Gain W., Hartmann J. *Strong Together! Developing Strength with a Partner.* Toronto: Sports Books Publisher, 1990.

◆ Sudy, Mitchell (Ed.). *Personal Trainer Manual: The Resource for Fitness Instructors.* Boston: Reebok University Press, 1993.

◆ Cantu RC and Micheli LJ. (Eds.). *ACSM'S Guidelines for the Team Physician.* Philadelphia: Lea & Febiger, 1991.

Chapter 9
Plyometrics

Premature plyometric framing may cause injury because plyometrics place considerable stress on the body. Plyometrics is an advanced training technique that should only be performed under the guidance of those with knowledge and experience with this type of training. It involves explosive types of activities (i.e., jumping onto and down from objects, bounding up and down stairs on one or both feet and high speed sending and receiving) to convert muscle strength to muscle power. Whenever you run, jump, catch or throw, you are performing a plyometric movement.

Box Jump   **Side Cone Jumps**

Plyometric exercises train the muscles to reach maximal strength in the shortest time possible. In other words, **muscle strength plus speed equals muscle power.** The rapid application of force is the goal of plyometric training. Plyometric exercises will not train an energy system as seen with aerobic or strength conditioning; rather such exercises train the *neuromuscular system* so that it may respond more quickly to increased loads. By making use of the inherent elasticity of the muscles and certain neuromuscular reflexes, plyometric exercises enhance the speed and distance an object moves (e.g., your body, shot put).

Plyometric training is very intense, highly specific, and if done improperly it may be injurious. It should not be routinely incorporated in the Naval Special Warfare physical training programs.

How Plyometrics Work

Plyometric exercises help to develop explosive strength and speed in fast twitch muscle fibers. These exercises use the inherent stretch-recoil properties of muscle (i.e., eccentric tension generated when the muscles are lengthened) to enhance subsequent shortening or concentric contractions. This is the dynamic action behind the rapid pre-stretch or "cocking" phase to "activate" these natural recoil properties. Examples of this phase include taking the arm back into position prior to throwing a baseball or bending the knees prior to jumping. Thus athletes that rely on explosive strength and speed, such as sprinters and basketball players, include plyometrics in their training programs. A plyometric movement can be broken down into three phases:

♦ Lengthening phase (eccentric contraction)
♦ Amortization phase
♦ Take-off (concentric contraction).

Figure 9-1. Three Phases of Plyometrics: Lengthening, Amortization and Take-Off

During the *lengthening* phase, the muscle creates tension like a spring being stretched. This type of contraction, called an eccentric contraction, occurs when performing movements such as jumping down from an object, running downhill, or lowering a weight. During an eccentric contraction, tension is built into the muscle as it lengthens. The *take-off* occurs via concentric contraction of the muscles. During this phase, the muscle shortens as it contracts, and actual work (i.e., movement of the body through space) is performed.

The *amortization* phase is the period of time from the beginning of the lengthening phase to the beginning of the take-off phase. This is the most important phase when it comes to plyometric training. During this phase, the muscle must convert the muscular tension generated during the lengthening phase to acceleration in a selected direction during the takeoff phase. The elastic properties inherent within the muscles and neuromuscular reflexes (the stretch reflex) are responsible for this conversion. Plyometric training may increase the efficiency of this conversion. The goal of plyometric training is to decrease the amount of time in the amortization phase and thereby increase speed.

Preparation for Plyometric Training

Plyometric exercises should be undertaken only once an adequate strength base has been developed. Most sources define an adequate strength base for lower body plyometrics as the ability to squat or leg press 1.5 to 2.0 times your body weight for one maximum repetition. For upper body plyometrics, larger athletes (weight greater than 115 kg or 250 lbs.) should be able to bench press their body weight and athletes weighing less than 115 kg (250 lbs) should be able to bench press 1.5 times their body weight.

Plyometric training should never be undertaken if you have any leg, hip, arm, or shoulder injury.

Safety in Plyometric Training

Several steps can be taken to ensure that plyometrics training is safe. These measures include using an appropriate surface, footwear, equipment, and proper technique.

Surface

Plyometrics should not be performed on hard surfaces such as concrete or steel, nor should they be performed on soft surfaces such as sand. **The best surface is a grass field, followed by artificial turf or wrestling mats.** Wrestling mats should not be too thick (> 15 cm) since they will increase the time in the amortization phase. The stored energy gained during the lengthening phase will be lost, and this will defeat the purpose of plyometric training.

Footwear

Recommended shoes are those that provide ankle and arch support, lateral stability, and have a wide, non-slip sole.

Equipment

Boxes that are used for in-depth or box jumps should have a non-slip top and should never exceed a height of 1.2 m (0.5 - 0.75 m is recommended: 1.5 to 2.5 ft. and less than 4 ft.).

Medicine balls are commonly used for many of the exercises. This is a ball that weighs no more than 10% of your typical training weight. For example, if you regularly train with a 200 pound bench press, then the medicine ball you use should be no more than 20 lbs. These balls can be covered with leather, plastic, rubber, or any type of fabric.

Technique

As with other exercises, attention should be paid to proper technique. For example, when performing lunges, the knee angle should not exceed 90°. Any movement beyond this angle will place undue stress on knee cartilage and ligaments. Keeping the knee directly over and in line with the big toe will help maintain technique. The step should be straight out, not to the side. The shoulders should always be over the knees during landing when performing in-depth jumps.

Fatigue from high-volume training can compromise technique and result in injury. When technique begins to fail, it is time to stop the exercise and rest.

Program Design and the Overload Principle

Plyometrics training should be tailored to account for individual characteristics and the activity for which one is training. More stress will be placed on the muscles, joints, and connective tissue of heavier individuals, therefore, bigger operators (weight greater than 90 kg or 198 lbs.) should not perform high-intensity plyometric exercises. **Persons with a previous history of injury should be cleared by a medical officer prior to plyometric training.** As previously stated:

Persons with any type of musculoskeletal injury should not consider plyometrics training.

A plyometrics program for the special operations community should incorporate those types of movements (i.e., linear, vertical, lateral, or a combination) required for operational performance. For example, downhill skiing would require diagonal movements, close-quarters battle (CQB) would require horizontal, vertical, and diagonal movements.

The overload principal is the basis for any training program whether it be cardiovascular training or the development of muscular strength, endurance, or power. The three basic variables used in the overload principal include the frequency, volume (or duration), and intensity of training. By increasing any one or a combination of these variables within a training program, one can continuously and safely overload the system that is to be trained (i.e., cardiovascular, muscular, neuromuscular).

Frequency

Frequency is the number of workouts per week (or other unit of time). For plyometric training, the range is usually from one to three sessions per week, depending on the sport and season. A plyometric training program for the Naval Special Warfare community should consist of two training sessions per week when operational demands require such training. Allow 2-3 days for recovery between workouts to avoid overtraining or injury.

Volume or Duration

The volume for plyometric training is defined as the number of foot contacts or landings per session.

- Beginners: 80-100 landings per session
- Intermediate: 100-120 landings per session
- Advanced: 120-140 landings per session

Intensity

The intensity for plyometrics training is the level of stress placed on the neuromuscular system, the connective tissue, and the joints and is determined by the type of exercises performed. For example, skipping is a low intensity exercise while in-depth box jumps are of higher intensity. Some guidelines are provided as follows:

- Vertical jumps are more stressful than horizontal jumps.
- One leg landings are more stressful than landings on two feet.
- The higher off the ground the body, the more forceful the landing and the more stressful the exercise.
- Adding external weight to the body also increases the stress.

When designing a program, it is best to increase only one variable per session to reduce the likelihood of injury. Generally frequency is held constant while either the volume or the intensity is increased. In advanced plyometrics, when high intensity exercises are performed, volume should decrease since these exercises place significant stress on the muscles, joints, and connective tissue. Table 9-1 provides an example of a 10-week progressive plyometric program. Remember: exercises that mimic the activity to be performed during the mission task should be selected.

Table 9-1. A 10-Week Plyometric Program

Weeks	Exercises	Volume
Weeks 1 and 2	4 Low Intensity	10 Reps: 2 Sets
Weeks 3 and 4	2 Low and 2 Medium Intensity	10 Reps: 2 Sets
Weeks 5 and 6	4 Medium Intensity	10 Reps: 2-3 Sets
Weeks 7 and 8	2 Medium Intensity and 2 High Intensity	10 Reps: 2-3 Sets 10 Reps: 2 Sets
Weeks 9 and 10	4 High Intensity	10 Reps: 2 Sets (Box Jumps)

Adapted from *"Speed Development and Plyometric Training"* by W. B. Allerheiligen, In: TR Baechle (Ed). *"Essentials of Strength Training and Conditioning"*, National Strength and Conditioning Association Champaign, ILL. Human Kinetics, (pp. 314-344), 1994.

Table 9-2 classifies plyometric exercises by their jump direction and intensity level. This table can be used in combination with Table 9-1 to develop a specific plyometric program. All exercises are described in detail in the following section.

Table 9-2. Plyometrics: Classified by Jump Direction and Intensity

Direction	Low Intensity	Medium Intensity	High Intensity	Shock
Vertical	Squat Jump, Split Squat Jump, Cycled Split Squat Jump	Pike Jump, Double Leg Tuck Jump	Double Leg Vertical Power Jump, Single Leg Vertical Power Jump, Single Leg Tuck	In-Depth Jump, Box Jumps (Single or Double)
Horizontal with a Vertical Component		Standing Triple Jump, Double Leg Hop, Alternate Leg Bound, Combination Bound, Front Hurdle Hops	Single Leg Hop	
Horizontal		4 Line Hop Drill	Double Leg Speed Hop, Single Leg Speed Hop	In-Depth Jump, Box Jumps
Diagonal		Double Zig-Zag Hop, 4 Line Hop Drill		
Lateral		Side Hurdle Hops		
Upper Body Plyometrics	Forward Ab Throw, Medicine Ball Chest Toss, Side Ab Throw, Medicine Ball Sit-Up, Plyometric Sit-Up	Medicine Ball Push-Up	Push-Up with a Clap	Drop Push-Up

Plyometric Training

Plyometric training should begin with a general warm-up followed by dynamic stretching (see Chapter 7 for stretching). Stretches should mimic the activity to be performed (e.g., 4-Way Lunges and Leg Swings for lower body plyometrics; Up-Back-and Overs or Press-Press-Fling for upper body plyometrics). Static stretches can also be added.

Two sessions of plyometrics per week is sufficient for SEALs.

This statement is true when operators have 8-10 weeks to train prior to a mission. If time is limited, a platoon may train three times per week if adequate time for recovery is allowed.

Heavy strength and plyometric training on the same body area should not be performed on the same day.

However, upper body strength training may be combined with lower body plyometrics and vice versa. Adequate time for recovery from each type of training is needed and can take from 1-3 days, depending on the intensity. If schedules are tight, the intensity of strength and plyometric exercises should vary from low to high to allow sufficient time for recovery. For instance, when high-intensity plyometrics is required (e.g., just prior to an operation) strength training should be of a lower intensity.

Plyometric Exercises

When performing jumps it often helps to think of "hanging in the air" for as long as possible, keeping shoulders parallel to the ground at all times. Emphasis should be on speed without sacrificing proper technique. Table 9-3 and Table 9-4 present a variety of plyometric exercises. Exercises are listed in increasing order of difficulty for each grouping in Table 9-3.

Table 9-3. Plyometric Exercises

Exercise	Intensity/Direction	Description
Jumps in Place and Standing Jumps		
Squat Jump	Low/Vertical	Start in squat position and explosively jump upward to maximum height. Land in squat position and immediately repeat jump until all repetitions are complete. Keep hands behind head during entire movement.
Split Squat Jump	Low/Vertical	Start in lunge position. Explosively jump off front leg using calves of back leg to propel body upward. Maintain same position when landing and immediately repeat jump until all repetitions are complete. Perform exercise with other leg forward. Keep arms at sides during entire movement.
Cycled Split Squat Jump	Low/Vertical	Start in lunge position. Explosively jump off front leg using calves of back leg to propel body upward. While in midair, switch legs so back leg is in front during landing. Land in lunge position and immediately repeat jump switching legs each time. Keep arms at sides during entire movement.
Single Leg Tuck	High/Vertical	Stand on one leg, arms slightly behind body. Using arms and leg propel body upward as high as possible. While in midair, bring knee of jumping leg toward chest and quickly grasp knee with hands and release. Land and repeat jump until all repetitions are complete. No extra jumps between repetitions are allowed.
Double Leg Tuck Jump (Cannonballs)	Medium/Vertical	Performed same as Pike Jump, but knees are brought toward chest while in midair and knees are quickly grasped with arms. Upon landing, repeat jump until all repetitions are complete.

Table 9-3. Plyometric Exercises

Exercise	Intensity/ Direction	Description
Double Leg Vertical Power Jump (Toyotas)	High/Vertical	Start in squat position, arms slightly behind body. Using arms and legs, explosively jump as high as possible while reaching upward. Land and repeat immediately; repeat jump until all repetitions are complete. No extra jumps in between repetitions are allowed.
Single Leg Vertical Power Jump (Michael Jordans)	High/Vertical	Stand on one leg, arms slightly behind body. Using arms and legs, propel body upward as high as possible while reaching upward with one or both arms. Land on one leg and immediately repeat jump until all exercise are complete. Perform exercise on other leg. No extra jumps in between repetitions are allowed.
Standing Triple Jump	Medium/ Horizontal with a Vertical Component	Start with legs shoulder-width apart, arms slightly behind body. Using legs and arms to propel body, jump upward and as far forward as possible. Land on right foot and immediately jump off right foot and land on left foot. Immediately jump off left foot and land on both feet. When performing next set, land on left foot first, switching to right and then both feet. Repeat until all repetitions are completed. Try to travel as far as possible between each jump.

Multiple Jumps and Hops

Exercise	Intensity/ Direction	Description
Double Leg Hop(Bunny Hops)	Medium/ Horizontal with a Vertical Component	Start with feet shoulder-width apart, arms at sides. Jump up and as far as possible forward. Bring feet toward buttocks while in midair. Land and repeat jump until all repetitions are completed. Goal: to achieve maximum distance.

Table 9-3. Plyometric Exercises

Exercise	Intensity/ Direction	Description
Front Hurdle Hop	Medium/ Horizontal with a Vertical Component	Begin with low obstacles, gradually increasing height with improvements in performance. Place 5 obstacles in a line approximately 1 meter apart. From a standing position, use both feet to jump over hurdles as quickly as possible, landing on both feet throughout.
Single Leg Hop (Monte Pythons)	High/ Horizontal with a Vertical Component	Place one foot ahead of other, as if taking a step. Rock onto front leg and push off (e.g., right foot). Bring knee of push-off leg up and as high as possible. Non-jumping leg is held in a flexed position throughout. Land on right foot and immediately repeat exercise until all repetitions using one leg are completed. Repeat exercise using other leg to push off.
Double Leg Speed Hop	High/Horizontal	Stand with feet together, arms at sides and slightly extended behind body. Jump up and out as far as possible while bringing feet toward buttocks. Land in starting position and immediately repeat jump until all repetitions are completed. Feet should be kept together throughout. Concentrate on speed, then distance, and last on height.
Single Leg Speed Hop	High/Horizontal	Begin with foot ahead of other. Rock onto front leg and push off (e.g., right foot). Bring knee of push-off leg up and as high possible while in midair. Non-jumping leg is held flexed throughout. Land on right foot and immediately repeat exercise until all repetitions using one leg are completed. Repeat using other leg to push off. Concentrate on speed, distance, and last on height.

Table 9-3. Plyometric Exercises

Exercise	Intensity/ Direction	Description
Side Hurdle Hops	Medium/Lateral	Place an obstacle on ground: height can be increased as performance improves. From standing position on both feet, jump sideways over hurdle, landing on both feet. Immediately jump sideways back over hurdle to starting position. Try to increase number of jumps performed within 30 sec.
Four Line Hop Drill	Medium/ Horizontal, Lateral, Diagonal	Draw a 5-ft. square on a flat surface. Start at point A facing out from square. Jump to point B then C then D and back to starting position. Perform as many jumps as possible in 30 sec. Develops speed and coordination in several directions: good drill for CQB training.
Double Leg Zigzag Hop (Ski Moguls)	Medium/ Diagonal	Set up course using about 10 cones, bags, or bodies 45-60 cm apart in a zigzag pattern. Start with feet shoulder-width apart, arms slightly behind body. Using arms and legs to propel body, jump diagonally over obstacles in place. Repeat until course is completed. Keep shoulders perpendicular to ground at all times.

Bounds

Exercise	Intensity/ Direction	Description
Alternate Leg Bound	Medium/ Horizontal with a Vertical Component	Begin with one foot ahead of other. Rock onto front leg and push-off. Bring knee of push off leg up and as high as possible while in midair. Think of hanging in air to increase distance traveled. Prepare legs and arms for landing. Land on opposite leg and immediately repeat bound, alternating legs with each bound until all repetitions are completed. Goal: to cover as much distance as possible.

Table 9-3. Plyometric Exercises

Exercise	Intensity/ Direction	Description
Combination Bound	Medium/ Horizontal with a Vertical Component	Begin with 1 foot ahead of other, as if taking a step. Rock onto front leg and push off (e.g., right foot). Bring knee of push-off leg up and as high as possible while in midair. Land on right foot and immediately explode off right foot and land on right foot again. Immediately explode off right foot and land on left foot. After landing on left foot, immediately jump off left foot and then land on right foot. Foot sequence is right-right-left. Repeat sequence until all repetitions using 1 foot are completed. Repeat using opposite leg.
In-Depth Jumps	Shock/ Vertical or Horizontal	Start on heels of both feet, toes slightly hanging over side of box, arms to sides and slightly back. Step off Shock/ box (do not jump) and land on balls of feet, almost Vertical or shoulder-width apart, knees flexed. Propel body Horizontal upward immediately (if vertical height is goal) or forward (if horizontal distance is goal) using arms and legs to propel body in desired direction.

In-Depth Jumps/Box Drills

Exercise	Intensity/ Direction	Description
Box Jumps (Single or Double Leg)	Shock/ Vertical or Horizontal	Place 4-8 boxes 1 to 2 m (3 to 6.5 ft.) evenly apart, depending on amount of horizontal movement desired; 1 box also may be used. Foot contact may be on 1 or both feet, but 1-leg lands are highly intense and should only be done by those doing advanced plyometrics and a body weight less then 100 kg (220 lbs.). Start about 0.6 m in front of first box, feet shoulder-width apart and slightly flexed, arms to sides and slightly back. Jump forward and up off both legs to land on first box. Foot contact may be double or single. Upon landing immediately explode off the box and onto ground. Upon landing on ground, immediately explode off ground and as high or forward as possible (if using one box) onto next box.

Table 9-4. Upper Body Plyometrics

Exercise	Intensity	Description
Forward Ab Throw	Low	Kneel on floor holding a medicine ball behind head with both arms. Use abdominals to throw it forward. Motion requires a bend at waist and follow through with arms.
Medicine Ball Sit-Up	Low	Starting position for lead partner is sitting on the deck, legs on the deck, shoulder-width apart and flexed at a 90° angle. Support partner stands 1.5 to 2 m (5 to 6.5 ft.) in front of lead partner holding medicine ball. Support partner passes medicine ball to lead partner at chest level. Lead partner catches medicine ball and allows the weight of the ball to push the upper body back and down. When the lower back touches the floor (do not wait till the shoulders touch), lead partner immediately sits up and performs a chest pass to support partner.
Medicine Ball Chest Toss	Low	This exercise may be performed using a partner or a wall and a medicine ball that rebounds. Holding medicine ball at chest level, throw ball forward with a pushing motion. Keep arms slightly extended following release. After ball rebounds off wall or your partner returns it, catch ball with arms extended, swing the weight and momentum of ball as resistance against flexing arms. Repeat throw.
Drop Push-Up	Shock	Starting position is kneeling on deck with torso perpendicular to deck. Keeping torso straight, lean forward, catching body with hands. Hands should be wider than shoulder-width apart and flexed.

Table 9-4. Upper Body Plyometrics

Exercise	Intensity	Description
Side Ab Throw	Low	This exercise may be performed using a partner or a wall and a medicine ball that rebounds. Stand with one side of the body toward the wall or partner holding the medicine ball on the opposite side. With a sideways motion at waist level, throw the ball across the body toward your partner or wall. The torque should come from the waist. Stay in this position to catch the ball when it is returned and swing back in starting position to repeat throw.
Plyometric Sit-Up	Low	Lead partner lies with back on deck, legs perpendicular to floor. Support partner stands with 1 foot on each side of lead partner's head while grasping his legs at ankle. Lead partner grabs ankles of support partner. Support partner pushes legs of lead partner forward and toward deck. Lead partner provides slight resistance to force while allowing legs to accelerate toward deck. Before legs touch ground, lead partner quickly lifts them back to starting position.
Medicine Ball Push-Up	Medium	Start in push-up position with hands supported by medicine ball. Quickly move hands off medicine ball and drop toward deck. Catch weight of body as it drops with arms slightly wider than shoulder-width apart and flexed. Chest should almost touch medicine ball. Rapidly extend arms to propel body upward. At maximal height, arms should be placed on medicine ball as in starting position. Catch weight of body and immediately repeat exercise.
Push-up with a Clap	High	Starting position is same for push-up. Flex arms, bringing body toward deck as if performing a push-up. Using arms to propel body upward, immediately push body off deck in time for hands to clap prior to landing in starting position. Repeat exercise.

Eccentric Downhill Training

Many SEAL missions *(e.g.* small unit patrolling) involve overland movement. Mountain and/or downhill hiking can result in severe muscle soreness, injury to muscle tissue, and strength loss that can last for several days if you are not accustomed to such activities. A recent Naval Health Research Center study found that as few as two downhill training runs (e.g., treadmill or mountainous terrain) one week apart could greatly minimize the muscle soreness and damage. This method of conditioning leg muscles is an effective way to prepare SEALs for future missions or events involving rugged terrain. Uphill and downhill training hikes with loads are also an effective means for conditioning legs.

Resources

◆ Allerheiligen, WB. Speed Development and Plyometric Training. In: T. R. Baechle (Ed.), *Essentials of Strength Training and Conditioning.* National Strength and Conditioning Association. Champaign IL: Human Kinetics, (pp. 314-344), 1994.

◆ Costello, F. Training for Speed Using Resisted and Assisted Methods. National Strength and Conditioning Association Journal. 1985;7(1):74-75.

◆ Chu, D. Plyometrics: The link between Strength and Speed. National Strength and Conditioning Association Journal. 1983;5(2):20-21.

◆ Chu, D. Plyometric Exercise. National Strength and Conditioning Association Journal. 1984;5(6):56-59, 61-64.

◆ Duda, M. Plyometrics: A legitimate form of power training? Physician and Sports Medicine. 1988;16(3):213-218.

◆ Law PL et al. (1994) Downhill Running to Enhance Operational Performance in Mountain Terrains. NHRC TR 94-36.

◆ Stone, M.H. Literature review: Explosive exercises and training, National Strength and Conditioning Association Journal. 1988;15(3):6-15.

◆ Wathen, D. Literature review: Explosive/plyometric exercises. National Strength and Conditioning Association Journal. 1993;15(3):16-19.

Chapter 10
Load-Bearing

Extended humping with a load is one of the most physically demanding tasks for a SEAL. As a SEAL, you must carry loads into rivers, jungles, deserts, and mountains as well as arctic areas and be prepared to engage in various styles of fighting and methods of infiltration. In the planning phase of these missions, Navy SEAL platoon leaders are frequently faced with decisions as to what type and how much equipment and ammunition to carry on a mission: common (minimum) and critical (mission specific) equipment need to be chosen wisely.

The development of multiple weapon systems and state of the art surveillance equipment has increased the firepower and protection of the individual warrior. However, the same equipment that is designed to provide a technological advantage in battle may also provide a load-bearing challenge.

Much remains to be learned about carrying heavy loads for both short and long distances. Moreover, weather, terrain, water discipline, acclimation status and other factors that impact load requirements must all be considered.

Both excessive fatigue and muscle strain during long humps can usually be explained by inadequate training for the unique physical demands of this task.

To assist you in maintaining readiness for tasks that involve carrying heavy loads, the following information is presented:

- ◆ Physiological and environmental factors
- ◆ Optimizing load-bearing
- ◆ Physical training for load-bearing
- ◆ Common medical conditions

Physiological and Environmental Factors

Body and Load Weight

Ideally, it is best to select the load-bearing weight as a function of body weight rather than selecting an absolute load-weight per man. You may not have the flexibility to tailor the load weight per man due to mission requirements. Therefore, an upper weight limit for load-bearing should be calculated so the load will not create a higher physical demand (energy cost) for individuals with smaller stature and lower lean body weight.

Determining the maximum weight of the load is a more important factor affecting load-bearing than the type of load carriage design. Numerous studies have examined the optimal load-bearing weight you should maximally carry before there is a disproportional increase in the rate of energy expenditure. This is calculated as a percentage of body weight.

Although those who are physically fit according to Physical Fitness Test Scores can typically carry 45% of their body weight for 8 hours at a pace of 4 mph, a lighter load is considered optimal.

"Rule of Thumb": A maximal load should be 40% of body weight. Example: 40% of 170 lbs. is 68 lbs.

The energy cost of the task rises steeply beyond this percentage. It has been reported that the energy cost of humping with a load increases proportionally with the weight carried. For loads more than 40% of body weight, the energy expenditure rises disproportionately and fatigue occurs sooner. **The key is to carry your load as close as possible to your body's center of gravity.** This will result in the lowest energy cost when you carry a load, which is evenly distributed, on your back.

Biomechanics of Load-Bearing

The duration of time your foot is on the ground during a normal gait does not increase until pack loads are greater than 50% of your body weight. However, the length of time your foot is in the air during the swing phase of your gait decreases with increasing load-bearing weight. This response occurs to increase the length of time both feet are on the ground for double support. As the load weight increases, your feet increase the ground force downward, forward, rearward and in lateral directions. Shorter stride lengths will increase stride frequency and help maintain normal walking patterns during moderate to heavy load-bearing.

Shorter strides may minimize strain and possibly reduce lower back and lower extremity injuries.

Load-Bearing and Walking Pace

Self-pacing during load-bearing results in a lower energy cost than a forced-pace. However, not all missions allow self-pacing. When the pace is forced, a self-selected decrease in walking pace will be observed as the load-bearing weight increases. The self-selected walking pace or exercise intensity during load-bearing depends on many factors. Some of the factors affecting the self-selected pace include:

◆ Load weight
◆ Aerobic fitness level (maximal aerobic capacity)
◆ Total distance walked

You will normally self-pace at 30%-35% of your maximal aerobic capacity when carrying a moderate load of 50 pounds.

With lighter loads, self-pacing normally results in an exercise intensity of around 45% of your maximal aerobic capacity. However, an exercise intensity of 60% or greater can be achieved when the load is light and the distance short. **Remember: walking pace and load weight carried during an infiltration or exfiltration contribute to the rate of exhaustion.** Figure 10-1 presents estimates of when exhaustion might occur at various walking speeds and loads. High rates of energy expenditure (900 to 1000 calories per hour) can be sustained for only 6 to 10 minutes. To be able to move quickly at this intensity, load weight must be light.

Figure 10-1. Workload and Energy Expenditure During Load-Bearing

Carrying a load at a walking pace that requires an energy expenditure in excess of 300 kcal per hour can compromise the energy reserves you will need at the desired destination. Figure 10-2 shows the speeds that you can expect to sustain with given loads at the designated paces: note these all result in an energy expenditure of 300 kcal per hour.

Figure 10-2. Effects of Walking Pace by Pack Weight and Terrain

Hydration Status

Appropriate water/fluid discipline must be observed at all times during load-bearing. Exercise without a load is severely compromised when dehydration occurs, and **when exercise is coupled to load-bearing, dehydration potentially becomes an even greater threat.** This is true regardless of the environmental conditions. *The Navy SEAL Nutrition Guide* provides information on optimal fluid ingestion, but in brief, **you should ingest at least one to two cups of fluid every 30 minutes during a hump.**

Fluid requirements are higher during exercise with load-bearing than during exercise without load-bearing.

Environmental Stress

◆ **Hot and dry or hot and humid environments** will increase the heat strain of individuals during load-bearing. Thermal heat load will be increased due to body heat production from load- bearing activities, and from the heat load from the sun and other heat sources in the environment. ALICE packs and double packs can restrict the body's ability to dissipate heat. Load-bearing vests with a nylon mesh body will trap less heat than backpack designs.

◆ **Cold environments** increase the energy cost of walking because the clothing worn is usually heavy and cumbersome. This can result in overheating and sweating, especially on the back where the load is carried. Hypothermia (drop in body temperature below 95°C) can also occur rapidly in cold environments if the inner layers of clothing are wet when you stop exercising.

◆ **Moderate to high altitudes** decrease exercise capacity since the available oxygen in blood decreases as altitude increases due to lower barometric pressure.

◆ **Sandy terrain** significantly increases energy expenditure up to 80% or greater as compared to walking on a firm surface. The energy demand increases with the difficulty of the terrain.

Sleep Loss

Lack of sleep can compromise your mental capacities, including attention, logical reasoning, and mental processing. In contrast, physically demanding skills seem little affected by up to 72 to 96 hours of sleep loss.

Protective Clothing

The type of clothing worn during load-bearing is an important consideration for dissipation of body heat. Mission Oriented Personnel Protection (MOPP) gear for nuclear, biological and chemical environments (NBC) is a very heat-restrictive garment.

Guidelines with estimates for work/rest cycles and hydration guidelines when in MOPP gear are available. With load-bearing activities in MOPP gear, work/rest guidelines should be adjusted downward and hydration requirements adjusted upward, since load-bearing activities have not been accounted for. The use of MOPP gear will be equivalent to adding 10° Wet, Bulb, Globe, Temperature (WBGT) to the existing ambient temperature. Therefore, the medical threat of heat illness will increase substantially in MOPP clothing.

Physical Training for Load-Bearing

Most regular home exercise programs and weekly NSW training programs are not adequate for the physical demands of moderate to heavy load-bearing. This section is designed to provide you with an appreciation of the physical demands of load-bearing and an approach to initiating load training.

Elements of a Load-Bearing Conditioning Program

The key elements for conditioning for load-bearing incorporate strength, speed, and endurance training while relying on the principle of specificity of training (see Chapter 1: Overview of Physical Fitness). These are as follows:

◆ **Load-bearing progressive marches:** Specificity of training is one of the basic training principles. To become better or more skilled at a particular event, the event must be practiced. To be able to carry heavier loads for longer periods of time, loads must be carried in training.

◆ **Resistance strength training:** Load-bearing requires strength. Strength training will help improve load-bearing ability and performance.

◆ **Aerobic training:** Aerobic capacity is very important with respect to load-bearing. Individuals with the highest maximal oxygen consumption are better able to tolerate the physical demand of moderate to heavy load-bearing and walk at a faster pace for longer durations with less fatigue than individuals with a lower aerobic capacity.

◆ **Anaerobic training:** Anaerobic power and muscular strength are needed for high intensity combat activities. Different muscle groups are used depending on the type of load-bearing tasks, whether it is a fast paced, short hump or a slower paced, long hump.

Strength training or endurance running alone will not improve load-bearing ability.

The best training for load-bearing is cross country marches with a pack.

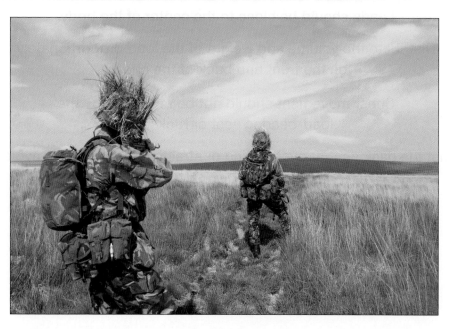

Initiating Load Training

Basic guidelines should be followed when beginning heavy load-bearing training.

◆ Start with loads 20% of your body weight and short distances (5 miles) once per week at the beginning.

◆ Progressively increase pack weight for each training session after two weeks: Loads should be increased to 25%, 30%, and 40% of body weight or greater (depending on the mission requirements).

◆ After achieving pack weight of 40% of weight, progressively increase distance: 7.5, 8, 9, 10, to at least 12.5 miles. Maintain distance for at least one month.

Maintaining Load-Bearing Fitness

To maintain fitness for humping a load equivalent to 40% of body weight for 10 miles would require at least:

◆ Upper and lower body weight training two days per week.

◆ Running three to four days per week for 30 minutes per session.

◆ One hump at least every other week, preferably once per week.

Optimizing Load-Bearing

The decision to calculate an optimal load-bearing weight per man is a difficult task. It is challenging to define an optimal load since no "hump" is going to be conducted under ideal

Table 10-1. Optimizing Load Carriage

Loads should be close to the center of the body.

Distribute the volume and weight of the load proportionately on the front and back of the chest.

Chest movement should not be restricted by the load-bearing vest or rucksack.

Adjust the pack so that overloading or straining of muscles is avoided.

Maintain normal posture and walking patterns.

A large padded waistbelt spreads 80% to 90% of the weight over the pelvic girdle.

Increase comfort by transferring most of the pack's weight to the waist belt by the use of a flexible frame.

conditions. Factors such as walking pace, weight carried, climate, grade, type of terrain, and clothing, etc., will all vary on any particular mission. Table 10-1 presents factors essential for ensuring energy conservation and comfort. These factors, combined with proper physical training, will serve to optimize your load-bearing.

Common Medical Conditions

A number of acute medical conditions are associated with load-bearing. Most are minor, but any one can potentially affect your ability to maneuver quickly and ultimately slow down the walking pace of the squad or platoon. By understanding the range of medical problems, you will be able to better prevent, assess, and treat these injuries. These medical conditions are all covered in Chapter 12: Training and Sports Related Injuries. The most common injuries incurred during load-bearing are:

- ◆ Foot blisters (See Appendix C)
- ◆ Back pain
- ◆ Stress fractures
- ◆ Rucksack palsy
- ◆ Dehydration
- ◆ Other minor lower extremity injuries, such as foot and knee pain

Conclusion

Appropriate aerobic and anaerobic training, along with bi-monthly training humps, will improve your ability for load-bearing, lower energy demands, and reduce the frequency of musculoskeletal injuries.

Acknowledgments

BMl Pete Vernia, USN, Advanced Training Department, SDV Teaml

LCDR Bruce Willhite, USN, J-5, Special Operations Command

Joseph Knapik, Ph.D.

Chapter 11
Training for Specific Environments

Physical training in extreme conditions, such as hot, cold, or high altitude environments, presents special challenges. Even highly accomplished athletes can be quickly overcome by "environmental exposure" injuries if proper preparation is overlooked or if signs and symptoms of impending illness are ignored. To compound matters, many extreme environments tend to be isolated and difficult to access. Proper planning and preparation before entering such areas can help ensure safe and beneficial training.

One way of adapting to a new environment is **"acclimation."** Acclimation is defined as *the continuous or repeated exposure to heat, cold, altitude, or some new environment so as to provoke physiologic or biochemical changes that allow you to better tolerate the new environment.* Thus, acclimation is the gradual change the body goes through as it adapts to a new environment. This chapter will focus on training under environmental conditions which require acclimation, and also under confined spaces.

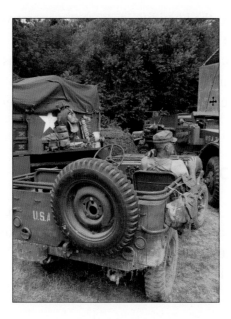

Training in Hot Environments

Exercising in hot, humid environment imposes a significant challenge on the body. The human body maintains tight control of body temperature through several different mechanisms. Under conditions which impose large heat loads (example: strenuous exercise or wearing protective gear in a hot environment), the primary mechanism for cooling is evaporation of sweat from the skin or evaporative cooling. Relative humidity is the most important factor governing evaporative cooling: when the humidity is high, evaporation is greatly limited.

Your skin is like the radiator of a car; as the temperature of the body core rises it warms the blood and pumps it to the skin to cool off. Sweat is released at the skin and absorbs the heat from the warmed blood. As sweat is warmed, it is vaporized the same way boiling water turns to steam and thus removes a large amount of heat from the body. Only sweat that evaporates can effectively cool the body; sweat that "drips" is essentially wasted fluid and provides little or no cooling effect. The body maximizes evaporative cooling by:

◆ **Increasing Heart Rate:** An increase in the heart rate increases blood flow to the skin and results in greater heat transfer to sweat and vapor.
◆ **Increasing Sweat Volume:** Beginning to sweat earlier and recruiting more sweat glands increases the rate of sweat production, therefore cooling.

How hot is too hot? The degree of danger posed by a hot environment is usually determined by the wet bulb-globe temperature (WB-GT). If the WB-GT is over 87° F (30.5° C) or if no WB-GT is available and the temperature is over 85° F with a relative humidity of 60% or above, exercise should be avoided or undertaken with caution.

Factors that Hinder Body Cooling in the Heat

◆ **Humid Heat:** As the humidity increases, evaporative cooling slows due to saturation of the air with moisture.
◆ **Skin Disorders:** Injuries such as deep thermal burns, sunburn, or rashes will prevent or hinder sweating.
◆ **Clothing:** Any clothing that is impermeable to water vapor will compromise cooling.

Heat Acclimation

Adapting to a hot environment can take one to three weeks; for physically fit individuals, 75% of acclimation occurs during the first week of heat exposure. During this time, sustained physical activity is more difficult and onset of fatigue occurs with minimal physical exertion. Acclimation involves two parts:

◆ **Cardiovascular adaptations:** Changes that gradually lead to a lower heart rate for a given workload or intensity of exercise. This is the most rapid change during acclimation to heat.

◆ **Sweating:** Sweating begins earlier with exertion; sweat rate is higher and can be sustained for longer periods of time. Sweat also becomes more dilute thus saving essential body electrolytes.

Maximizing Acclimation

Maintain Aerobic Fitness

A solid base of endurance training established before you enter a hot environment will ease the cardiovascular strain encountered during acclimation. Pre-acclimation endurance training must be rigorous enough to raise core temperatures for acclimation to be most beneficial. Aerobically fit individuals will retain heat acclimation longer once removed from a hot environment than less fit personnel. **Remember:** Aerobic fitness will help speed the acclimation process but is not a substitute for it.

Exercise in a Hot Environment

Any form of physical exercise will hasten acclimation. However, the intensity will be lower than what you are used to. Refer to your local medical officer for guidance. If the environmental conditions permit, gradually increase the intensity of exercise until you reach the desired workload or level of training.

Maintain Adequate Hydration

Acclimation results in an earlier onset of sweating as well as an increase in the sweating rate. These changes translate to an increased need for fluids. Acclimated personnel may produce as much as 8 to 10 liters (8.5 to 10.5 quarts) of sweat per day. Thirst cannot be used as a "measuring stick" for proper hydration. When training in hot environments, a minimum of 10 to 12 quarts of water per day should be consumed, but not more than 5 cups per hour. Drinking at frequent intervals will decrease the risk of a potentially fatal heat stroke.

Maintaining Acclimation

Heat acclimation cannot be maintained unless there is repeated heat exposure and even if repeated exposure is maintained, other factors may cause a loss of acclimation. Factors that lead to loss of heat acclimation include:

- Sleep loss
- Alcohol
- Dehydration
- Salt depletion
- Illness/Infections
- Cessation of physical activity

There is some disagreement as to how long it takes to lose acclimation to heat, but generally speaking after 2 weeks of working in a hot environment, it will take 3 to 4 weeks before most of the adaptations are lost.

Heat Injuries

There are many categories and subcategories of heat injuries. However, there are three classes of heat-induced injury that will be considered here:

- **Heat cramps** are painful contractions of muscles (usually in the extremities) following vigorous exercise. They occur most commonly in unacclimatized personnel. No specific cause is known (possibly depletion of electrolytes), but such cramps usually resolve when acclimation is complete.

◆ **Heat exhaustion** is a potentially serious injury resulting primarily from dehydration and electrolyte depletion. The affected individual may feel light-headed, dizzy, nauseous, fatigued, or develop a headache. If heat exhaustion is suspected, the injured individual should be placed in a cool location if possible and given replacement fluids by mouth or intravenously.

◆ **Heat stroke** is a **life threatening** injury in which the affected individual loses the ability to regulate temperature and is overcome by soaring body core temperatures (greater than 104° F). Such high temperatures can irreversibly injure vital organs and result in death if not rapidly treated. Many factors may contribute to heat stoke — even well hydrated personnel may become victims if they ignore the warning signs and symptoms (see the following Table).

Table 11-1. Warning Signs of Heat Stroke

Signs to Be Aware of	
Light-headedness	Headache
Confusion	Nausea/vomiting
Loss Of Consciousness	Combativeness

Immediate medical attention is necessary to prevent death. Always remember the basics of first aid and check the ABC's first (Airway, Breathing, and Circulation). If possible, move the injured person to a cool area and remove all of the person's clothing. Wet the body with a fine mist of water or pour cool water over the body and fan to facilitate cooling. If ice is available, apply bags of ice to the arm pits, groin, and sides of the neck. Medical personnel should start intravenous fluids and oxygen if possible and transport the individual to the nearest medical treatment facility.

Many drugs and chemicals can decrease your ability to tolerate the heat and knowing which ones may interfere with performance can be important on missions in hot environments. Table 11-2 presents some of the most common drugs that should be avoided in hot weather.

Table 11-2. Drugs and Chemicals to be Avoided in Hot Environments

Caffeine	Alcohol	Decongestants
Atropine and other anticholenergics		Antihistamines

Summary for Hot Environments

- Prepare by maximizing aerobic fitness — this will greatly help in sudden in-out ops where gradual acclimation is not possible.
- Plan work-out to avoid heat of the day.
- Optimize acclimation by a carefully scripted exercise program from the medical department.
- Plan for decreased physical performance the first two weeks.
- Maintain proper hydration.
- Be aware of any illness that may predispose to dehydration (diarrhea, vomiting, fever).
- Always be aware of the warning signs of heat illness: Pay attention to your body. Slow down or stop if signs or symptoms of heat injury become apparent.
- Avoid drugs and other substances that predispose to dehydration or heat injuries.

Training in Cold Environments

Cold climates represent the harshest environments and pose the greatest threat to survive that SEALs face. An unprotected man in an extremely cold environment will perish much faster than when exposed to extreme heat. In cold weather, the human body attempts to maintain a warm core temperature primarily by physiologic mechanisms and behavioral adaptations:

- **Increased Metabolic Heat Production:** This occurs as the body's fuels (carbohydrates, fats, and proteins) are metabolized or "burned" at the cellular level. Shivering represents involuntary muscle contractions that can increase the body's metabolic rate five to six times above normal.
- **Peripheral Vasoconstriction:** Blood vessels near the surface of the skin constrict or narrow in an effort to divert warm blood away from the cool surface of the skin.
- **Behavioral Adaptations:** Man's greatest asset in cold weather is his ability to create a warm micro-environment by wearing appropriate protective clothing or seeking shelter. He can also increase resting metabolic heat production by 10 times through vigorous exercise.

What is a cold environment? As with a hot environment, the temperature alone is not necessarily the best indication of coldness. In the heat, humidity, and in the cold, the wind, can greatly change your comfort level. In the cold, wind accelerates heat loss by replacing the warm layer of air surrounding the body with colder air. As a rule, you can be sure it is a cold environment when the ambient temperature is below 15° F and the wind speed is greater than 25 mph. Such environments pose potential dangers to those exposed for any length of time.

Factors that Compromise Adaptations to Cold

- **Inadequate Energy Intake:** Reduces the ability to generate "metabolic" heat.
- **Injury or Poor Physical Conditioning:** Inhibits ability to generate heat through vigorous exercise.
- **Dehydration:** Places greater demands on the heart and speeds up fatigue.
- **Low Percentage of Body Fat:** Subcutaneous fat has insulating properties which help protect against heat loss. This is a concern for SEALs, who usually have low body fat.
- **Excessive Sweating:** Dress appropriately using a layering system and ventilate as necessary to avoid excessive sweating. Sweat will destroy the insulating qualities of cold weather clothing and cause unwanted cooling by evaporation and freezing.
- **Alcohol:** Increases peripheral blood flow which promotes heat loss and causes core temperature to fall more rapidly.

Acclimation to the Cold

Unlike acclimation to hot environments, there is little evidence to suggest that in humans, there is a significant physiologic adaptation to the cold. There is evidence to suggest that hands which are exposed to the cold for 30 minutes per day for three weeks will receive more blood flow and gradually become more "functional." However, there is greater heat loss through hands conditioned in this manner.

Cold Injuries

The spectrum of cold injuries experienced in the SEAL community is broad but all can be avoided by wearing appropriate clothing and paying attention for signs and symptoms of cold injuries.

Hypothermia

A lowering of body core temperature below 95° F is not an uncommon cold injury of SEALs and mild hypothermia is a relatively easy injury to treat. Moderate to severe hypothermia is less common and should be treated as a medical emergency. Some warning signs of a falling body core temperature include:

- Uncontrollable shivering
- Slurred speech
- Clumsiness
- Slowed thought process
- If shivering stops but all other signs are present—it could be an indication of severe hypothermia

If any of the above signs occur, **immediate action** should be taken to prevent further injury or death. Always handle personnel suspected of having hypothermia gently—do not allow them to perform vigorous exercise to warm up as this may cause cardiac arrest. Remove wet clothing and place the individual in dry blankets or sleeping bag with one or two other dry and warm personnel. **Never completely immerse a hypothermia patient in warm/hot water as this may result in cardiac arrest.** Passive rewarming is usually satisfactory for mild hypothermia, but may not be adequate for severe cases.

Gentle rewarming is the safest method of restoring normal body temperature.

Frostbite

Frostbite is a freezing injury which most commonly affects the hands and feet. However, it can occur to any surface of the body that is not adequately protected. Symptoms often follow a progressive pattern to include the initial sensation of cold followed by numbness and eventually pain during rewarming. The skin may appear normal or appear pale. **If a frostbite injury is suspected, attempts to thaw the affected tissue should be avoided until there is absolutely no chance of it refreezing.** Frostbitten feet should not be thawed if it is necessary for the injured to walk unassisted to the extraction or medevac site. Rewarming is associated with severe pain and may turn walking wounded casualties into nonambulatory casualties. All cases of frostbite require evaluation at a definitive medical treatment facility.

How to avoid freezing injuries
◆ Dress appropriately and keep hands and feet as dry as possible.
◆ Do not touch metal with bare hands/skin. Tape frequently touched metals to reduce this risk.
◆ Wear protective goggles when exposed to high wind speeds such as in snowmobiles, aircraft, skiers.
◆ Use the "buddy system" to check each other for unprotected skin.

Immersion Foot

Also known as "trench foot", this nonfreezing foot injury results in tissue and nerve damage after prolonged exposure of wet feet to the cold (32 to 50° F). Immersion foot can be prevented by keeping feet as dry as possible and by avoiding tight fitting boots.

Nutritional Requirements

Special attention should be paid to nutritional requirements in cold environments. Energy requirements may increase several fold because of the increased work associated with performing physical tasks in cold weather and the caloric losses to shivering which can rapidly deplete glycogen stores. Carbohydrates are an excellent source of energy for replenishing depleted glycogen. Refer to the *U.S. Navy SEAL Nutrition Guide* for specific nutritional needs during cold weather operations.

Summary for a Cold Environment

◆ Check weather conditions and dress appropriately.
◆ Allow for a longer warm up.
◆ Avoid profuse sweating.
◆ Replenish body fuel (carbohydrates) during endurance events.
◆ Maintain hydration.
◆ Avoid drugs that cause dehydration: alcohol, caffeine.
◆ Be aware of the signs of cold injury.
◆ Use gentle rewarming for hypothermia victims.

Training at Altitude

An athlete's performance can suffer dramatically when he rapidly ascends to altitude. Several factors contribute to this decrement in performance but the most significant factor is the relative hypoxia or lack of oxygen available to do work at higher altitudes. Many changes occur during extended exposure to high altitudes; most occur after 2 to 3 weeks. The major adaptations that affect performance and ability to do work include:

- ◆ Increased oxygen carrying capacity of the blood
- ◆ Increased density of blood supply to and within muscle
- ◆ Increased oxygen carrying capacity of muscle
- ◆ Increased respiratory rate

Decreased oxygen at altitude reduces the maximal aerobic capacity of an athlete by 1% to 2% for every 100 meter (328 feet) rise above 1,500 meters (4,918 feet). Therefore, an elite endurance athlete may only be able to perform at 65% to 85% of maximal aerobic capacity at 10,000 feet when compared to sea level. Athletes that compete in anaerobic events, such as sprinters or weight lifters who perform brief (2-3 minutes) episodes of maximal effort events, may notice no initial difference in performance because sustained maximal oxygenation of muscle tissue is not necessary.

Acute Mountain Sickness

Acute Mountain sickness or AMS is typically a transient mild illness resulting from ascents to altitudes above 8,000 feet (2,440 meters) or ascents at a rate greater than 1,000 feet (305 meters) per day above 8,000 feet. Symptoms include headache, nausea, vomiting, fatigue, and poor appetite. The symptoms usually disappear within a few days. Some individuals, however, may have to descend to gain relief. Life threatening complications of AMS include High Altitude Pulmonary Edema (HAPE) and High Altitude Cerebral Edema (HACE); both require immediate descent. The incidence and severity of AMS may be reduced by taking

Acetazolamide (Diamox) 24 to 48 hours prior to and during an ascent. The dosage is 125 mg. by mouth, twice a day for two days, but this medication should only be given under the direction of a physician.

When participating in high altitude operations, you should report any of the following symptoms to your corpsman or medical officer:

◆ Cough or progressive shortness of breath
◆ Coughing up blood or frothy spit
◆ Progressive symptoms of headache
◆ Mental confusion or difficulty thinking
◆ Visual disturbances
◆ Lack of urination in excess of 8 hours
◆ Excessive irregular breathing

Other Factors that Hinder Performance at Altitude

Temperature

In general, temperature decreases 6.5° C for every 1,000 meter rise in elevation (or 11.7°F/ 3,280 ft.). At extreme altitudes (above 5,000 meters or 16,400 ft.), the combined effects of hypoxia and hypothermia may make sustained aerobic activity extremely difficult if not impossible.

Dry Air

Relative humidity falls as one ascends. Combined with the increased ventilatory rate experienced at altitude, significant water loss can occur from the normally moist respiratory passages. Cold temperatures will also cause an increase in urinary output and together these two sources of water loss can result in rapid dehydration. Thirst cannot be used as a "measuring stick" for hydration status and personnel must constantly replace fluids with frequent water breaks.

Weight Loss

Most people who ascend to 13,000 feet (4,000 meters) or higher will experience a weight loss of 3% to 5% in the first 2 weeks at altitude. Some of this loss is muscle mass and appears to result from a decrease in the size of individual muscle fibers. There are several reasons for this weight loss:

◆ Increased energy expenditure
◆ Decreased appetite due to a direct effect of hypoxia and a decreased sense of taste
◆ Loss of body water
◆ Acute Mountain Sickness—Please refer to *The Navy SEAL Nutrition Guide* for dietary recommendations at altitude

Acclimation to Altitude

Prolonged exposure to altitude will bring about several physiologic changes and result in improved exercise tolerance at submaximal effort levels. At levels above 10,000 feet (3,050 meters), maximal aerobic capacity is limited and is lower than what would be measured at sea level. Below 10,000 feet, maximal aerobic capacity may approach sea level values, but usually only after a 2 week acclimation period. Because of this inability to achieve maximal aerobic capacity above 10,000 feet, elite endurance athletes may experience mild to moderate aerobic deconditioning with extended stays at altitude.

Training in Confined Spaces

During deployments or extended training exercises it is not uncommon to be confronted with conditions which may limit physical training routines. Complete cessation of physical training will result in a significant and rapid reduction in both strength and endurance capacity (see section on Deconditioning). Submarines and small assault craft probably create the greatest challenge, but under almost all circumstances where time is not a limiting factor a reasonably well balanced training program can be maintained with a minimal amount of equipment. The following is a list of both aerobic and anaerobic training modalities for confined spaces:

- Calisthenics
- Pull-ups and dips
- Grip balls for grip strength
- Resistance equipment such as the Exergenie which imitate swimming strokes and are very light weight
- Therabands, another lightweight resistance tool to maintain strength in major muscle groups
- Jump rope
- Stair stepping (monotonous but good aerobic workout without need of special equipment)
- Plyoball
- Free weights
- Running in place

For larger platforms or forward operating bases with physical security limitations, the following equipment in addition to weights should also be considered:
- Climbers
- Cycle ergometer
- Rowing machine
- Stair climber

- ◆ Treadmill
- ◆ Ski machine
- ◆ Upper arm ergometer

Physical fitness equipment on a submarine should, at a minimum, include a cycle ergometer, a rowing machine, and free weights.

The stationary cycle and rowing machines should have a performance monitor to display time, distance, etc., so that progress on stationary equipment can be charted and monitored. Platoons deployed under confined circumstances can reduce the monotony of stationary equipment and boost training morale by creating competitions. Monitoring and charting each members daily PT progress will help demonstrate results, encourage physical training, and maintain physical fitness.

Deconditioning

When a person is unable to maintain his exercise program, for whatever reason, detraining or deconditioning occurs rapidly. Numerous studies have investigated the effect of detraining on cardiorespiratory fitness, and significant reductions in work capacity has been noted within two weeks. A 25% decrease in maximal oxygen uptake has been reported after three weeks, which is equivalent to a 1% decline in physiologic function for each day of inactivity. In addition, the proportion and size of the Type II fibers have been shown to decrease with detraining. In contrast, maximal muscle strength appears to be more resilient to periods of inactivity. **A reduction in maximal capacity only means that it will be harder for you to do a given task than prior to deconditioning.** You will still be able to do the work. Remember:

The benefits of training are transient and reversible.

Although maximal aerobic capacity is not maintained without training, other key factors can lead to a decrease in aerobic capacity which will ultimately reduce your work capacity. These include:

- ◆ Increasing age
- ◆ High altitude
- ◆ Dehydration
- ◆ Loss of lean body weight

Chapter 12
Training and Sports Related Injuries

One of the hazards of being a SEAL or an athlete is becoming injured. In BUDS training, 1 out of 3 potential SEALs sustain an injury that may curtail training or require them to drop out of training. Sustaining either a sudden injury or an overuse musculoskeletal injury can mean loss of work days, forced rest, and pain for a period of days to weeks. More severe injuries result in scar tissue formation at the site of injury. Thus, the purpose of this chapter is to describe:

- Treatments for training-related injuries
- Reconditioning for return to full activity
- Types of training injuries
- Common mission-related injuries
- When to seek medical care

The goal is NOT to have you treat your own injuries, but rather to be informed so that you will seek appropriate help when needed. Central to the rapid recovery from training-related injuries is a step-wise reconditioning program which starts immediately after the injury. Such programs are designed to arrest the inflammatory process, promote healing, and accelerate the return to full duty.

Treatments for Training-Related Injuries

Sudden, traumatic, or acute injuries to the musculoskeletal tissue quickly result in inflammation, a process characterized by localized warmth, swelling, redness, and pain. If left unchecked, however, the inflammatory process rapidly leads to:

- Tissue congestion
- Stiffness
- Weakness
- Decreased range of motion
- Loss of normal function

A highly successful Sports Medicine approach to accelerate the healing of any injury is to first decrease the inflammatory process (swelling, pain, and warmth), and then increase the range of motion at the joint. **RICE** and **ISE** are the approaches used to achieve these goals.

RICE = Rest, Ice, Compression & Elevation

After decreasing inflammation by RICE, range of motion at the joint is achieved through continued use of ice (I), stretching of the injured ligament or tendon (S), and weight bearing exercises (E).

ISE = Ice, Stretching & Exercise

Reduce Inflammation

RICE (rest, ice, compression, elevation) is appropriate for all strains and sprains. In general, if an operator cannot bear weight on the extremity, rest is indicated and x-rays to rule out a fracture should be completed as soon as practical.

- **"REST"** means applying no weight or only partial weight to the extremity; crutches should be used for locomotion. "Relative Rest" means decreasing activities that cause pain and replacing them with other activities that are pain-free.
- **"ICE"** means applying ice. This should continue until swelling has stabilized.
- **"COMPRESSION"** means applying an Ace wrap or similar compression wrap to the injured part for periods of 2-4 hours. Never sleep with a compression wrap applied unless medically advised.
- **"ELEVATION"** means placing the injured part above the level of the heart; this allows gravity to help reduce the swelling and fluid accumulation.

Application of Ice

Ice serves a variety of important roles in the treatment of training and sport injuries, including:

- Reduces swelling that accompanies inflammation
- Decreases muscle spasm and pain
- Allows for less painful range of motion
- Enhances blood flow back to the site after it has been removed

The operator should not wait for a medical evaluation before using ice.

All soft tissue or joint injuries, **except open wounds,** will benefit by **immediate application of ice** (See Table 12-1). Ice can be applied either passively or actively. Passive application is when you take some form of ice: crushed ice, ice slush, an ice pack, or snow and apply it to the injured body part. Active application is when you take the ice (perhaps in water frozen in a cup or bag) and massage the injured part with the ice. At home, a bag of frozen peas is an excellent way to passively ice the injured part, as the peas easily conform to the swollen area. After 20 minutes, the bag of peas can be tossed back into the freezer for reapplication later. The normal response to ice includes cold, burning, aching, and finally numbness over the affected part. This progression occurs over 7-10 minutes.

Table 12-1. Tips for Applying Ice: Passive and Active

- Apply ice to the area for 20 minutes as soon after the injury as possible.

- Repeat this every other hour the first day, then three times a day after the first day.

- Use ice until swelling decreases: usually 2-3 days.

Ice can be applied either passively or actively. Do not apply ice directly to the skin.

Caution: To prevent skin or nerve damage, do not keep ice on for more than 20 minutes, especially when applying to the elbow, wrist, or behind/side of the knee.

Range of Motion

The term range of motion is used to describe the extent to which a particular joint can be moved; achieving complete range of motion is the goal, but sometimes injuries restrict the range of motion. During the 20 minute icing session, you should attempt to move the injured part through a pain-free range of motion. Days later you can attempt a resistance activity which stresses the injured part while moving the joint through a range of motion that can be tolerated. An example would be moving the ankle up and down against resistance applied by holding a towel under the foot (Figure 12-1). Continued elevation and use of a compression wrap while doing these exercises will retard swelling.

Figure 12-1. Moving the AnkleThrough Its Range of Motion (ROM) with Resistance

ROM

Non-Steroidal Anti-Inflammatory Drugs (NSAIDs)

All of you have taken non-steroidal anti-inflammatory drugs (NSAIDs) at some point in your career, either as prescribed by a physician or on your own. NSAIDs are often used as the first treatment for overuse injuries because they are effective: NSAIDs decrease the symptoms due to inflammation (i.e., swelling, pain, tenderness, fever associated with injury). Although they are usually available over-the-counter, they are not a medication to take lightly. NSAIDs are used in training related injuries when there is inflammation caused by:

- Tendonitis
- Bursitis
- Sprains/Strains

In the case of an acute injury which involves bleeding (including bruising) or swelling, NSAIDs should not be started for 2 to 3 days or until the swelling has stabilized.

NSAIDs may cause side effects.

The most frequently reported side effects include:

- Gastrointestinal distress such as nausea, heartburn, or vomiting
- Gastrointestinal ulcers/bleeding
- Increased blood pressure
- Decreased ability of blood to clot
- Exacerbation of asthma
- Potential kidney damage with long-term use

Remember: NSAIDs should not be used, or should be used with extreme caution, in conjunction with alcohol, as both irritate the stomach. Table 12-2 provides a list of the most commonly prescribed (or over-the- counter) NSAIDs, with their generic and common brand name.

Table 12-2. Generic Names (and Common Names) for Various Non-Steroidal Anti-Inflammatory Agents

Generic Anti-Inflammatory Agents

Aspirin (Bayer, Aspirin, Ecotrin)	Ketoprofen (Orudis)
Diclofenac (Voltaren)	Meclofenamate (Meclomen)
Diflunisal (Dolobid)	Nabumetone (Relafen)
Etodolac (Lodine)	Naproxen (Naprosyn, Anaprox)
Fenoprofen (Nalfon)	Oxaprozin (Daypro)
Flurbiprofen (Ansaid)	Piroxicam (Feldene, Antiflog)
Ibuprofen (Advil, Motrin)	Sulindac (Clinoril)
Indomethacin (Indocin, Indocin SR)	Tolmetin (Tolectin 200,Tolectin 600)

If you have stomach or other gastrointestinal tract problems, Tylenol (acetaminophen) may be a better choice for relieving muscle soreness than Ibuprofen- and Aspirin-based products.

Reconditioning for Return to Full Activity

After the pain and swelling are reduced and the desired range of motion is achieved, ask the physician, therapist, or trainer to design a reconditioning exercise program with the overall goal of a **rapid return to full activity.** The exercises prescribed will be specific to the site and type of injury, and will work towards the following specific goals of maximizing:

◆ Flexibility	◆ Strength
◆ Endurance	◆ Power
◆ Speed	◆ Specific Duty Tasks

Each step should be successfully completed in a step-wise manner before returning to unrestricted activity. Definitions of most of these terms can be found in Chapter 1, however, the importance of each is described next.

◆ Strength and flexibility are closely linked. If flexibility is not balanced around a joint, or strength is maintained through only part of the range of motion, the risk of delayed healing or reinjury is high.

◆ With respect to endurance, the muscle quickly becomes deconditioned during the body's repair process and fatigues. Endurance is important in an injured ankle for example, as it may feel strong when rested but be prone to re-injury as the muscles and tendons around it become fatigued with activity.

◆ The strategies for any rehabilitation program include improving individual muscle endurance while maintaining cardiovascular or total body endurance.

◆ In terms of power, a weak, deconditioned muscle is prone to reinjury when called upon to perform a power move. Strategies for developing power include rapid motion against resistance, use of rubber bands, medicine balls or weight machines.

◆ Sustained speed provides for reconditioning the injured part to anaerobic (without oxygen) activity and coordination of movement. Interval training (e.g., sets of 440 yards over 90 seconds) several times per week is an excellent supplement to the rehabilitation of a lower extremity injury, provided the operator performs the activity below the pain threshold.

Continued use of ice and intermittent application of electrical stimulation, ultrasound and other therapeutic modalities will help accelerate the rapid return to full activity.

Return to Mission-Related Tasks

Ultimately, the operator must return to performing **specific tasks required to complete the mission.** This component of reconditioning MUST NOT be overlooked. Determine the specific mission-related tasks or training that puts the operator at risk for re-injury. These tasks should be practiced at slower speeds in a controlled setting and proficiency should be demonstrated prior to a return to full duty. The ultimate goal is to return the injured operator to controlled physical activity in 4-7 days for a mild to moderate injury and 1 to 2 weeks for a severe strain or sprain.

General Guidelines for Returning to Physical Activity

A number of general rules apply during the repair and reconditioning period. These include the following:

- ◆ If the operator has pain with flexibility work, vary the degrees of motion.
- ◆ If there is pain with strength and power work, vary the repetitions and/or weight.
- ◆ If there is pain with endurance or speed work, vary the distance and/or time.
- ◆ If there is pain with specific mission-related tasks, vary the quickness and/or time required to complete these tasks.

In summary, rehabilitation and reconditioning places its greatest emphasis on rapidly decreasing pain and increasing range of motion about the injured joint by using **"RICE"** and **"ISE",** followed by specific exercises to maximize flexibility, strength, endurance, power, and speed and using ice as necessary.

Types of Injuries

A variety of injuries can be encountered during SEAL and other forms of physical training. In this section we will start with those problems that may be relatively minor and cause mild discomfort, and then proceed to more serious injuries that may limit your activities.

Training-Related Muscle Soreness

Delayed soreness in a deconditioned muscle is normal and is caused by micro-injury. Pain and tenderness typically appear 12 to 48 hours after beginning a training session. Stiffness and soreness are worse after the cool down and resolve again after warming up. This normal process usually persists for 7-12 days and then disappears.

Table 12-3. A Process of Alleviating Muscle Soreness

Ice

Stretch

Extended Warm-Up

Work-Out

Stretch

Ice

Contusions

A blow to the muscle belly, tendon, or bony prominence may cause swelling and bleeding into the tissue and form a contusion. The blood may coagulate and eventually form scar tissue, impeding normal function. Passive ice therapy needs to be started as soon as possible. After swelling has stabilized, start with active icing and then use **Cross Friction Massage.** This is a simple technique used to reduce the swelling and congestion. The thumb or index and long fingers are used to apply firm pressure perpendicular to the long axis of the tendon or muscle (Figure 12-2). The injured part is rubbed in this manner for 10 minutes, four times a day.

Figure 12-2. Technique of Cross-Friction Massage

Sprains and Strains

Ligaments attach bone to adjacent bone and can be damaged in a fall, an accident, or through overuse. Such injuries are called sprains and include acute back sprains, knee sprains, or ankle sprains. Sprains are graded as mild, moderate, or severe. Mild sprains refer to overstretching and microtears of the fibers. A partial tear, with or without instability or looseness, is considered moderate. A severe sprain implies a complete or near complete tear of tendon fibers that results in looseness or instability at the joint.

A sprain is a damaged ligament.

Tendons attach muscle to bone. Muscle or tendon injury is referred to as a strain or tendonitis. Tendonitis, including achilles tendonitis, shoulder tendonitis, hamstring or quadriceps muscle strains, fall into this category.

A strain or tendonitis is an injury to a muscle or tendon.

Mild to moderate lower extremity sprains and strains heal without residual problems if treated early. Primary treatment includes ice and NSAIDs, partial weight bearing with crutches as necessary, and early therapy to maintain range of motion at the joint.

Muscle Cramps

Muscle cramps are common and may be precipitated by prolonged physical activity, high heat and humidity (black flag conditions), dehydration, and/or poor conditioning. Cramps are characterized by the sudden onset of moderately severe to incapacitating pain in the muscle belly and may progress to involve other adjacent muscle groups. The first treatment consists of immediate rehydration with a fluid containing electrolytes. After beginning rehydration, further treatment should consist of grasping and applying pressure to the muscle belly and immediately putting the muscle on stretch until the cramp resolves. The calf muscle, for example, would be stretched by flexing the foot toward the head, whereas a thigh cramp would be treated by flexing the knee, bringing the foot to the buttocks. Pictorial representations of procedures for treating these cramps are presented in Figure 12-3. In addition to these procedures, adequate rest should help prevent recurrences.

Fractures

A true fracture involves a break or chip in the hard outer surface of the bone. With few exceptions, true fractures of the lower extremity require a period of immobilization in a cast and supervised care by a medical officer.

Stress fractures differ from true fractures and are most commonly seen in the load-bearing bones of the lower extremities, i.e. pelvis, femur, tibia, fibula, and bones of the foot. They are caused by excessive strain on the bone. Bone constantly undergoes remodelling and repair in response to the stress of weight bearing. The repair process is accelerated by rest and is slowed in times of heavy exercise as with runs, hikes, marches, and prolonged training. When

Figure 12-3. Examples for Treating Painful Muscle Cramps in the Calf and Quadricep Muscles

Calf   Quadricep

the breakdown process exceeds the bone's ability to repair itself, a stress fracture may result. As the lower extremity bone becomes weakened, weight bearing activity, such as running, may cause a vague, achy pain at or near the weakened site. The first symptoms of stress fractures are initially poorly localized and often ignored. Later, as the process continues, the bone will become tender in a very localized area and will often ache at night or at rest. Ultimately, if left untreated, continued weight bearing may cause a true fracture within the weakened area of bone. Physical training factors which increase the risk for stress fractures include:

◆ A change in training surface (grass to asphalt, dirt to concrete)
◆ A change in shoe wear (worn out shoes or boots or new running shoes or new boots)
◆ An increase in physical activity (too much, too fast, too soon)

All suspected stress fractures should be evaluated and followed by the medical officer. Treatment for stress fractures include:

◆ Reduction or avoidance of impact and load bearing activities
◆ Partial weight bearing with crutches and advancing to full weight bearing when pain free

This process typically takes two to four weeks. Stress fractures are usually not casted when strict non-weight bearing or partial weight-bearing instructions can be assured. The reconditioning process should include swimming or water exercises (such as deep water running) to maintain flexibility and aerobic endurance. A program of lower extremity strengthening exercises should be started as soon as tolerated.

True fractures require a period of immobilization which varies depending on the bone involved. However, after the cast has been removed, the extremity should undergo a reconditioning program.

After the weight-bearing restriction has been lifted, the individual can begin a reconditioning program for running. A return to running should ideally be initiated on a treadmill. This allows the individual to customize increases in duration and speed while monitoring pain at the stress fracture site. A typical "return-to-running" program is presented in Table 12-4.

Table 12-4. Return to Running Post Injury

Return-to-Running

Run on soft and even surfaces-treadmill/track

Run 5 minutes at a slow pace

Increase time by 2 minutes every other day

When running pain-free for 15 minutes, increase pace

Advance to figure-of-eight runs: begin at 100 yard intervals and progress to tighter turns

Gradually increase distance (see Chapter 4)

Resume regular running program

Common Mission and Training Related Injuries

Given the nature of the SEAL's occupation, it is not surprising that injuries occur during training and mission-related scenarios. Clearly, the type of injury will depend on the specific physical tasks and the environments under which the tasks are performed. Table 12-5 presents a brief summary of some of the anticipated and common injuries that may occur during mission-related platforms. Other than these platforms, many of the injuries are a result of activities all SEALs participate in, namely swimming and running.

Table 12-5. Musculoskeletal Injuries Associated with Mission-Elements

Platform	Description of Injury
Steel Decks:	Knee Cap Pain (Patellofemoral Syndrome)
	Shin Splints
	Low Back Pain
High Speed Boats:	Knee Sprain with Effusion
	Back Pain
	Quadriceps Strain
	Tendonitis below Knee Cap (Patellar)
Parachute Jumps:	Fractures
	Patellar Tendonitis
	Low Back Strain/Sprain
	Muscle Strain
Confined Space (Submarine):	Header (Head Blow)
	Shin Contusions
Troop Transport:	Shin Splints
Rappelling/Rock Climbing:	Rope Burns
	Elbow Tendonitis
	Abrasions of the Fingers
	Biceps Tendonitis
	Back Strain
	Shoulder Sprain
Fast Roping:	Deep Heel Bruises

Swimming

Swimming is a non-impact activity involving maximum tension on the muscle-tendon unit. Most injuries result from overuse and over training, rather than from one traumatic event. Consequently, once an injury occurs, healing can prove difficult.

The older, experienced operator, despite a high skill level, faces the added challenge of tendons and joint capsules that are less resilient, muscles that take longer to warm up, and flexibility which is more difficult to maintain. All of these factors can lead to an increased risk of overuse and acute injury in this age group. The most common injuries arising from endurance swimming are sprains, strains, and overuse injuries of the shoulder, knee, and back.

Stroke-Associated Injuries

Freestyle, butterfly, and backstroke place a great amount of stress on the shoulder joint. Use alternate or bilateral breathing on freestyle and be sure to get plenty of roll on backstroke. Before beginning a butterfly set, be sure you are well warmed up. This will allow the shoulder to stay in a more neutral position during the activity of arm recovery and this neutral position helps prevent what is known as *"impingement syndrome"* (described later in Table 12-8).

Freestyle swimming and kicking with a kickboard places a great amount of stress on the low back because of hyperextension; doing the backstroke relieves the stress. A pullbuoy is also helpful as it raises the hips and allows the spine to assume a more neutral posture.

Kicking with fins may aggravate the knee (especially the knee cap) and result in a degenerative condition known as *patellofemoral syndrome*, which commonly afflicts athletic individuals (described later in Table 12-8).

The breaststroke kick helps balance the knee joint by increasing muscular tone on the inside of the quadriceps muscle and serves to balance the effect that running has: increasing muscular tone on the outside portion of the quadriceps muscle. However, the breaststroke may actually intensify *iliotibial band syndrome* (described later in Table 12-8). Swimmers may need to avoid doing the breaststroke if they feel increased pain over the outside of the knee.

Running and Hiking

Running and hiking work large muscle groups and enhance cardiovascular fitness in a short period of time. Hiking transmits a force to the spine of approximately three times load-bearing weight. Running transmits an impact force to the spine of up to five times load-bearing weight. These forces are minimized with good body mechanics, shock-absorbing shoes and cross-training for overall fitness. Table 12-6 outlines common running injuries.

Table 12-6. Common Running Injuries

Name of Injury	Description of Injury
Plantar Fasciitis	Inflammation and tightness of thick fibrous band on sole of foot.
Achilles Tendonitis	Inflammation of calf tendon or "heel cords" especially at insertion into heel.
Iliotibial Band Rub	Pain on outside or lateral aspect of knee or high on outside of hip.
Bursitis	Inflammation or irritation of various bursal sacs about inner or medial portion of knee, or behind the heel of the foot.
Shin Splints	Pain along medial aspect of lower third of tibia, worse in morning, resolves after warming up. Resolves with cooling down after running.
Back Strain/Sprain	Results from impact loading of spine.

Knee Sprains

A complete discussion of knee injuries is beyond the scope of this text. Medial and lateral collateral ligament sprains can be placed in a range-of-motion (ROM) brace to allow early flexion and extension while protecting the damaged ligament.

A knee immobilizer brace that extends and immobilizes the knee straight out should be used with caution. Within 72 hours of using this type of brace, the thigh muscle is weakened and atrophied (muscle wasting as a result of disuse). However, this type of brace must be used with patella (knee cap) fractures and patellar dislocations. While in this brace, strengthening exercises should be started as early as possible to avoid muscle atrophy.

Ankle Sprains

Ankle sprains are ideally treated in an aircast or similar splint. Ice, cross friction massage, partial weight-bearing, and early range of motion is allowed while protecting the injured ligament. Some severe sprains may require surgical intervention.

Overtraining Syndrome

The most common physical conditioning error for the SEAL operator is overtraining. Overtraining is exactly what the word implies, a condition caused by:

Too Much Physical Activity

Physical training for the operator differs from programs designed for elite athletes. The athlete in professional or college sports has an off-season to rest injured muscles and tendons, utilize physical therapy, maximize strength and flexibility, and finally cycle back into his sport. The SEAL team operator has no such luxury and training is a full time job. Typically he trains to peak levels year round. It is this repetitive, peak performance conditioning schedule that may lead to overtraining and overuse injuries.

The **OVERTRAINING SYNDROME** can present with a wide range of physiologic or psychological symptoms which vary widely among individuals (See Table 12-7). Overtraining is generally associated with endurance sports such as swimming or running.

There is no good laboratory or biochemical marker for overtraining syndrome. The **BEST INDICATORS** are resting heart rate in the morning and assessment of mood. Resting heart rate taken daily just before getLvg out of bed and monitored over time will give some indicator of fitness as well as fatigue. Individuals who are overtrained will show a resting heart rate which is 10-15 beats per minute higher than baseline when measured over a period of several days. A day or two of abstaining from physical activity should show a return to

Table 12-7. Characterization and Symptoms of Overtraining Syndrome

Major Symptoms of Overtraining	
Decreased performance and muscle strength	Decreased Capacity to make decisions
Burn-out or staleness	Difficulty with concentration
Chronically fatigued	Angry and irritable
Lacking motivation	Muscle soreness
Disturbances in mood	Increased distractibility
Feelings of depression	Difficulty sleeping
Change in heart rate at rest, exercise and recovery	Increased susceptibility to colds or other illnesses

baseline. The operator who continues endurance activities despite the baseline elevation in heart rate will only become more overtrained.

Changes in mood or mood swings may also be a signal that the individual is overtraining. Little data exists on mood assessment in the SEAL community. Typically, assessment of mood is accomplished with questionnaires. However, individuals who are overtraining and give an honest assessment of mood will consistently report feelings of frustration, anger, depression, or an inability to feel anything at all.

Cross-training, rest days, monitoring of morning heart rate, mood assessment, and taking time off from certain physical activities will reduce overtraining errors.

Overtraining differs from "overwork," which is the temporary deterioration of performance capabilities due to an increase in the volume or intensity of training. Overwork is what typically happens to BUDS students. Physical and mental performance deteriorates in the most demanding parts of the training schedule, only to rebound quickly as the schedule lightens up.

Unlike overtraining, the overworked individual is able to show an increase in physical performance when faced with a greater workload or physical challenge.

When to Seek Medical Care

Table 12-8 provides the symptoms, preventive measures, and selected treatment modalities for common training and mission-related musculoskeletal injuries. This list is presented for information and to help you determine whether you need to seek medical treatment. However, there are numerous conditions which demand immediate medical attention.

Conditions Requiring Immediate Evaluation by Medical Personnel:

◆ Back pain that radiates into the thigh, leg, or foot
◆ Severe pain
◆ Numbness
◆ Joint dislocation
◆ Suspected fracture
◆ Any lower extremity injury in which the individual is unable to bear weight
◆ Pain which limits activity for 3 to 5 days
◆ Any hip pain which causes a limp

Table 12-8. Symptoms, Prevention, and Treatment of Common Training- and Mission-Related Injuries

Injury	Symptoms	Prevention	Treatment
Plantar Fasciitis	Pain in sole of foot just in front of heel; stiffness in sole with first steps of morning.	Stretch Achilles and foot after runs, hikes; massage sole of foot; firm shoes; 1/4" heel lift; arch supports.	Stretch the Achilles tendon and foot on incline board; tape sole instep; massage, ice sore spot; place 1/4" heel lift in shoes.
Metatarsal Stress Fracture	Pain in long bones of foot, especially 2nd or 3rd; worse with weight bearing; aches at night.	Avoid training too much, too fast, too soon; take care when transitioning to new training surfaces (grass to asphalt); different footwear (old shoes, new boots).	Decrease amount of running or hiking; avoid full weight-bearing, use crutch or cane; seek medical evaluation.
Shin Splints	Pain at lower third inner tibia; worse with first steps of running or hiking; usually after long or hard runs or hikes.	Good shoe/boot wear; stretch before and after runs/hikes; pronators (flat feet) should use arch supports.	Ice to painful area before and after run, hike; ankle strengthening exercises, calf stretches, arch supports; medical evaluation for pain longer than 12 days.
Iliotibial Band Rub (ITB)	Pain at outside portion of hip or knee; gets worse several minutes into run.	ITB stretches; discard broken down shoes; use running shoes with wide heel base; check leg length differences.	Ice to painful sites. ITB stretches. Hamstring and quad stretches. Heel lift for leg length difference.

Table 12-8. Symptoms, Prevention, and Treatment of Common Training- and Mission-Related Injuries

Injury	Symptoms	Prevention	Treatment
Muscle Cramps	Sudden severe pain in muscle belly, causing stiffness and loss of motion.	Maintain hydration/ acclimatization protocols; stretch at first hint of muscle tightness.	Grasp and tightly compress muscle belly with both hands; stretch muscle to maximum tolerable length until cramp resolves.
Achilles Tendonitis	Pain at back of heel along heel cord; worse with running and climbing.	Incline board stretch of Achilles; over-the-counter arch supports; stretch after all runs.	Ice for 15-20 minutes, every hour when possible; incline board stretch; cross friction massage.
Patellofemoral Syndrome	Knee pain localized under or around the knee cap; worse with going up/down hills or after prolonged sitting.	Quadriceps stretching/ strengthening exercises; hamstring and ITB flexibility exercises; check foot for biomechanical abnormalities (over pronation).	Ice and range of motion to acute injury; NSAIDs for 5 to 7 days; stretching/ strengthening program. Arch supports or insert for over pronators.
Rucksack Palsy	Weakness, pain, and/ or numbness of upper extremities or shoulders.	Correct load distribution; adjustment of straps as needed. Correct padding.	Avoid heavy load-bearing for 2 to 3 weeks; NSAIDs for 5 to 7 days.
Foot Blisters	Localized pain and redness: "hot spots" caused by friction rub; clear fluid vesicle layer.	Shoe insoles (Spenco) Adaptive training to toughen skin; Change wet socks; Moleskin to blister-prone areas.	Cover blister with clean bandage and/ or moleskin; apply antiseptic to unroughen blister.

Table 12-8. Symptoms, Prevention, and Treatment of Common Training- and Mission-Related Injuries

Injury	Symptoms	Prevention	Treatment
Ankle Sprain	Pain, swelling, loss of function after turning the ankle.	Ankle stretching and flexibility exercises, ankle braces.	If unable to bear weight, seek medical evaluation. Ice 20 min. every hour; compression wrap from toes to lower leg; leaving no gaps. Elevation: elevate foot 18" off ground; motrin, aspirin for pain; partial weight bearing using cane or crutch; seek medical evaluation for pain lasting longer than 3 days.
Medial Epicondylitis	Pain at inner bony aspect of elbow; worse with wrist extension.	Caution with aggravating factors: narrow-based hand placement for push-ups or wrist extension under resistance; generalized wrist-strengthening program.	Ice to bony prominence; wrist stretching/ strengthening exercises; cross friction massage; avoid aggravating factors.
Heat Stroke	Hot, dry, flushed skin, high body temperature, altered level of consciousness, weakness, incoordination.	Hydration, stepwise acclimation to environmental conditions.	LIFE THREATENING MEDICAL EMERGENCY. Replace fluids; if possible, cool water immersion in the field; ice packs to arm pits, groin, temple; transport immediately to medical facility.
Heat Exhaustion	Cool, damp skin; nausea, weakness, fatigue, poor concentration.	Maintain hydration during exercise in all weather; avoid Black Flag conditions.	Remove excess clothing, replace fluids, cool body with water immersion, ice packs, transport to medical facility.

Chapter 13
Harmful Substances that Affect Performance

SEALs and other elite athletes are always looking for ways to improve their physical performance and gain a competitive edge to enhance their success in missions or competition. Often there is a temptation to seek other ways of increasing your capabilities, including trying various ergogenic agents or chemical substances, either natural or man-made, that promise to give an edge. This chapter reviews some of those chemicals that may give you a temporary edge, but the minor improvements you might see in the short-term can be harmful in the long-term. The goal of this chapter is to inform you of the detrimental effects and the legal consequences of using chemicals as performance enhancers. This chapter is not intended to support or promote the use of these chemicals for improving your performance.

Anabolic/Androgenic Steroids

Anabolic/Androgenic steroids, hereafter referred to as **AAS,** have been used by athletes to improve performance for more than 30 years. The non-medical use of AAS is widespread among athletes engaged in power sports such as power-lifting, bodybuilding, football, and rugby. Their popularity stems from their perceived contribution to increase muscle bulk and strength and to improve competitiveness. There are more than one million estimated users of AAS in the United States alone. Approximately 2% of athletes between the ages of 10 and 14, and 5% to 10% of high school athletes have used AAS, even though their use is prohibited. In addition, approximately 5% of college athletes currently use AAS. Because of legal and administrative issues it is difficult to estimate the number of Olympic and professional athletes currently using the drugs. However, a number of Olympic Gold Medalists have had their medals withdrawn for using such substances. The use of AAS for improved competitiveness violates ethical principles and is strictly prohibited by the military services as well as the United States Olympic Committee (USOC) and other national sports governing bodies.

How do Anabolic Steroids Work?

AAS are synthetic derivatives of the hormone testosterone, which is responsible for the development of male characteristics. The pituitary gland in the brain controls the production of testosterone in the male testes. Testosterone has both androgenic (masculinizing effects) and anabolic (tissue-building) properties. The main functions of testosterone in an adult are to:

◆ Promote secondary male sex characteristics, such as hair patterns and deepening of voice
◆ Increase muscle mass
◆ Initiate and maintain sperm production

Anabolic steroids were developed by structurally altering testosterone to reduce its breakdown and to maximize its tissue-building (anabolic) effects. The more commonly used anabolic steroids are listed in Table 13-1. This class of steroids was first used therapeutically to treat certain disorders of the blood, bone mass deterioration, protein wasting states, and as a replacement therapy for male children deficient in testosterone.

AAS should not be confused with corticosteroids which act as anti-inflammatory agents and are used to treat a variety of medical conditions.

Table 13-1. Commonly Used Anabolic/Androgenic Steroids

Generic Name	Street Name
Bolasterone	
Boldenone	Vebonol
Clostebol	Steranobol
Dehydrochlormethyltestosterone	Turnibol
Fluoxymesterone	Android F, Halotestin, Ora-testryl
Mesterolone	Androviron, Proviron
Metandienone	Danabol, Dianabol
Metenolone	Primobolan, Primonabol-Depot
Methandrostenolone	Dianabol
Methyltestosterone	Android, Estratest, Methandren
Nandrolone	Durabolin, Deca-Durabolin
Norethandrolone	Nilevar
Oxandrolone	Anavar
Oxymesterone	Oranabol, Theranabol
Oxymetholone	Anadrol, Nilevar, Anapolon 50
Stonozolol	Winstrol, Stroma
Testosterone	Malogen, Malogex, Delatestryl
Human Growth Hormone	Human Growth Hormone

How Anabolic Steroids Alter Metabolism

In a progressive weight training program, muscles are challenged to grow in size and strength in order to meet the increasing workload placed upon them. The structure of muscle consists chiefly of protein. Strength and size gains are achieved primarily by increasing the amount of protein inside the muscle. Protein requirements of the human body are determined by a complicated and difficult procedure called nitrogen balance. The body must ingest an adequate supply of protein in the diet to process, absorb, and retain nitrogen to support the weight training.

The stress of intensive strength training induces a catabolic state. In this state, muscle protein is broken down, but a state of anabolism or muscle protein formation follows. By an unknown mechanism, AAS enhance the anabolic processes. Anabolic steroids improve the body's nitrogen balance by reversing the catabolic state; thus muscle protein synthesis is supported. AAS are also believed to directly stimulate the growth of new protein within muscle cells and the cells of other tissues. A detailed description of protein needs is provided in *The Navy SEAL Nutrition Guide.* In brief, the daily requirement for protein is 0.6 to 0.8 grams per pound of body weight. Protein intakes in excess of 0.8 grams per pound do not cause an increase in protein stores, but such intakes do increase the work of the kidney. The kidneys are responsible for excreting the waste products from digestion of excess protein.

Purported Beneficial Effects of Anabolic Steroids

There are several purported effects of AAS which may be beneficial to athletes. The first is an increase in lean body mass. In muscle cells this would result in an increase in production of proteins responsible for muscle contraction, energy production, and energy storage. The second is strength. AAS may regulate the movement of calcium from within the cells, which could lead to an increase in the speed and force of contraction. Another potential benefit of AAS is an increase in aggression which may allow the athlete to do more work. At times this may be desirable whereas in other situations it may actually compromise a mission. Overall, the potential beneficial effects of anabolic steroids include:

◆ Increased muscle size
◆ Increased muscle strength
◆ Increased aggression
◆ A perception of improved performance
◆ Increased motivation
◆ Decreased fatigue

Adverse Effects of Anabolic Steroids

The use of anabolic steroids is strongly associated with numerous undesirable effects, many of which may not be predictable on the basis of the dose or frequency with which they are used. These potentially dangerous substances are usually taken without supervision, although this is illegal, and there have been many reports of serious illness or deaths resulting from their use. AAS may falsely increase the perception of strength and cause an individual to lift heavier weights than he should. This often results in torn muscle and ruptured tendons, in particular tears of the biceps and deltoids, because **the strength of muscles increases**

more rapidly than the strength of tendons. The immune system may be impaired, but this abnormality may not be detected until after its use. Importantly, transmission of hepatitis B and AIDS can occur from needle or drug sharing. Various cancers have also been associated with AAS use. Liver, cardiovascular, hormonal, reproductive, and nervous systems are most affected, but other systems may also be adversely affected.

The most frequently reported negative effects are listed in Table 13-2. Many of these are reversible when steroids are discontinued, but some can be permanent or irreversible. If used in young athletes, these agents limit final height because of the early termination of bone growth. Clearly, the health risks far outweigh any benefits anabolic steroids may confer. The most common problem includes liver dysfunction. This serious medical problem occurs frequently in users of oral AAS and causes jaundice. Peliosis hepatitis, a condition where blood filled cysts develop within the liver, has also been reported.

The cardiovascular effects of AAS in men and women include high blood pressure, increases in serum cholesterol concentration and serum LDL (the bad cholesterol), and a decrease in serum HDL (the good cholesterol). Heart attacks, strokes, and blood clots in the lungs have also been reported in AAS users.

The hormonal effects of AAS use in the male include decreased natural testosterone production, decreased sperm count, production of abnormal sperm, and shrinkage of the testes. Breast tissue enlargement is also common, as are acne, glucose intolerance, and baldness. Women AAS users have slightly different hormonal responses, including thickening of the vocal cords with resultant deepening of voice, male pattern baldness, facial hair growth, and enlargement of the clitoris, all of which are irreversible. Breast tissue shrinkage, menstrual irregularities, infertility, glucose intolerance, and acne are also common in women who use AAS.

Perhaps the most significant short-term adverse effects are the psychologic changes associated with AAS use. For both men and women AAS users, increased aggression, rage reactions ("roid rage"), altered libido, anxiety and panic disorders, psychosis ("bodybuilder's psychosis"), depression, mania, and addiction have been noted. Again, these effects are undesirable for tasks required by SEALs. It is extremely important to note that:

Many of the side effects may cause permanent impairment, and some are potentially, if not outright, lethal.

Table 13-2. Adverse Effects of Anabolic Steroids in Men: Physiologic and Psychological

Physiological Effects

Irreversible

Breast enlargement	Atrophy of the testicles

May Be Reversible

Decreased sperm production	Accelerated baldness
Decreased testosterone levels	Elevation of cholesterol
Liver tumors	High blood pressure
Acne	Liver dysfunction

Psychological Effects

Irritability	Depression
Mood swings	Addiction
Mania	Psychosis

Excessive aggressiveness

Legalities of Steroid Use

There are also legal ramifications associated with AAS use. Since early 1991, AAS and related compounds have been classified as drugs controlled by the Food and Drug Administration. These drugs have a high potential for physical and psychological dependence as well as their catabolic effects on various body systems. Transportation or distribution of these agents is punishable by fines of up to $500,000.00 and/or a prison sentence of up to 15 years. The military, as well as most sports governing bodies, (IOC, USOC, NCAA, NFL), ban the use of AAS. Users who are detected using such agents face significant penalties.

AAS screening is now performed in the military along with routine random drug screening. Oral AAS can be detected by urine drug screening from 2-14 days after use. Some forms may be detected for weeks to months after injection. There is zero tolerance for possession and use of AAS in the military, unless appropriately prescribed by medical personnel. Any violation would be punishable under Article 92 of the Uniform Code of Military Justice (UCMJ). If found guilty, that individual may also be processed for administrative separation from the military.

Medical Uses of Corticosteroids

As stated previously, AAS should not be confused with corticosteroids. Corticosteroids, or glucocorticoids, are a category of synthetic hormones used to restrain inflammation and to control itching. They are commonly used topically for skin disorders, and given by injection into joints which are inflamed. Corticosteroids have been classified by the USOC as subject to restrictions; a physician must declare the intent to treat prior to a competition.

Other Harmful Chemicals

Growth Hormone

Human growth hormone (hGH) is a hormone produced in the brain. The hormone is commonly used to increase the height of very short children and until recently to increase strength in the elderly. Athletes have been known to use hGH at a black market cost of about $2,000 for an 8-week course. The known effects of hGH in the athlete are shown in Table 13-3.

Table 13-3. Physiologic Effects of Growth Hormone

Increases muscle mass

Increases fat breakdown for energy

Conserves blood glucose and muscle glycogen storage

Increases height in the skeletally immature individual

Increases size of hands, feet, and jaw

Enhances healing of musculoskeletal injuries

Unfortunately, the increase in muscle mass does not increase muscle strength as much as strength training. No increase in height has been seen in a fully grown person, however, hGH may increase hand, foot, jaw, and body size. There is little known about the adverse effects of hGH use in the normal athlete, but the skeletal muscle growth may be abnormal and therefore the muscles may be weak. Given that hGH use is banned by the military, as well as the IOC, NFL, NCAA and most sports governing bodies, it should not be used.

Clenbuterol

Clenbuterol, a drug used by veterinarians to increase muscle mass in livestock, is being used by many athletes, primarily those in strength-related sports. However, increases in muscle strength have not been shown in humans. In addition, there are numerous adverse side effects, including rapid heart rate, muscle tremors, headaches, nausea, dizziness, fever and chills. Although technically classified as a ft2-agonist, it is officially considered an anabolic agent by the USOC, and is thus on their list of prohibited substances.

Stimulants

Stimulants are agents which increase arousal of the central nervous system (CNS). These agents are used medically in the treatment of various conditions, including depression, narcolepsy (sudden and irresistible onset of sleep), and in the treatment of diseases of the bronchial tubes. Athletes often abuse a number of stimulants because they think their performance will improve. Most stimulants are banned by the military as well as most sport governing bodies; these agents are also measured in routine random drug screening tests. The major classes of CNS stimulants are:

◆ Amphetamines
◆ Ephedrine
◆ Caffeine

This section will discuss only those agents which are illegal and can produce harmful effects.

Amphetamines

One class of stimulants is the **Amphetamines.** The term amphetamine also includes methylamphetamine, dimethy l-amphetamine, and benzylamphetamine which are metabolized to amphetamine after ingestion. In the 1960's, these drugs were "widely used by athletes in the belief that they improved strength and endurance. Stimulants such as amphetamines and many over-the-counter amphetamine "look alikes" have pronounced effects throughout the body. Taking these agents will result in the physiologic and psychological effects noted in Table 13-4 and Table 13-5. As can be seen, these effects are the same ones which occur normally without stimulants when you are asked to undertake dangerous missions.

Table 13-4. Reported Physiologic Effects of Amphetamines

Increases heart rate

Increases cardiac output

Elevates blood pressure

Increases conversion of glycogen to glucose

Elevates serum glucose

Elevates serum free fatty acids

Dilates blood vessels in muscles

Constricts blood vessels in the skin

Increases muscle cell excitability

Amphetamines can mask symptoms of fatigue. They may restore reaction time in a weary athlete but cannot improve reaction time or diligence in a well rested and motivated athlete. The potential beneficial effect is most marked when performance is reduced by fatigue or lack of sleep.

Exercise itself induces these same effects, so amphetamines have not been shown to make a net contribution to the physiological mechanisms which support athletic performance. They clearly make no difference in maximal aerobic capacity, but there is some evidence for small increases in speed and the time it takes to fatigue in endurance events. It could be that the primary performance enhancement benefit rendered by amphetamines lies in their psychological effects as listed in Table 13-5.

Table 13-5. Psychological Effects of Amphetamines

Delayed onset of the sensation of fatigue

Increased alertness

Mood elevation

Increased aggression

Improved self-confidence

Suppression of inhibitions

Perhaps more so than with many drugs, the use of amphetamines is associated with detrimental side-effects that cannot only erode athletic performance, but can also harm health and threaten life. These are listed in Table 13-6. Because of these side-effects and the illegality of their use, these drugs must be avoided.

Table 13-6. Adverse Effects of Amphetamine Use

Nervous System Effects		
Acute Effects	Irritability	Confusion
	Insomnia	Paranoia
	Restlessness	Delirium
	Dizziness	Uncontrolled Aggression
	Headache	Dry Mouth
	Vomiting	Abdominal Pain
Chronic Effects	Uncontrolled Involuntary Movements	Addiction
	High Blood Pressure	Cerebral Hemorrhage

Ephedrine and Pseudoephedrine

Ephedrine, and its most notable derivative, pseudoephedrine, are adrenaline-like CNS stimulants found in many over-the-counter cold and hay fever preparations as well as in many herbal products, in particular the herb known as Ma Huang. Like clenbuterol, ephedrine is a ft-agonist, and has properties similar to that of amphetamines. It is often combined with caffeine. At doses higher than found in over-the-counter medications, restlessness, muscle tremors, anxiety, and headaches are frequently produced. Ephedrine is not widely used in sports to improve performance and there is no scientific evidence that it does. However, many people have used ephedrine and Ma Huang to lose weight through an increase in resting metabolic rate and metabolism of fat. Recently a number of people have died from drinking tea containing ephedrine. Given that it is banned by the OSOC and a potentially life-threatening agent, it should not be used.

Erythropoietin

Erythropoietin (EPO) is used by endurance athletes to improve performance. One type of EPO, called rEPO or rhEPO, is used to treat a number of blood diseases. Athletes use rEPO because it increases the red blood cell count by stimulating red blood cell production and speeding red blood cell release from the bone marrow to the blood stream. The red blood cells carry oxygen to the muscles, so more red cells mean more oxygen. The effects of rEPO are actually similar to those seen in an athlete who trains at altitude. In order for these changes to occur, the athlete must have an adequate iron intake and maintain an aerobic training schedule.

The increase in red blood cell production can cause a number of significant adverse effects. High blood pressure, a flu-like syndrome, and a sluggish bloodflow are the most common. Bloodflow becomes sluggish when the percentage of red blood cells reaches 55%. Normal ranges are 40% to 48% in men and 36% to 45% in women. Sluggish blood flow causes a variety of complaints, including headache, dizziness, ringing in the ears, visual changes, and chest pain. Other possible complications are heart attack, seizure, or stroke due to a blockage of blood flow. Up to 18 deaths due to rEPO have been reported in cyclists. The use of blood doping or rEPO is prohibited by all sport governing bodies as well as the military.

DHEA

DHEA, or dehydroepiandrosterone, is a hormone released by your adrenal glands into your bloodstream each morning; from there it travels to other tissues and is converted into small amounts of testosterone (estrogen for women). It has been shown that levels of DHEA decline with age, and this finding has created a sensation among the manufacturing world. Although DHEA has been available for decades, it has only been on the market since about 1994. It is now being touted as the miracle drug of the 21st century. There is no question that it is a miracle drug to the companies producing and selling it, but the true benefits in humans has not been determined. The various claims being advertised for DHEA include:

- Lengthening of life
- Prevention of cancer, heart disease, and osteoporosis
- Burning of fat stores
- Stimulate libido
- Boosts energy levels and mood
- Enhances immune system

None of these claims have been demonstrated, and there are a number of reasons why it may be hazardous. As stated previously, DHEA is a hormone and it can be converted to testosterone. Increased testosterone levels could increase your risk of prostate cancer. The other potential dangers of DHEA will unfold as more research is conducted, and people who are taking it regularly are followed. To date it has not been banned by the USOC, but that may be only because it is so new on the market.

Summary

In conclusion, none of the chemical agents discussed above offer any guarantee that your performance will improve. However, there is a good chance you could compromise your military career by using them. The benefits of these agents are limited and the potential harmful effects are clear. Our advice is to keep up with your training according to the methods described in other chapters.

Resource

◆ Catlin DH and Murray TH. Performance-enhancing drugs, fair competition, and Olympic sport. Journal of the American Medical Association. Vol 276, pages 231-237, 1996

Chapter 14
Other Training-Related Issues

This chapter presents other issues important to SEAL training but may only pertain to certain subgroups of SEALs. For example, not all teams train for Winter Warfare and many individuals do not currently qualify as "High Mileage" SEALs (but will in the future). Also included is a section on nutritional ergogenic agents, since many athletes use these products in an effort to improve performance.

Winter Warfare Training

Winter warfare imposes some specific physical training demands on SEALs. During training and deployment, winter warfare operations challenge an individual's skill in protection from environmental factors and ability to move efficiently over snow and ice. Thus, cross country skiing is recommended for those involved in winter warfare operations. This section reviews training issues specific to the winter warfare mission.

Training for Skiing

A high skill level is essential if use of skis is contemplated. Under most operational conditions, cross country skiing provides the highest degree of non-mechanized mobility for travelling over snow and ice. Skiing becomes a very efficient form of man-powered transportation during long transits over flat terrain. However, the advantages of skiing only become apparent after acquisition of specific skills and fitness.

It is extremely easy to sustain a serious immobilizing injury while skiing heel free in non-release bindings and floppy loose boots. The potential for injury is magnified further when the skier is loaded down with gear. Thus, the operator participating in winter warfare must be a competent skier.

The overall fitness level of SEALs may be adequate for cross country skiing because fitness from running and aquatic training carry over to skiing. However, different muscle groups are used; thus SEALs should strive to customize their training programs in anticipation of winter warfare. Use of a ski machine does confer training specificity and assists with developing the coordination and muscle adaptations needed to ski efficiently. Other real training issues for skiing are skills and technique. There are several operational considerations to consider:

◆ Need to be able to stop and turn efficiently in a variety of snow and ice conditions.
◆ Need to be able to ski safely with a pack and weapons.
◆ Need to be familiar with gear modifications for maximum efficiency.

Turns, Stops, and Technique

Safe skiing with a pack demands aggressive unweighting and the use of parallel ski techniques. Forget about telemark turns while you are wearing a pack; the slow forward lunge required to initiate a turn in back-country snows while wearing a pack puts the skier in a vulnerable body position. This is an invitation to sustain a serious knee injury to the lead leg, particularly because of the extra weight transmitted to the leg due to wearing a pack.

Telemarking is useful when used to stop while traversing a hill. Instead of extending the uphill leg to initiate a downhill turn, extend the downhill ski and drift up into the hill. This maneuver is easy to control and is a useful tool for checking downhill speed while skiing heel free and wearing a pack.

Poles are essential tools for propulsion and balance while wearing a pack. It is important to use break-away wrist straps to prevent an injury to the arm or shoulder which can occur if the ski pole basket inadvertently catches on a stump or something else frozen solidly to the ground.

The High Mileage SEAL

Chronic overuse injuries and accumulated minor and major trauma to the musculoskeletal system have a cumulative effect on the "High-Mileage" SEAL approaching the age of 40. The most common chronic musculoskeletal injuries involve the neck, back, elbow, knee, ankle, and foot. Table 14-1 outlines the sites and causes of these various chronic conditions. It also presents selected recommendations for treating these conditions. Poor flexibility can be a major contributory factor in all of these conditions. A lifetime program of flexibility, strengthening, and cross-training for aerobic conditioning is essential for minimizing chronic injuries and pain. In the event of an injury, early self-referral for evaluation is an essential part of avoiding chronic injury.

For those having recurrent problems or nursing old injuries, fitness can still be maintained and rehabilitation can proceed. Aerobic activities that may help include the stationary cycles, indoor swimming, a rowing machine, a ski machine, or a climber. However, it is most important to emphasize flexibility, with a specialized PT program that includes stretching. We believe that the Physical Fitness and PT Programs presented in Table 14-2 and Table 14-3 may help restore function if carried out regularly. However, you must remember not to push yourself too hard so as to avoid a recurrence of previous injuries. Also, it is important to remember that you may need a longer time to recover than you did when you were 18. Listen to your body so it will be kind to you in the future.

Table 14-1. Sites, Common Causes of, and Recommendations for Chronic Musculoskeletal Pain

Site	Common Causes	Recommendations (After a Medical Evaluation)
Back	Ligament strain; instability; osteoarthritis; weak abdominal muscles; sacroiliac joint dysfunction; sciatica; poor flexibility.	Stretching program morning and evening; back and abdominal strengthening program; manipulations; avoid swimming with a kickboard and running until pain is manageable.
Neck	Ligament strain; Facet Syndrome; muscle strain; disc disease.	Isometric stretch; avoid freestyle swimming until pain-free.
Elbow	Tendonitis; epicondylitis.	Ice affected area; wrist and elbow stretching; avoid diamond push-ups until pain-free.
Knee	Patellofemoral Pain Syndrome; tendonitis.	Quad and hamstring stretching/ strengthening exercises; avoid extra trips up and down stairs; avoid jumping activities until pain-free; try stationary cycling.
Shoulder	Impingement Syndrome; instability; rotator cuff tendonitis.	Rotator cuff stretching/ strengthening exercises; ice shoulder after activity; avoid overhead activity, military press, butterfly stroke; do not swim train with paddles; breath on same side of injury during freestyle swimming.
Ankle	Old fractures with osteoarthritis.	Ankle flexibility exercises; calf stretching; avoid load-bearing and long runs; Try stationary cycling.
Foot	Plantar Faciitis.	Calf and foot stretching; heel lifts; steroid injection.

In the long run it is better to be conservative: injuries do not always go away. In fact, some lie dormant until you push just a bit too hard. Then it is too late. Seek medical care if there is any doubt, as your job depends on your health.

Table 14-2. Physical Fitness Program for High Mileage SEALs with Chronic Musculoskeletal Pain

Day of Week	Activities for the Day
Monday	PT/30 min Interval Work-Out (Rowing Ergometer)/Stretch
Tuesday	45 min Steady State Work-Out (Stationary Cycle)/Stretch
Wednesday	PT/45 min Fartlek Work-Out (Rowing Ergometer)/Stretch
Thursday	Cycle 15/Row 15/Cycle 15/Stretch
Friday	PT/30 min Slow Jog
Saturday and Sunday	Take one day off and use other day for low key training in whatever way you choose.
Two to Three Times/Week	Circuit or Free Weight Training

Table 14-3. A PT Program for High Mileage SEALs with Chronic Musculoskeletal Pain

Exercises*	Repetition (#)	Total Time in Seconds
Jumping Jacks	25	60
1/2 Jumping Jacks	25 - 2 count	60
Up-Back-and Overs	5	60
Crunches (All Variations)	25-50	60
Push-Ups (Regular)	20	60
Torso Prone Stretch	2	30
Butterflies Stretch	2	30
ITB Stretch	2 each side	60
3 Way Hurdler's Stretch	2 each side	180
Swimmer's Stretch	2	30
Push-Ups (Regular)	20	60
Sit-Ups	20	60
Supine Back Stretch	1	30
Prone Superman	10 each side	60
Vee-Ups	30	60
Donkey Kicks	20 each side	60
Posterior Shoulder or Upper Back Stretch	2	30
Triceps Stretch	2 each side	60
Iliopsoas Stretch (Russian Dancers)	2 each side	60
Standing Quad Stretch	2 each side	60
Standing Toe Pointers	30	60
Gastroc/Soleus Stretch	2 each side	60

* All exercises (described in Chapter 7: Flexibility or Chapter 8: Calisthenics) should be done in order.

Nutritional Ergogenic Agents

Ergogenic agents are by definition, substances or techniques that enhance performance. Because SEALs are required to perform at a high level both mentally and physically, many are looking for substances or techniques to improve performance and provide "an edge." To perform longer, to be faster, to be stronger, and to be leaner, if not a mission goal, are personal goals of many SEALs and elite athletes. People have been trying to accomplish these goals for centuries through the use of ergogenic agents. It is our goal to present information about certain products commonly found in retail stores or by mail order that claim performance enhancing effects. For a detailed discussion refer to *The Navy SEAL Nutrition Guide.* Specifically, this section will provide information on:

♦ Nutritional Products Advertised as Ergogenic Agents
♦ Protein-Carbohydrate Supplements

Nutritional Products Advertised as Ergogenic Agents

This section lists many of the nutritional ergogenic agents sold by manufacturers with claims to "enhance performance" or have "muscle building" properties. Some have valid claims whereas others do not. It is often difficult to differentiate false claims from valid ones if you haven't carefully researched each product individually. Many claims sound very scientific and convincing, but unfortunately, they are often false or unproven. For each agent described in Table 14-4, the claims, the usual dose used, and a comment are provided.

Table 14-4. Nutritional Ergogenic Agents

Agents	Dose	Comment	Claims
Choline	Enhances endurance performance	400 to 900 mg daily as choline bitartrate or citrate. Foods rich in choline include egg yolk, meat, liver, and peanuts.	No benefit reported—not known to be harmful at above doses. Most claims based on theoretical possibilities.
Octacosanol-Wheat Germ Oil	Improves endurance capacity.	100 to 6000 mg daily with expected results in 4 to 6 weeks.	Some benefit reported.

Table 14-4. Nutritional Ergogenic Agents

Agents	Dose	Comment	Claims
Arginine, Lysine, and Ornithine	Stimulate growth hormone release.	Variable. Ornithine— 500 mg a day or 250 mg one to three times a day. Arginine—500 mg one hour before meals and/or before workout. These items are sold separately or in combinations with varying amounts of amino acid content.	Ornithine— No benefit. Gastrointestinal disturbances are common. Arginine, Lysine—Some benefit reported.
Sodium Bicarbonate, ("Bicarb loading," "Soda loading")	Enhances anaerobic performance during high intensity exercise lasting 1 to 5 min.	0.3 grams of sodium bicarb per kg body weight mixed with 1 liter of water 1 to 2 hours before exercise.	Some benefit reported—Be careful...harmful if taken in large amounts. Discontinue use if abdominal cramps or diarrhea occurs.
Caffeine	"Fat burner," delays onset of fatigue, enhances performance.	4 to 9 mg/kg 30 mins to one hour prior to exercise.	Some benefits reported, but discontinue use if side effects noted (stomach pain, tremor) interfere with concentration or steadiness.
L-Carnitine	"Fat burner," delays onset of fatigue.	500 mg daily. Foods rich in Carnitine include meat and dairy products.	Little to no reported benefit—not harmful at above doses. AVOID D-carnitine—A carnitine deficiency may occur.

Table 14-4. Nutritional Ergogenic Agents

Agents	Dose	Comment	Claims
Chromium Picolinate	Increases muscle mass, growth stimulating.	50 to 1000 µg/day as a dietary supplement. Foods rich in chromium include beer, brewer's yeast, oysters, mushrooms, meats, and whole grain cereals.	Some benefit reported.
Coenzyme Q$_{10}$	Increases energy and cardiac performance. Potent antioxidant.	1.0 mg three times a day. Foods rich in CoQ$_{10}$ include beef, eggs, and spinach.	No benefit reported in athletes.
Dibencozide/ cobamamide— Coenzyme forms of B$_{12}$	Anabolic and growth promoting.	500 mg daily in tablet form.	Little or no proven benefit—no harmful effects at given doses.
λ-Oryzanol and Ferulic Acid	Increases testosterone and increases lean body mass.	Variable, but commonly found in 50 mg per day doses.	Little or no proven benefit—no harmful effects at above doses.
Glandulars (ground up animal organs; usually testes, pituitaries and hypothalamus)	Will elevate testosterone levels. The "extra" testosterone will make you more build up more muscle and get bigger.	As a dietary supplement mixed with protein/ carbohydrate powders.	Not recommended. Some products could be harmful.

Table 14-4. Nutritional Ergogenic Agents

Agents	Dose	Comment	Claims
Inosine	Energy enhancer; increases endurance, strength, and recuperation.	500 to 1000 mg 15 min prior to exercise.	No. People with gout should avoid inosine. Dubious effects not worth the risk.
Branched Chain Amino Acids (BCAAs)— Leucine, Isoleucine, Valine	Anabolic and growth hormone stimulator; may protect against mental fatigue of exercise.	There are various products with different amounts of BCAA in them. Example: Leucine 800 mg daily, Isoleucine 300 mg, Valine 200 mg. Usually consumed prior to working out. Foods rich in BCAAs include turkey, chicken, navy beans, and other meats.	Some benefits reported.
Sapogenins— Smilax Diascorea, Trillium, Yucca, or Sarsaparilla	Increases muscle mass and lean body weight by increasing testosterone levels. A testosterone precursor.	Sublingual or capsular as directed. Use prior to workout and before bed.	Little benefit reported. Some products suspended in 18% alcohol. READ the label.
Tyrosine	Reverses cold-induced working memory deficit. Positive impact on stress-induced cognitive performance degradation.	75 to 150 mg/kg of L-tyrosine 1 to 2 hours prior to exposure.	Some benefits reported in SEAL cold weather operations. Branched chain amino acids should not be taken with tyrosine since they interfere with tyrosine's action.

Summary of Ergogenic Agents

Below are brief comments on various ergogenic agents, grouped by purported benefit or effect.

Agent	Comment
Delays Fatigue/Increases Energy Levels	
Caffeine	Some benefit reported
Choline	Theoretically beneficial—remains to be tested
Coenzyme Q10	No proven benefit
Inosine	Little or no proven benefit
Octacosanol	Some reported benefit
Sodium Bicarbonate	Some reported benefit
Tyrosine	Some benefit reported during SEAL cold weather ops
Fat Burners/Lean Body Mass Increasers	
Carnitine	Little or no reported benefit
Chromium	Some benefit reported
l-Oryzanol/Ferulic Acid	Little or no benefit reported
Testosterone Enhancers	
Glandulars	Not recommended
Hot Stuff	Possible adverse effects
Smilax	Little or no reported benefit

Agent	Comment
Growth Hormone Releasers	
Arginine	Some benefit reported
Branch Chain Amino Acids	Some benefit reported
Lysine	Some benefit reported

Protein-Carbohydrate Supplements

Go into a retail or specialty store that caters to athletes and you may become overwhelmed by the number of different products available. One of the most highly visible and advertised group of products are the powdered protein and carbohydrate beverages. "Weight gaining," "anabolic," "muscle building"—these are just a few of the various claims made by manufacturers. They do share one thing in common however: they are sold as supplements to your diet. These products are intended to fortify your diet to meet the nutrient demands of your body. In general, there are three basic reasons why people take supplements:

◆ Compensate for less than adequate diets or life-styles
◆ Meet unusual nutrient demands induced by heavy exercise and/or
◆ Produce direct positive effects on performance

Your profession and life-style impose unique physical demands that require stamina, power, and strength. Consequently, your caloric (energy) expenditure is greater than the average person.

Supplements are a quick and convenient means for obtaining the nutrients you need. For example, some people find that after eating a normal breakfast they feel ill or nauseous during morning PT. If you can't tolerate exercising on a full stomach, then a powdered beverage may be the answer for your breakfast. You get the calories you need in the morning, but don't have that heavy feeling in your stomach. Remember that you may not need the full recommended serving size. Count the calories to suit your own energy requirements and goals.

It is also important to realize that it is not the supplement alone that leads to better performance. Success lies in addressing your goals and analyzing and adapting your diet to meet those goals. It will take some work on your part to calculate how much supplement, if any, you need to use. Read the labels and figure out how many calories you will expend before your next meal. Also, make sure you add up the vitamins and minerals you are getting from all the different supplements you are taking. Many products provide similar nutrients and you may be taking TOO much of one or several nutrients.

Another decision to make is whether or not to use a protein, carbohydrate, or combination beverage. Once again, it all depends on your goals. If you want to increase lean body mass through resistive training, then some protein may be the way to go. Remember that:

You only need 0.6 to 0.8 grams of protein per pound body weight per day.

This is equivalent to 105 to 140 grams for a 175 lb. SEAL. Keep in mind that there are food sources of protein that are very easy to come by and tend to cost much less money. For example:

◆ One 6 oz. can of tuna fish has 48 grams of protein
◆ One 4 oz. breast of chicken has 36 grams of protein
◆ One 8 oz. glass of milk (skim) has 10 grams of protein

Resource

◆ Deuster PA, Singh A, Pelletier PA. *The Navy SEAL Nutrition Guide,* 1994.

Chapter 15
Physical Fitness and Training Recommendations

The purpose of this final chapter is to provide a comprehen-sive training program that combines all the information presented in the preceding chapters. This chapter has been developed by group consensus and attempts to address the specific needs of SEALs.

The SEAL Physical Fitness Program

The ultimate SEAL physical fitness program will incorporate all aspects of physical training. After an initial warm-up, the overall workout will include exercises to develop and/or maintain:

◆ Cardiovascular Fitness (Aerobic/Anaerobic Capacity and Power)

◆ Flexibility

◆ Muscular Fitness (Strength, Endurance, and Power)

Aerobic fitness includes conditioning runs or swims whereas anaerobic activities would include interval or fartlek runs/swims. Flexibility is improved by stretching and muscular fitness by weight training, circuit training, or other such activities. The relative time spent on a particular aspect of fitness each day may vary, but every day incorporates exercises to improve or maintain: muscle strength, aerobic and anaerobic capacity, and flexibility. One point that has been stressed and should be remembered is that:

Strength and flexibility are closely linked.

Building strength tends to shorten muscles and limit flexibility; thus, stretching is essential for maintaining flexibility. The final recommendations are shown in Table 15-1. Some of the activities cannot accommodate the entire group, but rather must be done in smaller groups. For example, circuit weight training can be done in groups of 8 to 12, but not the entire team. These are recommendations, but alternate activities can be substituted. Table 15-2 provides some suggestions for alternative activities.

Table 15-1. The Navy SEAL Physical Fitness Program

Week Day	Activities for the Day
Monday	Stretch/1 circuit of O'COURSE/3 Mile Run/Stretch
Tuesday	PT/1.5 Mile Swim/Stretch
Wednesday	PT/4-5 Mile Run with Fartlek Workout/Stretch
Thursday	Run 3 Miles/Swim 1/Run 3/Stretch
Friday	Alternate 10 Mile Hike with Pack and Monster Mash
Saturday and Sunday	Take one day off and use other day for endurance training according to your preferences
Twice Each Week	2 Platoon hours with circuit/weight training

Table 15-2. Alternate Activities for a Fitness Program

Interval Sprints (Run or Swim)	Plyometrics	Total Body PT
Timed PRT	Cross Country Skiing	Bicycling
Running in Place	Pool Swim with Small Group (16/group)	
Jumping Rope	Rope Climbs for Grip Strength	

Physical training (PT) exercises are listed on two of the five days in the Recommended SEAL Physical Fitness Program. The PT program recommended for you (shown in Table 15-3) is called a Basic PT Program, and it will typically serve as a prelude to the main, more rigorous, activity(ies) of the day. It includes warm-up activities to loosen your muscles and exercises to increase your range of motion, muscle strength, muscle endurance, and power. Depending on the number of repetitions you perform, this PT can take as little as 10 or as many as 40 minutes.

Table 15-3. Basic Physical Training (PT) Activities for Warm-Up, Flexibility, and Strength

Exercises*	Repetition (#)	Total Time (Seconds)
Jumping Jacks	50	60
1/2 Jumping Jacks	50-2 count	60
Up-Back-and Overs	10	60
Crunches (All Variations)	60-100	60
Push-Ups (Regular)	30	60
Flutter Kicks	25	60
Butterflies Stretch	2	30
ITB Stretch	2 each side	60
3 Way Hurdler's Stretch	2 each side	180
Swimmer's Stretch	2	30
Push-Ups (Diamond)	30	60
Sit-Ups	30	60
Push-Ups (Wide Stance)	30	60
Supine Back Stretch	1	30
Torso Prone Stretch	2	30
Prone Superman	10 each side	60
Vee-Ups	30	60
Donkey Kicks	30 each side	60
Hand to Knee Squat	10	30

Table 15-3. Basic Physical Training (PT) Activities for Warm-Up, Flexibility, and Strength

Exercises*	Repetition (#)	Total Time (Seconds)
Posterior Shoulder or Upper Back Stretch	2	30
Triceps Stretch	2 each side	60
Iliopsoas Stretch (Russian Dancers)	2 each side	30
Standing Quad Stretch	2 each side	60
Standing Toe Pointers	30	60
Gastroc/Soleus Stretch	2 each side	60
Pull-Ups	MAX	60
Dips	MAX	60
Rope Climbs	1	-

*All exercises (See Chapter 7: Flexibility and Chapter 8: Calisthenics for descriptions) should be done in order.

For those interested in a more intensive PT program, a sample Total Body PT program is included for you. Alternatively, you can increase the number of repetitions of the exercises in the "basic" PT program. Both programs are very versatile, yet complete with respect to the whole body nature of the work-out.

Table 15-4. Total Body Physical Training (PT) Activities for Warm-Up, Flexibility, and Strength

Exercises*	Repetition (#)	Total Time (Seconds)
Jumping Jacks	50	60
1/2 Jumping Jacks	50-2 count	60
Up-Back-and Overs	10	60
Crunches (All Variations)	60-100	60
Push-Ups (Regular)	30	60
Flutter Kicks	25	60

Table 15-4. Total Body Physical Training (PT) Activities for Warm-Up, Flexibility, and Strength

Exercises*	Repetition (#)	Total Time (Seconds)
Dirty Dogs	20 each side	60
Butterflies Stretch	2	30
ITB Stretch	2 each side	60
3 Way Hurdler's Stretch	2 each side	180
Swimmer's Stretch	2	30
Push-Ups (Diamond)	30	60
Sit-Ups	30	60
Push-Ups (Wide Stance)	30	60
One Legged Squat	10 each side	60
Supine Back Stretch	1	30
Torso Prone Stretch	2	30
Prone Superman	10 each side	60
Vee-Ups	30	60
Donkey Kicks	30 each side	60
Hand to Knee Squat	10	30
Posterior Shoulder or Upper Back Stretch	2	30
Triceps Stretch	2 each side	60
Iliopsoas Stretch (Russian Dancers)	2 each side	30
Standing Quad Stretch	2 each side	60
Standing Toe Pointers	30	60
Gastroc/Soleus Stretch	2 each side	60
Repeat Starting at Crunches (2-3 times)		
Pull-Ups	MAX	60
Dips	MAX	60
Rope Climbs	1	

*All exercises (described in Chapter 7: Flexibility or Chapter 8: Calisthenics) should be done in order.

You should also include strength training at least twice per week. Details of a strength program are provided in Chapter 6.

A Physical Fitness Program for Confined Spaces

Maintaining fitness aboard a ship or submarine is possible. However, it requires motivation and discipline because usually the team spirit is missing. It is critical to maintain fitness so that when you reach your destination you have not become detrained. Table 15-5 presents a potential training program that could be followed on most ships. Most ships have stationary bicycles and rowing machines. However, if the ship has some other type of equipment, the schedule below could be modified to accommodate what equipment is available.

Table 15-5. Physical Fitness in Confined Spaces

Week Day	Activities for the Day
Monday	PT/30 min Interval Work-Out (Rowing Ergometer)/Stretch
Tuesday	45 min Steady State Work-Out (Stationary Cycle)/Stretch
Wednesday	PT/45 min Fartlek Work-Out (Rowing Ergometer, Jumping Rope)/Stretch
Thursday	Cycle 15/Row 15//Cycle 15/Stretch
Friday	Total Body PT
Saturday and Sunday	Take one day off and use other day for 60 minutes of low key training with whatever you choose
Two to Three Times/ Week	Circuit or Free Weight Training if Possible

A Physical Fitness Program for Coming Off Travel

When you first come back to shore or to your home base, you are not always in as good a physical shape as you were when you deployed. For this reason it is critical that you start back sensibly so as not to injure yourself. Both the PT and endurance components need to be modified so as to improve your overall fitness, not to put you in the doctor's office. Table 15-6 and Table 15-7 provide a reasonable Fitness and PT program for those coming off of travel. When you feel like you are back to your usual fitness level, then the Basic or Total Body Physical Fitness Programs can be started and/or worked into your schedule.

Table 15-6. Re-Entry Physical Training

Week Day	Activities for the Day
Monday	Modified PT/2-3 Mile Run/Stretch
Tuesday	1 Mile Swim/Stretch
Wednesday	Modified PT/3 Mile Run with Modified Fartlek Workout/Stretch
Thursday	Run 1.5 Miles/Swim 1/Run 1.5/Stretch
Friday	Alternate 5 Mile Hike with Pack and Monster Mash with Buddy Carries
Saturday and Sunday	Take one or two days off according to how you feel and your preferences
Two to Three Times/Week	Circuit or Free Weight Training

Table 15-7. A Re-Entry Physical Fitness Program

Exercises*	Repetition (#)	Total Time in Seconds
Jumping Jacks	25	60
1/2 Jumping Jacks	25-2 count	60
Up-Back-and Overs	5	60
Crunches (All Variations)	40-80	60
Push-Ups (Regular)	20	60
Flutter Kicks	15	30
Butterflies Stretch	2	30

Table 15-7. Re-Entry Physical Training

Exercises*	Repetition (#)	Total Time in Seconds
ITB Stretch	2 each side	60
3 Way Hurdler's Stretch	2 each side	180
Swimmer's Stretch	2	30
Push-Ups (Diamond)	20	60
Sit-Ups	20	60
Push-Ups (Wide Stance)	20	60
Supine Back Stretch	1	30
Torso Prone Stretch	2	30
Prone Superman	10 each side	60
Vee-Ups	30	60
Donkey Kicks	20 each side	60
Hand to Knee Squat	10	30
Posterior Shoulder or Upper Back Stretch	2	30
Triceps Stretch	2 each side	60
Iliopsoas Stretch (Russian Dancers)	2 each side	60
Standing Quad Stretch	2 each side	60
Standing Toe Pointers	30	60
Gastroc/Soleus Stretch	2 each side	60
Pull-Ups	MAX	60
Dips	MAX	60
Rope Climbs	1	-

*All exercises (described in Chapter 7: Flexibility or Chapter 8: Calisthenics) should be done in order.

Elimination of "Old" Exercises

As you may have noticed, some of your old favorites (or old foes) are no longer recommended. In May of 1994, a panel of experts convened to look at all of the different PT exercises currently in use by the SEAL community. A number of exercises were considered potentially harmful and were therefore eliminated. In addition, many exercises were modified to make them more effective (or potentially less harmful). Descriptions and diagrams for most of the exercises which are acceptable are provided in Chapters 7 and 8 (Flexibility and Calisthenics). Table 15-8 lists exercises that were eliminated and the reason for their elimination.

Table 15-8. Exercises Eliminated from SEAL PT

Exercise	Reason for Elimination
Windmills	Potential for injury to discs and lower back
Back Stretch	Potential for injury to cervical spine
Cherry Pickers	Potential for injury to discs and lower back
Cross-Overs (Hamstring Stretch)	Potential for injury to discs and lower back
Hand-toToe Sit-Ups	Mechanical stress on back; no benefit to abs.
Standing Head to Knee	Potential for injury to discs and lower back
Standing Hamstring Stretch	Potential for injury to back
2 Person Thigh Stretch	Potential for injury to knee

A Short Flexibility Program

Flexibility exercises are an important physical fitness component and may add years to your operational life. For those who have been injured, the "high mileage" SEAL (see Chapter 14), or someone with naturally short muscles, a short flexibility program is provided in Table 15-9.

Table 15-9. Selected Stretching Exercises for Improving Flexibility—A Short Program

Body Position	Flexibility Exercises*	
	Hold each for 15 to 30 seconds and perform two times on each side when appropriate.	
Standing:	Lateral/Forward Neck Flexion Upper Back Stretch	Posterior Shoulder Stretch Triceps Stretch
Sitting:	Swimmer's Stretch 3-Way Hurdler's	ITB Stretch
Back:	Supine Back	Hipstretch
Stomach:	Torso Prone	Prone Quad
Kneeling:	Kneeling Lunge with Pelvic Tilt	Achilles Stretch
Standing:	Gastroc Stretch	Soleus Stretch

*All exercises are described in Chapter 7: Flexibility

The Navy SEAL Physical Readiness Test (PRT)

The Navy SEAL Physical Readiness Test (PRT) is conducted in one session in a continuous manner with no less than two minutes or greater than 15 minutes rest between exercise and no more than a 30 minute break between the run and swim. Failure to successfully complete all events constitutes failure of the PRT. The PRT events, in order performed, include:

- Pull-Ups
- Sit-Ups
- Push-Ups
- 3 Mile Run
- 0.5 Mile Pool Swim

The first event, the pull-ups, has no time limit, whereas the sit-ups and push-ups have a three minute time limit. All three events are performed in clearly designated ways, and points are assigned to each event based on age and the number completed. The 3 mile run and 0.5 mile swim are timed events, and the time to completion and age are used to assign points. When all events have been completed, points for individual events are summed and an overall score is assigned. Table 15-10 provides a sample PRT test.

Table 15-10. PRT Score for a 34 year old SEAL

Event	Number or Time Completed	Points
Pull-Ups	18	80
Sit-Ups	105	85
Push-Ups	100	90
3 Mile Run	18:00	94
0.5 Mile Swim	15:00	90
	Total Points	439

The greatest number of points for any event is 100; thus the highest possible composite score is 500. The overall score is used for classification purposes: you can fall into one of five categories:

- Outstanding   425 - 500
- Excellent   350 - 424
- Good   275 - 349
- Satisfactory   200 - 274
- Fail   < 200 or < 40 for any event

In the example in Table 15-10, the overall score was 439; this would be rated as OUTSTANDING. Please refer to COMNAVSPECWARCOMINST 6110.IB for further information with respect to the Navy SEAL PRT and the tables describing points for each event.

Final Comments From: RADM Smith

This manual is a superb guide covering all the major focus areas required to maintain fitness as a SEAL. I offer as a final piece of SEAL culture, my version of "burn-out PT" in Table 15-11. The progression of the program is as follows: start at Stage 1 and cycle through the first set of each exercise, followed by the next sets. Next, move on to Stage 2 and use the same sequence. Begin with lower reps per exercise, with the goal of eventually completing the PT as set forth in Table 15-11. Those who have done it, know it is not what a modern fitness expert would necessarily approve of e.g., no stretching (do it on your own time), over repetition of the same exercises, and several stomach exercises clearly not beneficial for the lower back (an understatement!). Having said that, you can do it practically anywhere (if you have two or more hours), it exercises the vast majority of muscle groups, and finally, it imposes great pain and discomfort on the body—an instinct carefully nurtured, although sometimes avoided, (what's the water temp?) by even the most driven of us.

Its origin stems from a legendary SCPO in UDT-12 - Frank Perry, who reigned supreme among the West Coast teams for at least 15 years. I have omitted one of his favorite exercises — the eight-count body builders — invoking the principle that if you do my PT fast enough (it's structured to do that), you will get the requisite cardiovascular benefit without the 100 eight counts we did every Friday morning (one set-non-stop). Enough is enough! While I suspect it was only Frank Perry's way of reminding us who WAS "the king" in those days, I certainly don't recall any challenges to his reign!

I've also picked up many of these exercises from working out with the various SEAL teams. I've attempted to incorporate unusual or esoteric exercises to provide the more easily-bored SEAL with a bit of variety. I've also attempted to work opposing muscle groups—my one compromise to modern-day fitness.

Of course, do not feel constrained with what I offer—add your own or modify mine as you see fit. However, if you can do this program in less than 2 hours 15 minutes, you might try marketing the program to the public (plenty of former SEALS are already doing so with their programs)!

More importantly, do it with your platoon! It makes for great brotherhood when one shares pain with one's teammates!

Hoo-Yah!

RADM Smith

Table 15-11. RADM Smith's PT Program

Exercises	Repetitions (#)	Exercises	Repetitions (#)
Stage 1		**Stage 10**	
Up-Back-Over	10/20	Bicycle	50/40/30
Trunk Twist	10/20	Lunge (R)	20/20/15
Trunk Side Stretch	10/20		
Stage 2		**Stage 11**	
Push-Ups	10/15/20/25	Sit-Kneesbender	100/80/60
Neck-Up	30/40/50	Shoulder Crunch	120/100/80
Stage 3		**Stage 12**	
Cross Sit-Up	50/30/30	Sitting Flutter Kick	150/80/70
Diamond Push-Ups	30/25/20	Dirty Dawgs	40/40/50
Stage 4		**Stage 13**	
Side Crunch	50/40/30	Backnecks	100/80/60
Toe Raise	100/80/60	Narrow Squat	30/25/20
Stage 5		**Stage 14**	
Push-Ups	50/40/30/20	Sit-Ups	100
Side Snapper	30/20/10	Squats	50
Stage 6		**Stage 15**	
Jumping Jacks	20/20/20	Hand/Toe Sit-Ups	30/20/15
Wide Grip Push-Up	40/30/20	Push-Ups	10/25/40
Stage 7		**Stage 16**	
Back Exercise	50/40/30	Back Flutter Kick	300
Thigh Crunch	50/40/30	Wide Squat	50
		Push-Ups	50
Stage 8		**Stage 17**	
Push-Ups Side	50/40/30	Handstand Push-Ups - In Pairs	6/10/12/16
Neck	50/40/30		
Stage 9		**Stage 18**	
Stomach Crunch	200/125/100	Pull-Ups	100 reps
Lunge (L)	30/20/15	Dips	100 reps
		In Stage 18 vary with Pyramids/ Reverse Pyramids/Etc.	

Many of the exercises in the RADM Smith's PT program have been described previously in the Calisthenics chapter (Chapter 8), but some are new. So you don't have an excuse not to try this program, diagrams for the new exercise are provided in Table 15-12. Have fun!

Table 15-12. Examples of RADM Smith's Exercises

Exercises	Exercises

Stage 2 - Neck-Up

Stage 7 - Back Exercise

Stage 3 - Cross Sit-Up

Thigh Crunch

Stage 4 - Side Crunch

Stage 8 - Side Neck

Stage 5 - Side Snapper

Stage 11 - Shoulder Crunch

Table 15-12. Examples of RADM Smith's Exercises

Exercises	Exercises
Stage 12 - Dirty Dawgs	**Stage 13 - Back Neck**

Summary

Physical fitness is a critical component of SEAL training, and being in shape is essential for mission readiness. A comprehensive whole body conditioning program has been provided for you to use in your training. In addition, RADM Smith's PT program and a training program for confined spaces and for SEALs coming off travel have been included. Alternative exercises have also been provided to maintain motivation and optimize the concept of cross-training. Try it, you may find yourself in better "all around" shape.

Appendix A
Weight Lifting Techniques

Exercise	Instruction	Diagram
Hips and Legs		
Squats	1. Place barbell across shoulders on upper back. DO NOT place bar directly on neck. 2. Keep head up, back straight, and feet slightly wider than shoulder width. Point toes out. Keep back perpendicular to floor. 3. Squat in a controlled motion until upper thighs are parallel to floor. 4. Pause. Return to standing position. 5. Inhale squatting down, exhale standing up.	
Lunge	1. Stand with feet shoulder-width apart, bar resting on back of shoulders. 2. Lunge forward with one leg, bending it until thigh is parallel to floor. Do not let front knee bend so it moves in front of toes. 3. Pause. Return to standing position. Repeat with other leg. Inhale lunging, exhale standing up.	

Exercise	Instruction	Diagram
3/4 Squat	1. Place barbell across shoulders on upper back. Do not place bar directly on neck. 2. Keep head up, back straight, feet slightly wider than shoulder width. Point toes out. Keep back perpendicular to floor. 3. Squat in a controlled motion, until knees are at a 120° angle. 4. Pause. Return to standing position. Raise up on toes and return to starting position. 5. Inhale squatting down, exhale standing up.	
Stiff Legged Dead Lift	1. Place barbell on floor. 2. Bend at waist, head up, back arched, knees slightly bent. You should feel stretch in back of legs, not in lower back. 3. Straighten-up lifting barbell off bench until barbell is at arms length. 4. Pause. Return to upright position. 5. Inhale bending over, exhale straightening up.	
Leg Press	1. Make sure hips and back remain flat against support pad during exercise. 2. Slowly lower platform until legs achieve a 90° angle. 3. Without pausing, return platform to starting position. NOTE: DO NOT LOCK KNEES AT TOP OF THIS MOVEMENT. 4. Pause. Repeat steps 2,3. Exhale raising platform, inhale lowering platform.	

Weight Lifting Techniques

Exercise	Instruction	Diagram
Leg Curls	1. Place heels, with feet flexed, under foot pads with pads at back of heels, not calves. 2. With a smooth motion, curl legs up to complete full range of motion. 3. Pause. In controlled motion, return to starting position. 4. Exhale curling legs up, inhale extending legs. 5. Do not lift hips or arch back while curling.	
Leg Extensions	1. Sit on machine with feet under foot pad. Lightly hold seat handles for stabilization. 2. Keeping feet flexed, raise weight up until legs are parallel to floor. Make sure to flex quadriceps. 3. Pause. Slowly lower weight to starting position. Do not let weight drop. 4. Repeat steps 2,3. Exhale extending legs, inhale lowering legs.	
Seated Calf Raises	1. Place balls of feet on calf machine's foot piece, pads resting on top of knees. 2. Raise up on toes as fully extended as possible. Pause and hold. 3. In a controlled manner, return to starting position and move heels down as low as possible for maximum range of motion. 4. Repeat motion. Exhale lifting up, inhale lowering weight.	
Standing Calf Raises	1. Place shoulders under pads of calf machine and balls of feet on floor pad. 2. Standing straight with knees slightly bent rise up on toes as fully extended as possible. 3. Pause. Return to starting position, in a smooth motion. 4. Exhale lifting up, inhale lowering weight. 5. Do not lock knees during exercise.	

Exercise	Instruction	Diagram
	Back	
Curl Grip Pulldowns	1. Sit with back flat, arms extended. Grab pulldown bar using underhand curl grip. 2. Keep hands a shoulder width apart, pull bar down until it touches top of chest. Let bar follow elbows. Do not swing or rock lower back during movement. 3. Pause. Return to starting position and repeat. 4. Exhale pulling down, inhale returning up.	
Reverse Barbell Rows	1. Start by standing with barbell 4-6 inches in front of you on floor. 2. Grab bar using an underhand grip. Hands shoulder width apart, head supported by resting it against a padded bench. 3. Knees slightly bent, lift bar off floor at arms length, a few inches from floor. 4. Slowly pull elbows back and slightly out, lifting bar until it reaches upper abdomen. 5. Pause, Return to starting position. 6. Repeat steps 4,5. 7. Exhale when raising barbell, inhale when lowering barbell.	
Lat Pulldowns	1. Hold special handles so that your palms are facing each other. Fully extend arms and stretch your back. 2. Begin pulldown by bringing elbows down to your sides until the bar touches your upper chest. NOTE: Do not swing or rock your lower back to begin or complete this lift. 3. Pause, then return to starting position with a smooth and controlled motion. 4. Repeat steps 2,3,. Exhale while pulling, inhale while raising weight.	

Exercise	Instruction	Diagram
Seated Rows	1. Place feet against a stationary object or foot rest. Knees slightly bent. 2. Hold pulley handle at chest height, arms extended. Shoulders will roll forward, back remains straight. 3. Using upper back, pull handles to middle of chest, keeping forearms parallel to floor. Do not rock backwards or forward during movement. 4. Pause, then return to starting position. Exhale pulling, inhale extending. Repeat steps 3,4.	
One Arm Dumbbell Rows	1. Place left knee and hand on bench, right leg held straight. Keep back straight. 2. Hold dumbbell with right hand. Pull straight up to rib cage. 3. Lower dumbbell to starting position. Exhale raising dumbbell, inhale lowering dumbbell. 4. Repeat steps 2 & 3. 5. Reverse position and repeat movement on opposite side.	
Hyper extensions	1. On a hyperextension bench, lean hips forward on lower flat pad until top of hips are over front end of pad. 2. As you slowly lean forward and bend down, let ankles lock under back of the rear pads. 3. Pause, then slowly return to starting position. 4. Exhale when raising torso, inhale when lowering torso.	

Exercise	Instruction	Diagram

Shoulders and Arms

Exercise	Instruction	Diagram
Incline Dumbbell Press	1. Lie on 20° incline bench. Feet flat on floor. 2. Bring the dumbells to front of shoulders as if holding a bar. 3. Press dumbbells up until arms are extended, elbows slightly bent. Keep lower back on bench and do not arch back. 4. Pause. Lower dumbbells to upper chest, repeat movement. 5. Exhale raising dumbbells, inhale lowering.	
Dumbbell Flys	1. Lie on bench with feet flat on floor. 2. Hold dumbbells at arms length above upper chest with palms facing each other. 3. Keeping elbows slightly bent, lower dumbbells out to each side of chest in semi-circular motion. Dumbbells should be even with sides of chest and slightly back. 4. Pause. Return dumbbells to starting position using same path of movement. 5. Repeat steps 3,4. Exhale raising dumbbells, inhale lowering dumbbells.	
Behind the Neck Press	1. Sit with back straight and against support pad, keeping feet flat on the floor. Bench should be inclined 5-10°, if possible. 2. Raise dumbbells to shoulder height, palms facing forward. If using barbell, remove from safety holder. Keep elbows out. 3. Raise dumbbell/barbell to arms length, overhead. Use a careful, controlled motion. 4. Pause. Lower weights to starting position. Exhale raising weights, inhale lowering them.	

Exercise	Instruction	Diagram
Cable Flies	1. Lie on bench with feet flat on floor. 2. Arms extended, palms up, gripped firmly on handles, elbows slightly bent, bring arms to front, and cross-over your chest. 3. Pause. Return with a controlled motion to starting position. Keep upper arms in line with shoulders and collarbone during movement. 4. Exhale pulling cables, inhale extending arms.	
Upright Rows	1. Hold barbell with narrow overhand grip. An E-Z curl bar is suggested. Hands should be no more than 6" apart. 2. Stand straight, hold barbell against upper thighs at arms length. 3. Keep bar close to body and back straight throughout this movement, pull bar upward until just under chin. 4. At top of movement forearms are almost parallel to floor. Keep elbows out and up. 5. Pause. Slowly return bar to starting position. Exhale raising bar, inhale lowering bar. Repeat steps 3,4,5.	
Rotating Dumbbell Curls	1. On incline bench, hold dumbbells at arms length, arms extended down-ward, palms facing toward the rear. 2. Begin curl by lifting dumbbells up. Slowly rotate hands until they pass thighs. Palms must be facing up. 3. Bring dumbbells up to shoulder level. DO NOT SWING dumbbells up, use a controlled motion. 4. Pause. Lower dumbbell with palms up, passing upper thigh. Begin rotating arm until palms are facing back. Arms should be fully extended. 5. Pause. Repeat 3,4,5. Inhale lowering dumbbell, exhale raising dumbbell.	

Exercise	Instruction	Diagram
Barbell Curls	1. Stand, feet shoulder width apart, back straight. Grab barbell (hands shoulder width apart) with underhand grip. 2. Hold barbell against upper thighs at arms length. 3. Controlling motion, curl barbell through natural range of motion. Keep elbows and arms close to sides. Do not throw weight up by arching back and swinging barbell. Do not rock elbows forward. 4. Pause. With a smooth motion, lower barbell to starting position. 5. Pause. Repeat steps 3 & 4. Exhale raising barbell, inhale lowering barbell.	
Internal Rotators	1. Lie on side on bench. Place and keep working elbow on bench in front of waist for support. 2. Hold dumbbell in lower hand. Lower dumbbell towards floor at a comfortable angle. 3. Pause. Raise dumbbell toward upper arm. 4. Lower dumbbell to starting position. Repeat steps 3 & 4. 5. Reverse position, repeat on opposite side. 6. Exhale raising dumbbell, inhale lowering.	
External Rotators	1. Lie on side on bench. Place lower arm and elbow on bench in front of waist for support. 2. Hold dumbbell in upper hand. Upper arm is across upper body, working elbow resting against side for support. 3. Raise dumbbell towards ceiling. Use elbow as pivot point. 4. Pause. Lower dumbbell across upper body. Repeat steps 3 and 4. Exhale raising dumbbell, inhale lowering	

Exercise	Instruction	Diagram
Wrist Curls	1.Sit on bench. Place elbows on bench between knees holding dumbbell. Let wrist hang over end of bench. 2. Begin by lowering hands towards floor; as you open up hand, dumbbell will be resting in fingers. 3. Pause. Curl fingers back around barbell as you raise hand in a semi-circular motion towards chest. Keep forearms flat against bench through entire exercise. 4. Pause. Lower dumbbell back to starting position. 5. Repeat 2,3,4. Exhale raising dumbbell, inhale lowering it.	
Reverse Wrist Curls	1. Sit on bench. Place elbows on bench between knees holding dumbbell, palms face down. Let wrist hang over end of bench. 2. Begin exercise by raising hands in semi-circular motion towards body. 3. Pause. Lower hands down toward floor. Keep forearms flat against bench through entire exercise. 4. Pause. Raise dumbbell back to starting position. 5. Repeat 2,3,4. Exhale raising dumbbell, inhale lowering.	

Diagrams have been adapted from *Strength Training for Sports*, from Applied FuturisticsSM 1994 with permission Fred Koch.

Appendix B
Common Anatomical Terms and Diagrams

Common Terms for Muscle Groups	Muscles	Function
Chest Muscles	Pectoralis major*, pectoralis minor*, serratus anterior, subclavius	Flexion, adduction, extension, and rotation of shoulder girdle (pushing, bench pressing)
Abdominals	Transverse abdominal*, rectus femoris, external oblique, internal oblique, psoas major	Spinal flexion, lateral flexion, and rotation of trunk
Back Extensors	Erector spinae* (iliocostalis, longissimus, spinalis)	Move vertebral column backward
Hip Flexors	Iliopsoas*, rectus femoris*, sartorius, pectineus, tensor facia latae, adductor muscles, anterior part of gluteus medius	Move leg forward and toward the chest at the hip joint

Common Terms for Muscle Groups	Muscles	Function
Hip Extensors	Gluteus maximus*, semitendinosus, semimembranosus*, biceps femoris*	Extends leg backward at hip joint
Hip/Thigh Adductors	Adductor magnus*, adductor longus*, adductor brevis*, pectineus, gracilis	Moves leg toward midline
Hip/Thigh Abductors	Gluteus medius*, gluteus minimus*, tensor fasciae latae, sartorius	Moves leg away from midline
Knee Flexors	Biceps femoris*, semimembranosus, semitendinosus, gracilis	Flexes or bends leg at knee joint
Knee Extensors	Quadriceps femoris*, (vastus lateralis*, vastus intermedius*, vastus medialis, rectus femoris), sartorius	Extends leg forward at knee joint. Vastus medialis muscle plays important role in prevention of overuse injuries of knee
Calf Muscles	Gastrocnemius, soleus	Extends foot at ankle
Tibialis	Tibialis anterior, tibialis posterior	Flexes or extends foot at ankle

*Major muscles involved in movement

Figure B-1. Selected Muscles of the Chest

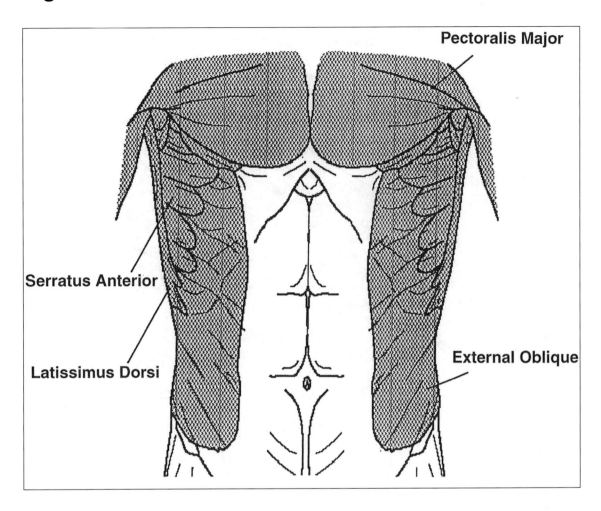

Pectoralis Major

Serratus Anterior

Latissimus Dorsi

External Oblique

Figure B-2. Selected Muscles of the Back

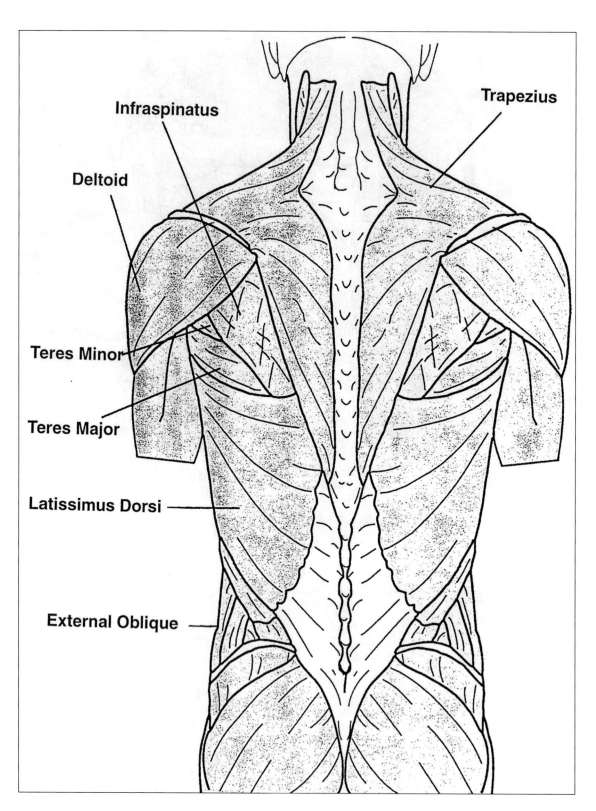

Trapezius

Infraspinatus

Deltoid

Teres Minor

Teres Major

Latissimus Dorsi

External Oblique

Figure B-3. Selected Muscles of the Front Part (Anterior) of the Upper and Lower Leg

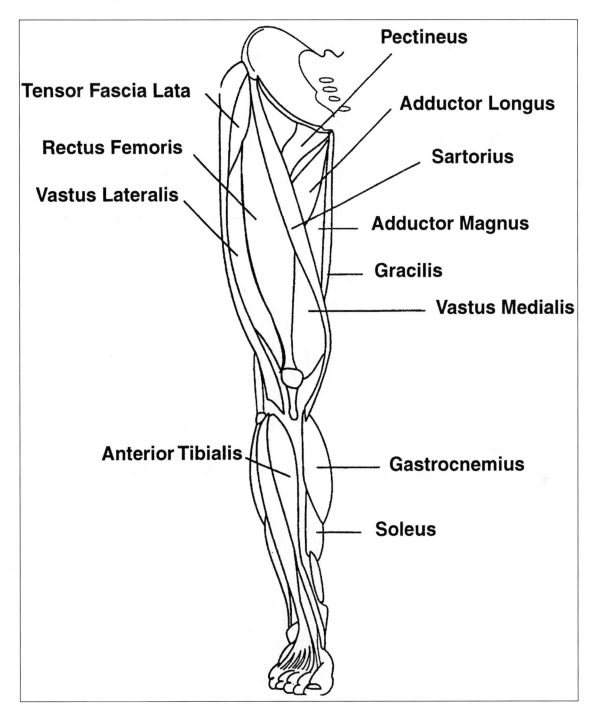

Pectineus

Tensor Fascia Lata

Adductor Longus

Rectus Femoris

Sartorius

Vastus Lateralis

Adductor Magnus

Gracilis

Vastus Medialis

Anterior Tibialis

Gastrocnemius

Soleus

Figure B-4. Selected Muscles of the Back Part (Posterior) of the Upper and Lower Leg

Gluteus Medius

Gluteus Maximus

Gracilis

Adductor Magnus

Biceps Femoris

Semimembranosus
Semitendinosus

Soleus

Gastrocnemius

Common Anatomical Terms and Diagrams

Appendix C
Foot Care for Load-Bearing

Foot hygiene and sanitation are important for preventing injuries during prolonged walking, particularly when carrying heavy loads. Injuries to the feet that should be considered during prolonged load-bearing include:

- Blisters
- Abrasions
- Foot Perspiration Problems
- Athletes' Foot
- Trench Foot
- Immersion Foot

Proper care of feet should occur before, during, and after load-bearing activities. Foot care involves frequent and thorough cleaning of feet, use of foot powder, wearing properly fitted footwear, and correctly trimming toenails.

Before any load-bearing hump, trim toenails short, square, and straight across. Keep feet clean and dry, and use foot powder. Wear clean, dry, well-fitting socks (preferably cushioned-soled) with seams and knots outside. Socks that have been previously mended should not be used. A nylon or polypropylene sock liner can reduce friction and add protection. Carry an extra pair of socks. Carefully fit new boots. When getting used to new boots, alternate with another pair; tape known hot (red skin) spots before wearing.

When possible during a rest period, lie down with feet elevated. If time permits, massage feet, apply foot power, change socks, and medicate any blisters. Cover open blisters, cuts, or abrasions with absorbent adhesive bandages. Obtain relief from swelling feet by loosening bootlaces where they cross the arch of the foot.

After completing the load-bearing exercise, procedures for care of feet, wash and dry socks, and dry boots stated above should be repeated. Medicate any injuries on feet. Sides of the feet can develop red, swollen, tender skin during prolonged humping with a load, which could become a blister. Thus, feet require airing, elevation, rest, and wider footwear. Prevent major foot problems by keeping feet clean. The combination of abrasions with dirt and perspiration can cause infection and serious injury. If possible, give feet a daily foot bath. In the field, cool water seems to reduce the sensation of heat and irritation. After washing, dry the feet well.

Photo Credits

All photos purchased from Thinkstock.com.

iStockphoto	7, 25, 26, 58, 63, 69, 71, 103, 162, 163, 164, 175, 181, 185, 190, 221, 229, 235
Hemera	8, 199
Mike Powell, Digital Vision	11
Stockbyte	18, 187
Stocktrek Images	23, 37, 53
Jupiter Images, Getty Images, liquidlibrary	24, 93, 113
Photodisc	37
Ryan McVay, Photodisc	42
Digital Vision, Photodisc	43
Dorling Kindersley RF	72, 79
Zoonar	76
George Doyle	85
Pixland	109
Ryan McVay, Digital Vision	116
Siri Stafford, Lifesize	133
Comstock Images, Comstock	142
Jupiterimages, Polkadot	194

Part II — Nutrition

Preface to Part II Nutrition

The demands imposed by SEAL training are profound, and success requires the mustering of all your strength—physical and mental. One factor that may bring you closer to success is nutritional interventions. It is well known that appropriate nutritional habits and interventions can enhance your ability to perform, and we want you to be familiar with those successful habits. This manual is for you to read, participate in, and use as a resource when you have questions about nutrition and no one is available to give you answers.

The first five chapters are very basic—they provide background information about nutrition concepts in general, and little to nothing about performance. However, they are very important for fully understanding the information in subsequent chapters. In the remaining chapters, we have tried to be as specific as possible in terms of what we think you should and shouldn't do, and given you reasons for our recommendations. For example, in Chapter 8: Restaurants, Fast Foods, and Eating Out, we have given you sample menus at Fast Foods places so you can select a high-carbohydrate diet. In the chapter on Mission Recovery, we target three areas you need to focus on and provide ways to ensure a rapid recovery. In Chapter 15, Ergogenic. Agents, we discourage the use of some products because not only is there insufficient information, but there may be potential risks and adverse effects associated with using them. Again, our objective is to make you more informed so you can make educated choices about foods and supplements. Many commercial products sold in stores and through magazines make claims so you will purchase them. With some products you are wasting your money, and with others, possibly hurting yourself. Other products may actually give you the "edge" and improve your performance, but it takes information to make the appropriate decision. This manual should help you do that.

You men are a select group—we know that from our years of working with SEALs and SEAL trainees. For that reason you must be treated as such. This manual has been prepared with that in mind: we want to help you perform to the best of your abilities under the

---

rigorous conditions you confront in training and during missions. We certainly don't have all the answers to nutritional enhancement of performance, because the answers are not all available yet. However, we will continue searching for answers and encourage you to continue asking questions that relate to nutrition and performance so we can help you find those answers. We wish you the best and hope you will let us know when you can't find answers to your questions.

Patty Deuster, Anita Singh, and Pierre Pelletier
Bethesda, MD

Foreword to Part II

Many people consider the U.S. Navy SEALs the toughest, most versatile, and fittest warriors on the planet. Because of the incredibly challenging demands placed on Navy SEALs, their fitness requirements as well as their nutritional requirements are of critical importance to the Navy and to the Naval Special Warfare community.

SEAL is the acronym for Sea, Air, and Land. Navy SEALs train and operate in every environment the planet has to offer, from parachuting into enemy and hostile terrain to swimming in rough seas, diving in icy waters, and conducting maritime operations launching from submarines, small craft, ships, fixed wing aircraft, and helicopters. They operate in arctic, mountain, desert, and jungle terrain. A Navy SEAL can function efficiently anywhere in the world and can insert or extract from the area of operation (AO) using every possible means the military or civilian community has to offer. Navy SEALs must be able to work under any condition and in any environment; to do so, they must have access to up-to-date information on the most state-of-the-art physical fitness, nutritional, and fluid requirements.

From its early beginnings, SEALs and their predecessors faced some of the most physically challenging operations in the history of the military. The Navy has always required its operators to be in top physical condition to meet the rigorous demands placed on them. To achieve such physical shape, SEALs must consume the most nutritionally well-balanced meals available, whether it be whole foods, MREs, or freeze-dried foods. For the majority of a Navy SEAL's career, he will consume between 2,000 and 4,000 calories each day. These calories must be energy-efficient fuel.

SEAL training and missions require strength and endurance. Navy SEALs must be able to operate in adverse conditions at various altitudes for long days and sometimes weeks. During these arduous periods, they must be able to perform at a high level of efficiency, which a proper diet will facilitate. One of the most critical components of fitness is diet. Failure to replace nutritional fuel, electrolytes, and fluids will undoubtedly weaken a SEAL's performance level.

The Navy Special Warfare (NACSPECWAR) community remains focused on the objective of keeping its personnel as physically fit as possible and understands that the better their nutritional intake, the better their performance. What SEALs eat on a daily basis helps determine how much energy they will have for intense, rigorous performance.

An updated extensive SEAL-specific nutritional study was required to ensure Navy SEALs were receiving optimum nourishment and meeting hydration requirements during training, during deployment, and while engaged in combat. It is of critical importance to the Navy to ensure the SEALs receive the most up-to-date information available and then to modify it to meet the specific requirements of the SEALs so they can operate at their maximum performance levels.

The U.S. Navy SEAL Guide to Nutrition was written specifically for the SEAL community by a team of Navy SEALs, dieticians, and physicians who specialize in exercise, sports nutrition, and exercise physiology. Numerous basic off-the-shelf nutritional resources and guides exist and are readily available to the public, but those books lack the specific nutritional requirements of the Navy SEAL.

The objectives of *The U.S. Navy SEAL Guide to Nutrition* are to introduce appropriate nutritional guidelines and interventions to the Navy SEAL operator. The Guide addresses:

◆ nutritional concepts,
◆ energy expenditure,
◆ energy intake,
◆ macro and micro nutrients,
◆ essential vitamins and minerals,
◆ supplements,
◆ fiber intake,
◆ fluid replacement,
◆ snacking,
◆ military rations,
◆ ergogenetic and ergolytic rations, and
◆ nutritional requirements when operating in extreme environmental conditions.

Most importantly, this book discusses nutrition for optimum performance, as well as "The Naval Special Warfare 10 Commandments of Nutrition."

SEALs require more calories to replenish their energy than most people or other athletes. It is important that the diet of a SEAL consists of adequate amounts of protein, carbohydrates, fat, and the more than fifty nutrients the body requires. These cannot be provided in any one food or supplement. The Navy SEAL Nutritional Guide details how this can most effectively be accomplished.

In this book, the authors discuss how consumption of supplements, vitamins, and minerals is typically unnecessary, provided that the SEAL is following a well-balanced nutritional diet. The key to nutrition and athletic performance is moderation and control of the daily consumption of required foods. With the additional stress that SEALs place on the nervous system, it is critical to ensure that SEALS consume at least the minimum required vitamins and minerals and have proper control over their daily diets.

SEALs must consume adequate calories to meet the needs of intense training. They are encouraged to get most of their nutrients from "real" food rather than supplements. Their diet should be rich in complex carbohydrates to provide the energy source to fuel the high demands of their daily routines. Consumption of fruits, vegetables, and whole grains are the best insurance for getting the necessary vitamins and minerals required for optimum health. SEALs must also pay close attention to the quality of the produce and meats they eat. Foods that are less refined are best, but organic is optimal. SEALs should attempt to get nutrition from as close to the original food source as possible.

It is just as important to be well-hydrated, especially in high temperatures. Performance can decrease dramatically when the body is depleted of fluids. Optimal performance during extended exercise sessions occurs when the rate of fluid intake equals the rate of fluid loss through sweating. The authors of this guide stress the importance of always staying hydrated, regardless of SEAL status.

The U.S. Navy SEAL Guide to Nutrition emphasizes that nutritional misinformation can do as much harm as proper nutrition can help. The authors also state that good, life-long nutritional habits must be emphasized from a young age. This guide has been a tremendous resource to the Naval Special Warfare Community throughout the years. This edition includes the latest research as it applies to the SEAL community. If you are interested in a comprehensive guide on nutrition and SEAL-specific nutritional requirements, this guide is for you.

Don Mann
CWO3/SEAL/ret

About the Authors

The U.S. Navy SEAL Guide to Nutrition

Dr. Patricia Deuster is an Associate Professor and Director of the Human Performance Laboratory in the Department of Military and Emergency Medicine at the Uniformed Services University of the Health Sciences, School of Medicine in Bethesda, Maryland. Her credentials for writing this book are many. She has been conducting research in the area of sports nutrition and exercise physiology for over 14 years, has published numerous papers on the nutritional needs of U.S. Navy SEALs, and has given many sports nutrition seminars to high school, college, and professional athletes, recreational athletes, SWAT teams, dietitians, and other health professionals. She is also an athlete herself. She was a tennis professional for 5 years and has competed in several triathlons and over 20 marathons; her best marathon time was a 2:48 in the Boston Marathon. Dr. Deuster was a nationally ranked runner for several years and a qualifier for the First Women's Olympic Marathon Trials. She is an avid sportswoman and a former sky-diver who has logged over 100 jumps. With her combination of athletic abilities and interests, professional training, and research endeavors, she is clearly one of the few persons prepared to develop this guide.

Dr. Anita Singh received her Ph.D. in Nutrition in 1986 from the University of Maryland, where she was selected as an Outstanding Graduate. She is an Assistant Professor in the Department of Military and Emergency Medicine at the Uniformed Services University of the Health Sciences in Bethesda Maryland. She is also a registered dietitian and has been working in the area of Sports Nutrition for about 10 years. In addition to looking at nutritional needs of U.S. Navy SEAL trainees, she has studied women who qualified for the First Women's Olympic Marathon Trials, triathletes, ultramarathoners, and recreational athletes. Dr. Singh has presented her research work at various national and international meetings and has published extensively in scientific journals. She is a runner, tennis player, and avid hiker.

Pierre A. Pelletier ENS, MC, USNR will be graduating in 1995 from the Uniformed Services University of the Health Sciences (USUHS), School of Medicine in Bethesda, MD. He received his undergraduate degree from Norwich University in Biology and Chemistry. ENS Pelletier has always been active in athletics both as a participant and teacher. He was a competitive skier and instructor for eight years and a kayaking instructor in New England. He is also active in the Potomac Rugby Union in Maryland and most recently was invited to play with the US Navy Rugby Club. His personal interest in nutrition as it relates to athletics has been nurtured while at USUHS and culminated in a clinical year of research in the Human Performance Laboratory at USUHS where he assisted in writing the manual. He plans to practice Operational Medicine as a Diving Medical Officer with the US Navy SEALs.

Chapter 1
Energy Balance = Energy Expenditure - Energy Intake

Balancing energy intake and expenditure can be difficult when activity levels are very high, as in SEAL training, and when activity levels are very low, such as during isolation. Typically, body weight remains constant when energy intake equals expenditure.

Intake=3000 kcal Output=3000 kcal Weight Gain=0

Intake=4000 kcal Output=2000 kcal Weight Gain= +

Intake=2000 kcal Output=3000 kcal Weight Gain= −

Units of Energy

The unit commonly used for describing energy intake and energy expenditure is the Calorie. The term Kilocalorie (kcal) is also used as a measure of energy intake and expenditure and **1 kcal = 1 Calorie. Throughout this book we will use the terms kcal and calorie interchangeably.**

Sensitivity of Energy Balance

The energy balance equation can be "unbalanced" by changing energy intake, energy expenditure, or both. To gain or lose 1 pound it takes approximately 3500 extra kcal consumed or burned. Believe it or not, the energy balance equation is very sensitive, as is shown in the following example.

Example 1:

If you ate one extra chocolate chip cookie (65 kcal) each day for one year, this would be 65 X 365 or 23,725 extra kcal.

This small daily increase in energy intake would result in a gain of ~ 6.8 pounds in one year.

Energy Balance = Energy Expenditure - Energy Intake

Example 2:

If you ate one less chocolate chip cookie per day and started running 1 extra mile per day 5 days per week, you would lose 14 pounds. This number is obtained by adding the 6.8 pounds from not eating the cookie and the 7.4 pounds/year for running (100 kcal/mile X 5 miles/week X 52 weeks/year = 26,000 kcal or 7.4 pounds/year). **You see? It works both ways!**

Components of Energy Expenditure

The three major contributors to energy expenditure are:

◆ Resting energy expenditure
◆ Physical activity
◆ Energy for digesting foods

The first two are of interest here and will be discussed in detail.

Resting Energy Expenditure

Resting energy expenditure (REE) is the amount of energy required to maintain life, such as breathing, beating of the heart, maintenance of body temperature, and other life processes. Measurements are usually made in the morning after waking with the body at complete rest. REE can be estimated by a formula and used to predict your daily energy/caloric requirements. The only information needed is your body weight in pounds.

Table 1-1. Determining Resting Energy Expenditure (REE) of Men from Body Weight (in pounds)

Age (years)	Equation to Derive REE (kcal/day)
18–30	6.95 X Weight + 679
30–60	5.27 X Weight + 879

Energy Expenditure For Physical Activity

The amount of energy you expend during physical activity is different each day, depending on your training. Some days are very strenuous and involve running, swimming, calisthenics, cold water exposure, sleep deprivation, and carrying heavy loads. Some days you are in the classroom sitting a good portion of the day. Thus, determining your actual energy expended during activity is more difficult, but there are ways to estimate it. You would usually take your REE and multiply it by a number (or factor) as shown on the next page to get a rough estimate of your total energy/calorie needs. Lets try out an example.

Energy Balance = Energy Expenditure - Energy Intake

Total Energy Expenditure

Table 1-2. Estimating Total Daily Energy Needs of Men at Various Levels of Activity

Level of General Activity	Activity Factor (X REE)
Very Light - Seated and standing activities, driving, playing cards	1.3
Light - walking, carpentry, sailing, playing ping-pong or pool, golf	1.6
Moderate - carrying a load, jogging, light swimming, biking, calisthenics, scuba diving	1.7
Heavy - walking with a load uphill, rowing, digging, climbing, soccer, basketball, running, obstacle course	2.1
Exceptional - running/swimming races, cycling uphill, carrying very heavy loads, hard rowing	2.4

Example: You are 21, weigh 175 lbs, and activity is moderate

REE = 6.95 X Weight + 679 = 6.95 X 175 + 679 = 1895 kcal/day

Total Energy Needs = 1895 X 1.7 = 3222 kcal/day

The formula for REE came from Table 1-1.

The 1.7 is the Activity Factor for "Moderate" from the table above.

Worksheet 1-1. Estimate Your Total Daily Energy Needs

Weight:_____ Age:_____ Activity Factor:_____

Determine Your REE:_____ kcal/day

Energy Needs = REE X Activity = _____ X_____

My Estimated Energy Needs = _____ kcal/day

Body Size and Body Mass Index

The BODY MASS INDEX, or BMI is a measure commonly used to rapidly assess body composition and then classify and identify individuals as under-, overweight or overfat. The BMI is actually a ratio: weight/height^2, with weight in kilograms and height in meters. Reference standards have been developed for the United States population as a whole, broken down by race and gender, so that individuals at risk for obesity can be identified. However, the reference values for the U.S. population as a whole do not always apply to special populations, such as SEALs. As a result, unique populations often develop their own standards and references based on individuals within that population. A reference range based on a survey of over 800 SEALs was recently developed. For all the SEALs combined, the average BMI was 25, and the average body fat was 13%. What is important to remember, is that this index is a screening tool. You can use the BMI to assess and keep track of changes in your body composition. If your BMI is high, have your body fat checked, and if your body fat is more than 20%, you need to take some action to lower your weight. Reference BMI values for you are provided below:

Reference BMI Values for SEALs	
Lean	<20
Typical SEAL	20 to 29
Check Your Body Fat	29 to 32

Energy Balance = Energy Expenditure - Energy Intake

Use the normogram below to find your BMI and see where you fall relative to the reference values. To use the normogram, place a ruler or straight edge between height (right side) and body weight (left side); then read BMI from the central scale. NOTE: Even with these reference values, the BMI can misclassify some large frame, very strong men as overweight. Check your body fat; that will be the deciding factor.

Worksheet 1-2. Normogram for Body Mass Index

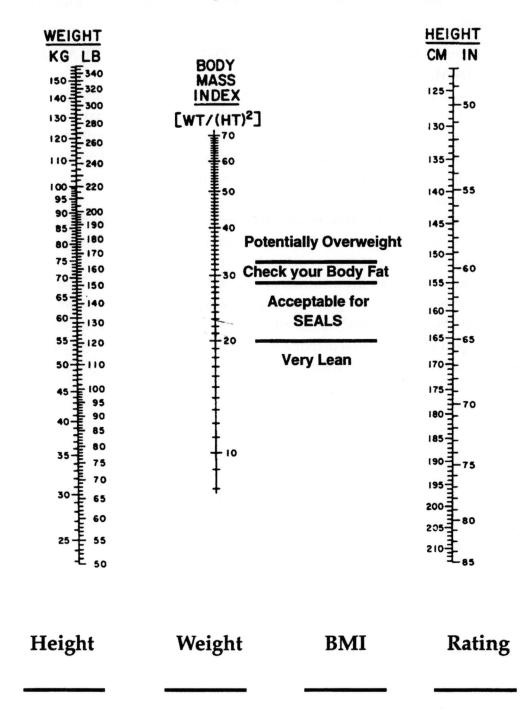

Height	Weight	BMI	Rating
_____	_____	_____	_____

How To Calculate Energy Expenditure

You will need a calculator to complete this exercise.

Over a 24 hour period you will expend different amounts of energy in each activity in which you engage, be it watching TV, eating, running on the sand, paddling, or listening to your teammates. The objective of this activity is to make you aware of the energy you actually do expend.

♦ Record your name and date on your **ENERGY EXPENDITURE ACTIVITY FORM.**

♦ List all the activities you participated in over the last 12 hours and the approximate length of time (in minutes) you spent on each activity on the form.

♦ Go through the alphabetical list of activities provided in **Appendix 4,** and find the activity that most closely approximates each one you listed on the form.

♦ Write down on the form the kcal/minute (not per hour!) value in the appropriate column (**Energy Value**).

♦ Multiply the energy value by the total time in minutes. For example, if you ran in the sand in boots for 25 minutes, then your energy expenditure for that activity would be 15 (energy value) X 25 (time) = 385 kcals.

♦ Do this for at least five activities, or preferably all the events in 12 hours. Then add up the numbers to get an actual energy expenditure estimate. How did you fare? You were probably surprised by some of the numbers, but this experience should give you a good overview of energy balance. Keep track of your weight if you are in doubt—it is the most accurate way to monitor energy balance.

Energy Balance = Energy Expenditure - Energy Intake

Worksheet 1-3. Energy Expenditure Activity Form

Name:		Date:	
Activity	**Time in Minutes**	**Energy Value (kcal/min)**	**Total Calories**
Obstacle Course	30	10	300
4 mile run, 8 min/mile pace	32	14	448
5 Mile Ocean Swim	175	9	1575
Calisthenics	30	8	240
Weight Lifting	45	11	495
14 Mile Run in boots	140	12	1680
5 Mile Hike w/80 lb load	100	14	1400
GRAND TOTAL			

Chapter 2
Carbohydrate, Fat, and Protein: The Energy-Providing Macronutrients

You have heard the saying *"You are what you eat."* Although this statement has not been proven, we do know that what you eat makes a difference in how you perform, how long you survive, and the quality of your life. The *macronutrients,* or energy-providing nutrients, are extremely important in this respect. Also, without energy you would starve, and your ability to perform would be greatly reduced. Our three main sources of energy are:

◆ Carbohydrate or **CHO**
◆ Fat
◆ Protein

These fuels are called *macro* because they are eaten in "large quantities" unlike the micronutrients we will discuss later. This chapter will provide basic information about these *macronutrients.*

Carbohydrate

Carbohydrates, commonly abbreviated CHO, are foods we want to become very familiar with since they are the preferred foods for endurance activities, competitive athletic events, and healthy living. In fact, CHOs are the basic source of energy for humans. Luckily, CHOs are also foods you are encouraged to eat, not foods you are urged to restrict, such as fat.

Definition, Composition, and Classification

Carbohydrates are composed of three elements: carbon, hydrogen, and oxygen. They exist in many forms, but the two major types of CHOs are simple and complex.

- Simple CHOs have one (mono) or two (disaccharides) sugar molecules hooked together.
- Types of simple CHOs include glucose (dextrose), table sugar (sucrose), honey (fructose and glucose), fructose (sugars in fruit), maltose (sugars in malt), lactose (sugar in milk), brown sugar, corn syrup, maple syrup, refined sugar products, raw sugar, corn sweeteners, high-fructose corn syrup, and molasses.
- Complex CHOs have three or more simple sugar molecules hooked together; polysaccharides are long strands of simple sugars.
- Complex CHOs are found in grains, fruits, seeds, potatoes, pasta, macaroni, seaweed, algae, and legumes such as peas and beans, and all other vegetables.
- The main forms of complex CHOs are starches and fibers; they come from plant materials. Starches are digested by the body whereas dietary fiber cannot be. Fiber will be discussed in Chapter 5.
- The only CHO stored in animals is "glycogen" which is found in liver and muscles.
- The amount of glycogen stored in liver and muscle is limited: muscle glycogen stores can be depleted after 3 to 4 hours of heavy exercise and a 24-hour fast could use up liver glycogen stores.

Functions of Carbohydrate in the Body

CHOs are used in the body mainly as:

◆ *Fuel in the form of glucose*—glucose is the most important source of energy in our body, and it is stored in the liver and muscle as glycogen. The complex CHOs you eat are digested into simple sugars, mostly glucose, and then used by the muscles, brain, heart, and other organs for energy.

◆ Building blocks to make chemicals needed by the cells of your body.

◆ Chemical cement for repairing structures of your body.

Carbohydrate in the Diet

CHO foodstuffs are the largest part of the world's food supply. In Mexico the CHO staples are corn tortillas and beans; in Brazil—black beans and rice; in India—chickpeas (garbanzo beans), lentils, rice, and whole grain unleavened breads; in Japan—rice, tofu, and vegetables; and in the Middle East—hummus (chickpeas) and tahini (sesame seeds). In the United States our classic CHOs are bread, potatoes, noodles, and macaroni.

Unfortunately, many people think starches are unhealthy and lead to weight gain. That notion came about because most people add high-fat toppings and/or sauces to their starchy foods. For example, many individuals put lots of butter or margarine on their bread, sour cream on their baked potato, cream cheese on bagels, and cream sauces on their macaroni or pasta! Look below to see what kinds of foods provide simple and complex CHOs.

Energy From Carbohydrate

> ### One gram of CHO supplies 4 kcal

EXAMPLE: One Fig Newton contains 10 grams of CHO and provides 60 calories. Calories from CHO and percent of calories from CHO are:

$$4 \text{ kcal} \times 10 \text{ grams} = 40 \text{ kcal from CHO}$$
$$40/60 = 0.67 = 67\% \text{ of energy from CHO}$$

Table 2-1. Ideas For Selecting Foods/Food Combinations High In Complex CHO

Below are some suggestions for foods to eat at meal and snack times. Fruits are always good—especially since they also provide water which is very important.

Breakfast Cereals	Grains	Fruits
Oatmeal	Bagel with Jam	Orange
Wheaties	Whole Wheat Bread	Banana
Cornflakes	English Muffin	Cantaloupe
Wheatena	Pancakes	Peach
Cheerios	Rice	Apple
Raisin Bran	White Potatoes	Pineapple
Grape-Nuts	Sweet Potatoes	Grapefruit
Granola	Macaroni/Noodles	Strawberry
	Tortilla	
	Waffles	
	Muffins, bran, blueberry etc.	

Vegetables	Beans/Legumes
Tomato/Tomato Sauce	Kidney Beans
Carrots and Peas	Lentil Stew
Eggplant	Chickpeas

Vegetables	Beans/Legumes
Squash	Black-eyed Peas
Broccoli	Lima Beans
Cauliflower	Pinto Beans

Sandwiches and Fillings	Other Ideas
French Roll w/ Tuna, Lettuce, Pickles	Pasta with Turkey and Veggies
Pita w/ Turkey, Lettuce, Mustard	Rice with Chicken and Veggies
Chicken, Lettuce, Mustard on Rye	Pasta with Tuna, Celery, Onions
Bagel with Peanut Butter and Jelly	Fruit Salad
Pita w/ Mashed Beans, Onions	Spaghetti and Sauce
Tortilla with Beans, Lettuce	Chicken Noodle Soup
Chicken Burrito	Potato Salad

Low-Fat/High-CHO	High-Fat/High-CHO
Any Kind of Fruit	Most Cookies
Raisins, Dates, Prunes	Most Cakes
Popcorn, Pretzels	Candy Bars
Bagel with Jam	Ice Creams

Fat

Monounsaturated Fats
(Canola and Peanut oils)

Saturated Fats
(Animal fats and tropical oils)

Polyunsaturated Fats
(Corn and Safflower oils)

Believe it or not, fat is an essential part of your diet, even though you hear everyone say "Don't eat that, it's high in fat!" Fat adds taste to foods and satisfies your sense of hunger. However, not all fats are created equal. By understanding the different types of dietary fat, how fat works in the body, and using guidelines for daily fat consumption, you can eliminate excess fat from your diet and eat for better health.

Definition, Composition, and Classification

Fat is an essential nutrient for your body, and is usually classified according to its chemical form. There are three major types of fats or fatty adds:

♦ Saturated
♦ Monounsaturated
♦ Polyunsaturated

Saturated fats ("fatty adds") which are solid at room temperature, have no room for any additional hydrogen atoms. Saturated fats are found primarily in animal foods—red meats, lard, butter, poultry with skin, and whole milk dairy products. Palm, palm kernel, and coconut oils are also highly saturated.

Mono- and polyunsaturated fats, which remain liquid at room temperature, have room for additional hydrogen atoms. Monounsaturates have room for only one hydrogen and are found in olives, olive oil, avocados, and peanuts. Polyunsaturated fats, which have room for more than one hydrogen, are found primarily in fish, corn, wheat, nuts, seeds, and vegetable oils, such as peanut, sunflower, corn, and safflower oils.

Functions of Fat in the Body

Fats, or fatty adds, serve several important roles in the body. Fat:

◆ Is our major form of stored energy; it provides energy during exercise, in cold environments, and when you don't have enough to eat
◆ Insulates the body
◆ Helps carry other nutrients to places in the body
◆ Protects organs
◆ Serves a structural role in cells

Despite its bad reputation, fat is very important, and some fats/fatty adds are essential.

How Much Fat Should We Eat?

A little of all the different types of fats is desirable, but TOO much fat is the primary dietary problem in our country. A high intake of fat is associated with many diseases, including:

◆ Heart disease   ◆ Many forms of cancer

◆ Obesity   ◆ Diabetes

The average American consumes 42% of his or her daily calories as fat (40% carbohydrate and 18% protein). **Most health experts agree that Americans should decrease their fat intake to no more than 30% of the total daily calories, and saturated fat should provide no more than 10% of the total daily calories.** In our country, more than 15% of our calories are from saturated fat. The key to this is knowing which foods are high in fat and which are low. Once you have that information, it is up to you to start changing your dietary behaviors.

Energy from Fat

> **One gram of FAT supplies 9 kcal**

Fat provides more than twice the energy supplied by carbohydrates.

Example 1:

A 1-ounce bag of potato chips contains 10 grains of fat, so the calories from fat are:

9 kcal X 10 grams = 90 kcal of energy

Example 2:

One hot dog supplies 17 grams of fat, so calories from fat would be:

9 kcal X 17 grams = 153 kcal of energy

Determining Your Daily Fat Allowance

Everyone talks about grams of fat, but what does that mean on a practical level? How does one translate "grams" of fat to percent fat and how many grams of fat should you allow yourself each day? You know that only 30% of your calories should come from fat, so with that in mind, you will learn how to determine your daily fat allowance. Let's take an example first:

Example: Determining A Fat Allowance

If estimated energy need (EEN) = 3222 calories

Step 1. Multiply EEN by 0.3 to get calories from fat
3222 X 0.3 = 967 fat calories

Step 2. Divide fat calories by 9 to get grams of fat.
967/9 = 107 grams of FAT per day

Where Did the Numbers Come From?

◆ Estimated energy need was provided in the example. You know your EEN from the previous chapter.

◆ **0.3** in Step 1 is for calculating 30% of calories from fat.

◆ **9** in Step 2 is the number of calories in one gram of fat.

◆ **107** is the number of grams of fat that should not be exceeded to ensure that the diet provides no more than 30% of calories from fat.

Worksheet 2-1. Figure Out Your Fat Allowance

Refer back to your Estimated energy needs (EEN) exercise (Chapter 1, page 6) and write your EEN in the box below.

> **Estimated Energy Need (EEN) =**
>
> **STEP 1. EEN X 0.3 =**   X 0.3
>
>   **Calories from Fat =**
>
> **STEP 2. Calories from Fat/9 =**   /9
>
>   **Grams of Fat per Day =**

Now that you know how to do this, just take whatever percent fat you want, multiply it by your energy needs, and then divide by 9.

You can also use the above method to determine the percent of fat in particular foods. If you read a food label and it shows the item provides 270 calories, of which 15 grams are fat, then to calculate the percent of calories from fat you would do the following:

Total Calories = 270
Total Fat = 15 grams
Calories from Fat = 15 grams X 9 kcal = 135 kcal
% Calories from Fat = (135 X 100)/270 = 50%

Worksheet 2-2. Calculating Percent of Calories from Fat

Food	Total Calories	Grams of Fat	Fat Calories	% of Calories
Hot Dog	183	16.6	$16.6 \times 9 = 149.4$	$149 \times 100/183 = 81.6\%$
Double Cheese Pizza, 1 slice	370	19	$19 \times 9 = 171$	$171 \times 100/370 = 46.2\%$
Barbecue Potato Chips	278	18.4	$18.4 \times 9 = 166$	$166 \times 100/278 = 59.7\%$
Tootsie Roll	112	2.5		
BLT Sandwich w/ Mayo	282	15.6		

Worksheet 2-3. Select A "Lower Fat" Alternative

Below is a list of foods that are high in fat. Look at each food item and determine a suitable replacement that you think would be much lower in fat.

FOOD	REPLACEMENT
French Fries with Ketchup	Boiled Potatoes
Chicken Drumstick w/ Skin	Chicken Breast w/o Skin
Beef Hot Dog	Chicken or Turkey Dog
Tuna Packed in Oil	Tuna Packed in Water
Whole Milk	Skim or 1% Milk
Regular Cottage Cheese	1% Fat Cottage Cheese
Regular Ice Cream	Ice Milk or Italian Ice
Ground Beef	Ground Turkey or Extra Lean Beef
Baked Potato and Sour Cream	Baked Potato with Yogurt
Bagel with Cream Cheese	
Whole Milk Yogurt	

Carbohydrate, Fat, and Protein: The Energy- Providing Macronutrients

FOOD	REPLACEMENT
Cheese Sandwich	
Turkey Sandwich with Mayonnaise	
Pizza with Double Cheese	
Salad with Blue Cheese Dressing	
Potato Chips with Dip	
Bologna and Cheese Sandwich	

Protein

Many people like to eat high-protein foods because they think protein makes them grow "big and strong." Are they correct? Let's take a look at protein and what it really does.

Definition and Composition

Unlike carbohydrates and fats which contain only carbon, oxygen, and hydrogen, protein also contains **nitrogen** and other elements essential for life. Proteins are made up of several **amino acids**—small building blocks that are hooked together. Although there are many different amino acids (at least 20), only 9 are called *essential amino acids* because the body cannot make them; they must be obtained from the diet. That's why we must eat protein—to take in the essential amino adds.

Functions of Protein in the Body

Proteins vary in size, depending on how many amino acids are linked together, and each one performs different functions in the body. Although they can provide energy, they are not a main source of energy like carbohydrates and fat. Some functions of protein are:

◆ Form muscle, hair, nails, skin, and other tissues
◆ Direct energy production
◆ Repair injuries
◆ Carry fats, vitamins, and minerals to different parts of the body
◆ Muscle contraction
◆ Serve a structural role for every part of the body

How Much Protein Should I Eat?

Many people eat 150 to 200 g of protein each day which is more protein than is actually needed by the body. Protein needs are determined by age, body weight, and activity level. Many athletes think that if they eat more protein their muscles will get larger, but this is not true. Excess calories from protein can be converted to fat and stored. Additionally, the liver and the kidneys are put under a lot of strain when processing large quantities of protein.

Table 2-2. How Much Protein Do I Need?

Grams of Protein Per Pound of Body Weight

Activity Level	Protein Factor
Low to Moderate	0.5 grams
Endurance Training	0.6 - 0.8 grams
Strength/Weight Training	0.6 - 0.8 grams

Example

Suppose you weigh 175 pounds and are training to be a SEAL. Then you are "IN TRAINING" for sure—both endurance and strength training. Your protein needs would be 0.6 to 0.8 grams per pound of body weight, as shown in the figure above.

Protein Needs = 0.8 X 175 = 140 grams

Worksheet 2-4. Calculate Your Protein Needs

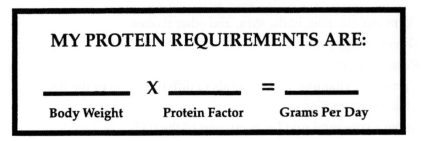

MY PROTEIN REQUIREMENTS ARE:

_____ X _____ = _____
Body Weight   Protein Factor   Grams Per Day

Energy from Protein

One gram of PROTEIN supplies 4 kcal

Protein supplies about the same energy as carbohydrates.

Example 1:

One hard boiled egg contains 6 grams of protein; calories from protein are:

4 kcal X 6 grams = 24 kcal of energy

Example 2:

One small hamburger supplies 24 grams of protein; calories from protein would be:

4 kcal X 24 grams = 96 kcal of energy

Chapter 3
Micronutrients:
Vitamins and Minerals

Micronutrients are substances required by or essential to the body in very small amounts and include both vitamins and minerals. Taking in either too little or too much of these nutrients can interfere with normal bodily functions. It is difficult to consume excessive amounts through a typical diet. However, it is possible to obtain too little of selected vitamins and minerals if proper food selections are not made.

Vitamin E

α-TOCOPHEROL

Vitamin C

ASCORBIC ACID

Pro-Vitamin A

β-CAROTENE

What Are the Recommended Dietary Allowances?

The amounts of particular vitamins and minerals a normal person should eat to prevent a deficiency are known as the Recommended Dietary Allowances (RDA). The RDA are periodically updated to reflect new information, with the most recent revision taking place in 1989. Since there are individual variations in nutrient requirements, the RDA are based on the average nutrient requirements of most people with a safety factor added. Thus, the RDA are expected to meet the nutrient requirements of most people in a healthy population.

The Military has its own set of RDA known as the Military Recommended Dietary Allowances (MRDA). The MRDA are designed to meet the nutrient needs of most 17–50-year-old moderately active, military personnel. In some cases the allowances are similar but in others the MRDA are slightly higher. This is because the last version of the MRDA was in 1980. Neither the RDA nor the MRDA considers the nutrient needs of special populations, such as SEALs who are extremely active and train and operate under diverse, often gruelling, environmental conditions. Therefore, both sets of recommendations can serve only as guidelines for your minimal intake. In most instances your micronutrient needs will be met through increased food intake provided you eat a variety of foods.

What Are Vitamins?

Vitamins are organic compounds that do not provide calories. They are broadly classified into two categories:

◆ Fat soluble vitamins
◆ Water soluble vitamins

Fat soluble vitamins, which include vitamins A, D, E, and K, are absorbed with dietary fat, can be stored in various tissues such as the liver, and are not excreted in the urine. In contrast, water soluble vitamins, which include all B vitamins and vitamin C (ascorbic acid), are not stored in the body in appreciable amounts and small amounts are excreted in the urine each day.

What Functions Do Vitamins Serve?

Vitamins perform a wide variety of functions, including the release of energy from macronutrients (carbohydrate, fat, and protein), tissue growth and repair, maintenance and support of reproductive function, and production of an immune response. Some functions

---

may be specific to only one vitamin, whereas some functions may require more than one vitamin. For example, several B vitamins and some minerals are required for releasing energy from macronutrients as shown below.

Table 3-1. Recommended Intakes and Functions of Vitamins

Vitamin	RDA for Men*	Important Functions
Vitamin A (retinol, retinoids)	1000 μg Retinol Equivalents (RE) or 5000 International Units (IU)	Antioxidant. Important for making proteins in tendons and bone. Protects the skin from sun ultraviolet damage. Protects lungs against pollutants. Needed for dark adaptation. May reduce risk of cataracts. Enhances resistance to infections. Supports immune function.
Carotenes: beta-carotene converts to vitamin A in healthy people		Water soluble, safe form of vitamin A that is not stored. Same functions as vitamin A. Stronger antioxidant than vitamin A.
Vitamin D	10 μg or 400 IU	Regulates calcium metabolism and bone mineralization.
Vitamin E	10 mg α-Tocopherol Equivalents (TE) or 10 IU	Antioxidant. Protector of cell membranes. Protective against detrimental effects of environmental toxins. Enhances immune function.
Vitamin K	1μg/kg body weight	Assists in blood clotting. Participates in calcium metabolism.
Vitamin B$_1$ (thiamin)	1.5 mg	Participates in energy production, CHO metabolism, and growth. Supports muscle and cardiovascular function.
Vitamin B$_2$ (riboflavin)	1.7 mg	Energy production from CHO, fat, and protein metabolism. Needed for growth and tissue repair.

Table 3-1. Recommended Intakes and Functions of Vitamins

Vitamin	RDA for Men*	Important Functions
Vitamin B_3 (niacin, niacinamide, nicotinic acid)	19 mg of Niacin Equivalents (NE)	Energy production from CHO, fat, and protein metabolism. Essential for aerobic metabolism.
Vitamin B_5 (pantothenic add)	4–7 mg	Essential for energy production from CHO and fat metabolism. Maintains normal growth and function of cells. Needed for proper function and production of anti-stress actions.
Vitamin B_6 (pyridoxine HCl, pyridoxal 5'-phosphate)	2 mg	Essential for protein metabolism and immune function. Supports red blood cell production. Promotes healthy skin and connective tissues. Helps prevent and treat repetitive motion injury such as carpal tunnel syndrome. Required to release glucose from CHO stored in muscle as glycogen.
Vitamin B_{12} (cobalamin)	2 µg	Required for red blood cell synthesis. Promotes growth and energy production.
Biotin	30–100 µg	Participates in fat and glycogen metabolism.
Folate (folic acid, folacin)	200 µg	Vital for red blood cell synthesis. Essential for the proper division of cells.
Vitamin C (ascorbic acid, ascorbate)	60 mg	Antioxidant. Primary role in growth and repair of connective tissues and bone. Increases resistance to infection and supports optimal immune function. Essential for proper function and production of stress hormones. Accelerates wound healing and repair. Increases resistance to environmental toxins.

* From the 1989 RDA for normal healthy men 19 to 50 years. **CHO** = carbohydrate.

Micronutrients: Vitamins and Minerals

What Foods Are Good Sources of Vitamins?

No one food is a good source of all vitamins and as such a variety of foods should be consumed. Some foods are very high in selected vitamins whereas some contain precursors or substances that serve as building blocks for making the vitamin in the body. For example, beta-carotene and other carotenoids from plant foods are converted by an enzyme in the body to vitamin A. Some processed foods provide many vitamins because they have been fortified with nutrients. Other foods will contain few, if any, vitamins. Make sure you READ FOOD LABELS to see how much of the RDA the food contains.

Food preparation techniques can affect the final amount of a particular vitamin in a food; this is specially true when cooking vegetables. Of all vitamins, vitamin C is most easily destroyed during cooking and as such raw fruits and juices are preferred sources of this vitamin. Steps you can take to increase the retention of vitamins while preparing a meal include:

- Avoid soaking vegetables in water
- Cook vegetables in just enough water to prevent burning
- Use the shortest cooking time by cooking vegetables to a crisp and tender stage
- Steaming and stir frying result in the best vitamin retention
- Use leftover cooking water in soups and sauces whenever possible to use the water soluble vitamins that were leached out
- Cut and cook vegetables shortly before serving or refrigerate in an airtight storage container.

If you are not responsible for cooking your meals or if you eat in the galley, the key is to eat a variety of foods when possible. If you are eating field rations during training or deployment, eat the entrees as well as the other food and beverage items provided in the pack. For example, cocoa in the MRE ration is a source of vitamin B_1, calcium, and magnesium. Good food sources of the vitamins are provided in Appendix 5.

What Are Minerals?

Minerals are inorganic compounds found in all body tissues and account for 4 to 5% of a person's total body weight. Typically they are classified as minerals, trace minerals, and electrolytes, depending on how much is found in the body and the functions they serve. For example, calcium and magnesium are minerals, whereas zinc, copper, and iron are trace minerals, because the body contains small amounts of them. Sodium, potassium, and chloride are the primary electrolytes.

What Functions Do Minerals Serve?

Minerals carry "charges," either positive or negative, which help determine their functions. Like vitamins, minerals are essential for a variety of important physiological functions, such as regulation of fluid balance, conduction of nerve impulses, muscle contraction as well as others. Selected functions and the Recommended Dietary Allowances for most of the essential minerals are presented in the next table.

Table 3-2. Recommended Intakes and Functions of Minerals

Mineral	RDA for Men	Important Functions
Boron	Unknown	Important in bone retention.
Calcium	1200 mg	Essential for growth and structural integrity of bones. Important to nerve conduction and muscle contraction-relaxation.
Chromium[1]	50–200 µg	Participates in CHO and fat metabolism. Works with insulin to promote proper glucose utilization. May have an anabolic effect on body composition.
Copper[1]	1.5–3 mg	Essential for oxygen-carrying hemoglobin synthesis. Involved in energy production, cardiac function, and regulation of inflammation. Essential for the antioxidant enzyme super oxide dismutase (SOD).
Iron	15 mg	Essential for the production of hemoglobin in red blood cells and myoglobin in skeletal muscle. Essential cofactor for detoxification and energy producing enzyme systems.
Magnesium	350 mg	Essential for nerve impulse conduction and muscle contraction-relaxation. Essential for CHO metabolism. Essential for proper calcium utilization and metabolism.

Mineral	RDA for Men	Important Functions
Manganese[1]	2–5 mg	Essential to formation and integrity of connective tissue. Important in normal immune and nervous system function.
Phosphorous	1200 mg	Essential for energy production. Involved in most physicochemical reactions in the body. Integral component of all cell membranes, nerve tissue, and bone. Needed for transfer of nerve impulses. Involved in calcium balance.
Potassium	2000 mg	Essential for nerve impulse conduction. Important for regulating water balance in the body. Important in regulating acid-base balance. Essential for normal heart beat and rhythm.
Selenium	70 µg	Antioxidant. Works with vitamin E to reduce oxidation damage to tissues. Supports proper cardiovascular and immune function.
Sodium[2]	500–2,400 mg	Essential for nerve impulse conduction and muscle contraction. Essential for fluid balance and acid-base balance.
Zinc	15 mg	Participates in formation of proteins. Involved in skeletal muscle metabolism. Important for proper neurologic functions. Supports immune function and increases resistance to infections. Enhances wound healing.

[1]Estimated safe and adequate daily intake range—meets requirements of individuals and avoids the danger of toxicity (Food and Nutrition Board, 1989).

[2]The minimum daily requirement for sodium is 500 mg or 1250 mg of salt. Salt is 40% sodium and 60% chloride. 1 teaspoon of salt (sodium chloride) = 5 g provides 5 X 40/100 = 2 g of sodium; 2 g is the same as 2000 mg. The minimum daily requirement for potassium is 2000 mg.

What Foods Are Good Sources of Minerals?

As with vitamins, a variety of foods should be eaten in order to meet your mineral requirements. The amount of a particular mineral that will be absorbed from foods varies widely and depends upon a number of factors. Absorption of minerals can be influenced by:

◆ Other dietary constituents, such as dietary fiber, oxalates and phytates

◆ The amount of other minerals in the diet

- ◆ Medications
- ◆ The body's need for the mineral
- ◆ Chemical form of the mineral
- ◆ Integrity of the intestinal tract

Even though foods may contain certain minerals, other food constituents can influence the actual amount absorbed. For example, insoluble materials like dietary fiber, phytates (chemicals found in high-fiber foods), and oxalates (chemicals found in certain foods such as spinach, chard, and rhubarb) bind minerals including iron, calcium, and zinc to make them less available for absorption. In contrast, the presence of vitamin C improves the absorption of calcium, iron, and zinc. The absorption of iron is dependent on its particular form: heme or non-heme. Heme iron is found in animal foods and is better absorbed than non-heme iron from plant foods. Finally, excessive intakes of some minerals can interfere with the absorption of others: high intakes of supplemental zinc can decrease copper absorption and high iron intakes can decrease zinc absorption. Good food sources of minerals are listed in Appendix 6.

What Substances May Interfere with Microrutrients?

Many things you take or do can affect your losses of vitamins and minerals. In particular, substances that act as "ANTI" vitamins/minerals and may interfere with the amounts of vitamins and minerals in your body include:

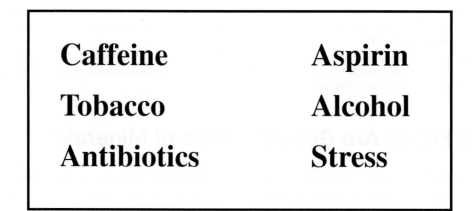

Caffeine	Aspirin
Tobacco	Alcohol
Antibiotics	Stress

Summary

The key to meeting your vitamin and mineral needs is eating a diet containing a variety of foods. Remember, food preparation can affect micronutrient content, and that simple changes, such as drinking water or juice instead of tea or coffee with meals can increase absorption of many minerals. If you do not eat a lot of fresh fruits and vegetables, then try to eat fortified, ready-to-eat breakfast cereals in the morning and for snacks. If you are in doubt about the nutrient content of a processed food, just look at food labels. Most unprocessed foods are nutritious. The following practices will help ensure that you meet your daily vitamin and mineral needs:

Eat A Variety of Foods

Be Savvy in Your Food Selections

Use Good Food Preparation Techniques

Chapter 4
Vitamin and Mineral Supplements

Vitamin and mineral supplements are being widely used by physically active people because of all the performance enhancing claims made by supplement manufacturers. It is estimated that about 40–50% of athletes use some form of vitamin/mineral supplements. These include single vitamins (such as vitamin C) or minerals (such as iron) and multivitamin-mineral combinations in doses that range from amounts that are similar to the Recommended Dietary Allowances (RDA) up to levels many times the RDA (see Chapter 3 for information on the RDAs).

Role of Vitamins and Minerals in Physical Activity

Vitamins and minerals are required in micro (very small, minute) amounts by the body to perform vital metabolic and physiologic functions. Some of the functions related to physical activity that vitamins and minerals are involved in include:

◆ Production of energy: many vitamins and minerals are involved in producing energy from carbohydrates (CHO), fats, and proteins.

◆ Formation of red blood cells: some vitamins and minerals are also required for the formation of red blood cells. Red blood cells contain hemoglobin, an iron-containing protein that carries oxygen.

◆ Providing oxygen to the exercising muscles: hemoglobin and myoglobin are iron-containing proteins which transport and deliver oxygen to exercising muscles.

◆ Maintenance of healthy muscles and joints.

◆ Recovery from exercise: some vitamins and minerals may help in recovering from exhaustive exercise.

Because of all the functions served by vitamins and minerals (see Chapter 3 for additional information), the supplement industry has embarked on a promotional campaign to encourage the use of supplements by physically active people. Whether all the hype about supplement use and performance is justified is discussed below.

Benefits of Supplementation

Supplements are useful under a variety of conditions. Some conditions where benefits of supplementation have been found are when:

◆ There is an existing vitamin or mineral deficiency

◆ Individuals have poor nutrient intakes and dietary habits

◆ Individuals are exposed to extreme environmental conditions, such as altitude

Supplement Use and Performance

Vitamin Supplements

Taking a general multivitamin supplement appears to be without measurable performance enhancing effects in healthy, well-nourished, physically active men on measures of maximal aerobic capacity, heart rate, submaximal endurance running performance, and muscle glycogen stores. Similarly, no improvements in muscle strength or endurance have been noted in strength athletes, such as body builders, who tend to use megadoses of vitamin and mineral supplements.

We don't know yet whether supplementation with various nutrients will have other more subtle beneficial effects that may allow you to perform at an optimal level for extended periods of time. For example, supplementation with selected vitamins or minerals may accelerate recovery and/or reduce susceptibility to infections. Some information to confirm these possibilities is available, but confirmatory studies have not been conducted in military populations. As such, if you elect to take supplements, you should monitor your overall health and performance to determine whether the expense is justified. Also, be sure not to take more than 2 to 3 times the RDA; preferably take a supplement that provides nutrients in amounts that meet the RDA (see Chapter 3 for the RDAs).

Vitamin C

> **Supplementation with 600 mg/day of Vitamin C may decrease the incidence of upper respiratory infections during extended missions and/or prolonged activities.**

When selected individuals participate in prolonged competitive athletic events, supplementation with vitamin C has been shown to be beneficial for reducing the incidence

---

and or severity of upper respiratory infections. This may help in BUD/SEAL training, especially during the first phase and Hell Week, when upper respiratory tract infections and cellulitis are frequently noted. Infections, such as an outbreak of pneumococcal pneumonia, have also been noted during Ranger training.

Vitamin E

> **Supplementation with 400 IU/day of Vitamin E may protect cell membranes from damage by free radicals produced during strenuous exercise.**

For conditions of altitude exposure, one recent study indicated that mountaineers who took vitamin E supplements minimized altitude-induced performance decrements by being able to maintain adequate blood flow and protect their cell membranes from "oxidative" damage.

Mineral Supplements

As with the vitamins, there is no clear-cut evidence to indicate that mineral supplements will enhance physical performance in normal, healthy individuals. However, some minerals may be useful and others may be harmful.

Chromium

Chromium is becoming increasingly popular among athletes because of purported muscle-building or anabolic effects. The results from studies to date are not consistent, and more work is required before definitive recommendations can be made. Meanwhile, if you take chromium supplements, limit the amount to the current recommendations (200 µg/day); do not take more than 1000 µg/day.

Zinc

Supplementation with zinc has also been studied. Taking a zinc:copper supplement (25 mg to 2 mg) twice a day also seems to minimize the production of free radicals generated during prolonged exercise. However, if zinc supplements are taken, they should provide no more than 100 mg per day, and copper should be taken to prevent a copper deficiency.

Iron

Iron is commonly used by physically active people looking for the performance edge. However, iron supplements do not improve performance in non-deficient individuals. If your diet provides any meat, fish or poultry, it is unlikely you need iron supplements. Moreover, excessive iron intakes can be detrimental (see risks) and **the use of prenatal supplements to boost iron stores is not recommended.**

Vitamin and Mineral Supplements

Antioxidants

As SEALS, you are continually exposed to hazardous environments, extensive sunlight, and other situations which result in a process called "oxidation." Oxidation results in the formation of "Free Radicals" or "Superoxide Anions." Because you are exposed more than the average person, taking an antioxidant supplement may be protective (see Chapter 3 for food sources of antioxidants). If you chew tobacco, this may be particularly important to your future health.

Types of Antioxidants

Vitamin E	**Vitamin C**
Beta-carotene	**Selenium**
Cysteine	**Glutathione**
Flavonoids	

♦ Several multivitamin and mineral supplements contain antioxidants—CHECK labels for amounts.

♦ Antioxidant vitamins and minerals are also available as single nutrient supplements, e.g., vitamin E is sold separately. So even if you do not take multivitamins and minerals, you may choose to use an antioxidant.

Risks of Supplementation

The indiscriminate use of high potency vitamins and minerals is of concern since excessive amounts of vitamins and/or minerals can be harmful and may result in nutrient imbalances. Excessive intake of some vitamin and mineral supplements can result in multiple side effects. Harmful side effects of nutrients which are frequently taken in excess are provided on the next page.

Vitamin A

Daily intake of large amounts of vitamin A over several months is extremely toxic. Symptoms of overdosing with retinol indude nausea, vomiting, abdominal pain, weight loss, hair loss, cerebral edema (swelling of the brain), and liver failure.

Vitamin B₆

Chronic megadoses of vitamin B_6 have resulted in neurological problems, including loss of muscle coordination and loss of sensation in hands and feet; some individuals may develop these neurological problems with even lower doses of vitamin B_6 (~100 mg/day).

Iron

Chronic use of iron supplements can be a problem, especially in individuals genetically predisposed to iron overload (hemochromatosis); damage to multiple organs including the liver has been observed. Thus, supplemental iron is not indicated unless an iron deficiency anemia has been diagnosed.

Zinc

High intakes of zinc interfere with copper absorption. Daily zinc intakes of >150 mg/day may increase the risk for cardiovascular disease by decreasing serum high density lipoprotein levels and increasing low density lipoprotein levels.

Although some people take excessive amounts of nutrients on a regular basis, it is important to distinguish between excessive and toxic. Intakes of nutrients at their potentially toxic levels can result in significant adverse effects quite readily. Table 4-1 list the toxic values of many nutrients, and these amounts should never be taken. Preferably, intakes will be well below these numbers, even over a one-week period.

Table 4-1. Nutrients and Their Toxicity Values

Nutrient	Toxicity (units/day)	Nutrient	Toxicity (units/day)
Vitamin A	> 25,000 IU	Magnesium	> 6,000 mg
Carotene	None	Boron	>100 mg
Vitamin D	>50,000 IU	Chromium	>10 mg
Vitamin E	>1,200 IU	Copper	>35 mg
Vitamin B₆	>2,000 mg	Iron	>100 mg
Vitamin C	Rare	Selenium	>1 mg
Calcium	>2,500 mg	Zinc	>150 mg

What to Look for When Buying Supplements

The better informed you are about marketing practices of vitamin and mineral supplements the more likely you will be to save money and still use a good supplement. For example, did you know that most supplement manufacturers get their initial supply of vitamins and minerals from the same small group of suppliers? After that they formulate their various combinations, label them, and sell them. Listed below are some factors you should consider when buying supplements.

Natural Versus Synthetic Vitamins

Both forms are used the same way by the body so why pay more for a "natural" product? Also manufacturers often add a few plant extracts or a bit of the natural vitamin and sell the product at a higher price by labeling it as natural.

Presence of Starch, Sugar, and Other Additives

Many supplements contain starch, binders, and other additives. These additives are present in very small amounts and in very rare instances they may cause headaches and other reactions in some people.

Disintegration Rate

If a supplement does not dissolve in the gut, it won't be absorbed and it won't do you any good. One way for you to insure you are taking the right kind of supplement is to look for supplements that meet the U.S. Pharmacopoeia (USP) standards which say that water-soluble vitamin supplements should disintegrate in 30 minutes if uncoated and 45 minutes if coated. This standard does not apply to time-release or chewable supplements. Standards for fat-soluble vitamins, minerals, and multivitamin are currently being prepared but several companies are already marketing multivitamin-mineral supplements that dissolve within 45 minutes. Look at supplement labels or call the manufacturer for information.

When to Take?

Fat-soluble vitamins are better absorbed when taken with food, so if you take a multivitamin/mineral supplement, it is best to take it with a meal.

Tea or coffee will reduce the absorption of several nutrients in supplements.

In general, the body can only absorb and use a certain amount of nutrients at one time and the rest will be excreted. Do not take a vitamin/mineral supplement with a carbohydrate-protein drink that is already supplemented with vitamins and minerals as you would literally be wasting the supplement and your money.

Amount of Nutrient

Be especially careful about the amount of fat-soluble vitamins in the supplement.

Daily supplements should not contain more than 10,000 IU (RDA is 5,000 IU) of Vitamin A as retinol palmitate or acetate.

This form of vitamin A in excess is very toxic. If you use several supplements that each contain retinol palmitate or acetate, you will very quickly exceed safe levels. Also, excessive amounts of the water-soluble vitamin, vitamin B_6, can be harmful. Read labels and watch your supplement intakes.

In general, you can safely take 2–3 times the RDA of most vitamins and minerals without harming yourself.

Nutrient Balance

Besides the potential for toxicity, excessive amounts of single nutrient supplements can upset your overall nutrient balance and cause a deficiency in other nutrients. Iron, zinc and copper are good examples since all three are absorbed by the same pathway. An excessive intake of one of these minerals can prevent the proper absorption of the others. This could eventually cause a deficiency and defeat the nutritional enhancement being sought through supplementation.

Expiration Date

The expiration date on labels refers to the length of time a particular supplement is expected to hold its vitamin and mineral potency. Check the expiration date on the label and avoid buying supplements that are due to expire within 6 months since the potency of vitamins may be on the decline.

Summary

◆ Vitamin and/or mineral deficiencies can impair performance. Restoration to a sufficient level reverses performance decrements. However, deficiency states are rare in otherwise healthy males.

◆ Vitamin and mineral supplementation does not improve aerobic capacity, endurance performance, or muscle strength in healthy, nutritionally adequate individuals.

◆ Megadoses of vitamins and/or minerals can be harmful.

◆ CHECK LABELS to make sure you are not taking too much of any single nutrient.

◆ Under most circumstances you should be able to obtain adequate amounts of vitamins and minerals from your daily diet.

Chapter 5
Fiber and Health

Dietary fiber is a food constituent you should be familiar with as it is important for health. Many of the nutritional approaches discussed in this manual will, in fact, promote good health. Although health is important when performance is your end result, you should be aware that dietary fiber should assume a definite BACK SEAT role during mission and training operations/scenarios. In this chapter we will discuss the role of fiber in overall health and during special operations.

What Is Dietary Fiber?

Dietary fiber is a form of carbohydrate we get from fruits, vegetables, grain products, beans, nuts, and other plant foods. A more meaningful definition of dietary fiber would be: the structural components of plant foods that cannot be digested by the human body. Because fiber is neither digested or absorbed, it really can't be considered a nutrient, like vitamins, minerals, proteins, fats, and other carbohydrates, but it is still an essential part of your diet.

Typically, dietary fibers are classified as soluble or insoluble, but most fiber-rich foods contain some of both types. These two types of fibers function differently in the body. Insoluble fibers are known for their ability to absorb water in the gastrointestinal tract and promote regular elimination of stools. An increase in stool weight and a faster transit time are common when diets high in insoluble fiber are ingested. Transit time is the time it takes for your meal to be digested and be excreted in your stools. Insoluble fibers are the predominant fiber in most foods. In contrast, soluble fibers appear to help lower serum cholesterol, a risk factor for heart disease and they also help regulate blood sugar levels. These special effects of dietary fiber have prompted many health promotion agencies to make specific recommendations regarding how much dietary fiber our diet should provide. In a nutshell, fiber serves a very important role in health.

Why Should I Eat More Fiber?

The National Cancer Institute, the American Heart Association, the National Academy of Sciences, and the United States Department of Agriculture have all come out with dietary recommendation for fiber. There are many reasons to increase your daily intake of fiber, and they are all related to risk factors for chronic disease. A lack of fiber in the diet has been associated with gastrointestinal diseases, hypertension, diabetes, heart disease, and several types of cancer, including colon cancer, whereas a high fiber intake is associated with a decreased risk. For these reasons, increasing your intake of dietary fiber may be very important with respect to your future health.

Recommendations for intake of dietary fiber include:

◆ Consume at least 3-5 servings of various vegetables, 2 or more servings of fruit, and 6 or more servings of grain products, or
◆ Increase dietary fiber intake to 20 to 35 grams per day

The first recommendation is the easiest to follow since it is extremely difficult to know how much fiber is in each food. Moreover, what the above-mentioned organizations use as a typical serving is probably only a quarter of what your portions are. For example, one serving of fruit would be one apple, one banana, one orange or one pear. One serving of grain products would be one slice of whole wheat bread or one bagel. Furthermore, one serving of vegetables would be 1/2 cup of peas, one small potato, or 1/2 cup of carrots. It is likely that you are eating more than one serving at each meal.

How Can I Get More Fiber in My Diet?

Eating more fruits and vegetables, whole wheat breads, whole grain cereals, beans, rice, nuts, and seeds is the best way to add fiber to your diet. Foods that provide the most soluble fiber include kidney beans, avocados, green beans, baked potatoes with their skin, sweet potatoes, oatmeal, oranges, bananas, and watermelon. A list of some foods and their total dietary fiber in grams (g) is provided below.

Table 5-1. Serving Sizes and Dietary Fiber Content (in grams) of Selected Foods

Fruits			Vegetables		
Apple	1 medium	2.0	Asparagus, cooked	4 spears	1.5
Banana	1 medium	1.5	Green Beans, cooked	1 cup	2.4
Cantaloupe	1/2 medium	1.9	Broccoli, cooked	1 cup	5.4
Grapefruit	1/2 medium	0.6	Brussels Sprouts, cooked	1 cup	6.4
Grapes	20 each	1.0	Carrots, raw	1 medium	1.8
Orange	1 medium	2.5	Corn, cooked	1 ear	1.6
Pear, Bartlett	1 medium	4.6	Green Pepper, raw	1 whole	1.3
Plum	1 each	0.8	Potato, baked with skin	1 medium	5.1
Raisins	1/2 cup	2.6	Potato, french fries	20 fries	4.6
Watermelon	1 cup	0.6	Sweet Potato, baked with skin	1 medium	3.4

Table 5-1. Serving Sizes and Dietary Fiber Content (in grams) of Selected Foods

Breads, Cereals, and Grain Products			Legumes, Nuts, Seeds, and Miscellaneous		
Bread, French	2 slices	1.9	Almonds	2 tbsp	2.5
Bread, Whole Wheat	2 slices	1.3	Avocado	1/2 medium	4.7
English Muffin	1 whole	0.9	Black-eyed peas, cooked	1 cup	7.1
Saltine Cracker	10 squares	1.7	Green Peas, cooked	1 cup	6.0
Taco Shell	2 each	4.4	Kidney Beans, cooked	1 cup	5.8
Corn Flakes	1 cup	1.0	Lima Beans, cooked	1 cup	7.1
All Bran	1 cup	9.1	Peanut Butter	2 tbsp	2.0
Shredded Wheat	1 cup	5.5	Walnuts	2 tbsp	1.1
Rice, cooked	1 cup	0.7			
Spaghetti, cooked	1 cup	1.9			

When Should I Minimize My Fiber Intake?

Dietary fiber is very important to your health: it promotes regularity by increasing stool bulk and weight. However, during extended operations, you will most likely want to avoid "regular eliminations" for as long as possible. A low-fiber diet may be preferred for these occasions. Also, many high-fiber foods can cause bloating and gas if you are not accustomed to eating them or if you don't drink enough water. Make sure to try such foods during training so you can find out how your system reacts. That way you can make dietary modifications where necessary before the actual event.

For Special Operations You May Want to Minimize Your Intake of Dietary Fiber

Chapter 6
Fluid Replacement: Water and Other Beverages

Water is an essential nutrient and the most abundant component of the human body. Believe it or not, approximately 60% of your total body weight is water. Since lean body/muscle mass requires more water than fat, the leaner you are, the more body water you have. As you may imagine, water must be consumed regularly to ensure normal functioning of your body.

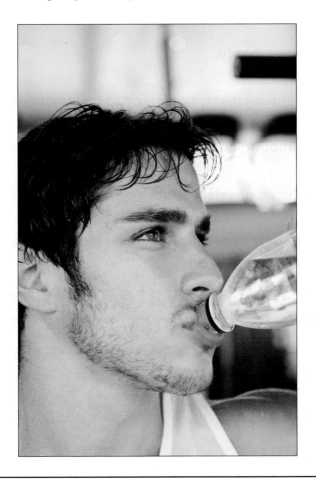

Distribution and Functions of Water

Water is found both inside and outside cells, but most water is inside cells, especially muscle cells. The lowest concentration of water is in bone and fat. Water in the body serves many important roles, including:

◆ Participates in digestion and absorption of nutrients
◆ Participates in excretion of wastes
◆ Essential for maintaining blood circulation throughout the body
◆ Maintains body temperature

A loss of 20% of body water can result in death, and if 4% of your body weight is lost because of sweating, large decrements in decision-making, concentration, and physical work occur. In addition, being well hydrated during operations is absolutely critical, since adequate fluid volume will help compensate for blood loss when wounded. For these reasons, consumption of water is absolutely critical, and maintenance of water balance is essential to SEAL performance. Below are signs and symptoms you might experience as you become dehydrated.

% of Body Weight Loss	
0	Feeling Great
1	Feeling thirsty
2	Increasing thirst; beginning to feel uncomfortable
3	Dry mouth; urine output reduced; blood volume declining
4	Reduced physical performance; feeling sick
5	Hard time concentrating; sleepiness; headache

How to Maintain Water Balance

Water balance is determined by water/fluid output and input. In order to maintain performance, it is critical that a fluid deficit, or dehydration, does not occur. With dehydration, water output exceeds input and balance becomes negative. The average man loses 1,000 ml to 2,300 ml (0.9 to 2.4 quarts) of water/day. This water is lost:

- In the urine
- Through breathing
- By sweating
- Through the stools

When activity level is low, most fluids are lost through the urine. However, when activity level or the outdoor temperature is high, most fluid is lost by sweating. In fact, up to 2,000 ml (1.8 quarts) per hour can be lost through sweating, depending on outside temperatures.

All fluids lost must be added back to the body each day to maintain fluid balance. Sources of fluid for the body are:

- Water in food
- Water in beverages (like orange juice, coffee, sodas, and beer)
- Water from the metabolism or chemical breakdown of foods

The easiest way to restore fluid balance is by drinking water, and this is VERY important to remember. The figure on the next page graphically depicts water output and input for normal temperature conditions, hot weather, and with prolonged exercise. Notice how sweat output increases dramatically with both hot weather and prolonged exercise—these amounts would be even greater if exercise were performed in the heat. The only way to match this great output is to drink fluids.

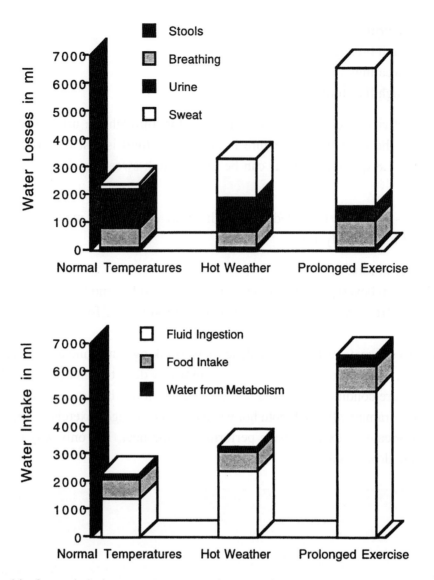

In this figure it is important to note that exercise and heat exposure increase sweat losses and reduce urine losses. In addition, the only good way to replace those "lost fluids" is by drinking fluids: fluid intake MUST go up to accommodate losses.

Although eating fods high in water will help restore or maintain water balance, drinking fluids is preferred. Some foods that are over 90% water include watermelon, strawberries, grapefruit, cucumbers, and many other fresh fruits and vegetables. If you eat many of those foods and drink lots of beverages, it is less likely you would be in negative water balance.

What Conditions Will Increase Water Losses?

The primary factors which could cause dehydration are:

◆   Exercising for over 30 minutes

- Working in a hot environment—wet or dry
- Working in a cold environment—wet or dry
- Going to high altitudes
- Drinking too much alcohol
- Exercising in the heat, cold, or at altitude
- Exercising with a hangover

How Can You Make Sure to Get Enough Fluids?

Several points about fluid intake should be considered:

- Do not rely on thirst as a good indicator of fluid needs; body weight losses are better
- Before any exercise or simulated mission, you should drink fluids in anticipation of losing fluid
- Before you start, make sure your urine is clear (unless you take B vitamin supplements)—this is a sign that you are well hydrated. The more dehydrated you are, the darker (and smellier) your urine will be
- Drink regularly or whenever possible during your workouts and operations
- Weigh yourself before and after an event to determine how much fluid you have lost—for every pound of weight lost, you should drink 16 ounces of fluid (2 cups or 500 ml)

What You Should Drink

Many beverages—both regular and sports drinks—are commercially available. These include:

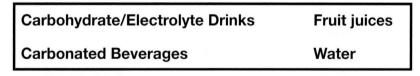

Carbohydrate/Electrolyte Drinks	Fruit juices
Carbonated Beverages	Water

Although the type of activity you participate in will determine what you drink, the beverage you select should:

- Taste good
- Cause no gastrointestinal/stomach discomfort
- Be rapidly absorbed
- Contain sodium and potassium especially when exercising for a prolonged period in the heat
- Have an osmolality of less than 350 mOsm/L

Osmolality refers to the number of particles in solution. If it is high (> 350), the beverage can cause stomach distress and not be absorbed well if you drink it shortly before or during physical activity. Note in the chart below that the osmolality of some beverages is greater than 350. Thus, if you choose to drink those beverages as sports drinks, you should dilute them appropriately or drink an equal amount of water. For example, orange juice should be mixed with an equal amount of water.

Table 6-1. Comparison of Fluid Replacement Beverages

Beverage*	CHO Source[1] & Concentration	Sodium (mg)	Potassium (mg)	Other Nutrients	Osmolality (mOsm/L)
Gatorade®	6% Sucrose/ Glucose	110	25	Chloride, Phosphorus	280–360
Exceed®	7.2% Glucose Polymers/ Fructose	50	45	Chloride, Calcium, Magnesium, Phosphorus	250
Body Fuel®	4.2% Maltodextrin/ Fructose	80	20	Phosphorus, Chloride, Iron, Vitamins A, B, & C	210
10-K®	6.3% Sucrose/ Glucose/ Fructose	52	26	Phosphorus, Vitamin C, Chloride	350
Quickick®	4.7% Fructose/ Sucrose	116	23	Calcium, Chloride, Phosphorus	305
Coca Cola	11% High Fructose Corn Syrup/Sucrose	9.2	trace	Phosphorus	600–715
Sprite	10.2% High Fructose Corn Syrup/Sucrose	28	trace	—	695
Cranberry Juice Cocktail	15% High Fructose Corn Syrup/Sucrose	10	61	Vitamin C, Phosphorus	890
Orange Juice	11.8% Fructose/ Sucrose/ Glucose	2.7	510	Calcium, Niacin, Iron, Vitamins A & C, Thiamin, Phosphorus, Riboflavin	690
Water		low	low	low	10–20

* Serving Size = 8 fluid ounces.
[1] Sucrose = fructose and glucose; Maltodextrin = a mixture of short chains (2–3 molecules linked) of glucose; high fructose com syrup = a 54:46% mixture of fructose and glucose derived from processed and converted com starch; glucose polymers = long chains (> 3 molecules linked) of glucose.

If the exercise is of long duration, it may be advisable to ingest a beverage that provides energy in the form of carbohydrate (CHO) to the working muscles. Beverages with "glucose polymers," which are complex CHOs are usually preferred over the glucose and sucrose drinks, which are simple CHOs. However, the important message is to drink. Below is a list of beverages, some of which are currently used as "fluid replacement beverages" by athletes and others that are popular with many individuals.

Table 6-2. Fluid Intake Recommendations for Before, During, and After an Event or Mission

	TYPE OF FLUID	FREQUENCY	VOLUME
High intensity activities shorter than 1 hour (soccer game, PT test, 10k run)			
BEFORE[1]	5–8% Beverage with CHO[2]	1–2 hours before	8–16 oz. (1–2 cups)
DURING	Water	As needed	16–32 oz. (2–4 cups)
AFTER	5–8% Beverage with CHO[1]	0–2 hours after	16–32 oz. - Check your weight since you may need more
Moderate to high intensity activities lasting 1 to 3 hours (long run, swim, or march)			
BEFORE[1]	Water	0–2 hours before	8–16 oz. per hour
DURING	5–8% Beverage with CHO and electrolytes	Every 20–30 minutes	12–24 oz. per 30 minutes
AFTER	5–8% Beverage with CHO and electrolytes	0–2 hours after	8–16 oz. per 30 minutes - Check your weight since you may need more
Low to moderate intensity activities lasting over 3 hours (land warfare scenario)			
BEFORE[1]	Water	0–2 hours before	8–16 oz. per hour
DURING	5–8% Beverage with CHO and electrolytes	Every 20–30 minutes	8–16 oz. per 30 minutes
AFTER	5–8% Beverage with CHO and electrolytes	0–6 hours after	8–16 oz. every 30 minutes - Check your weight since you may need more

Table 6-2. Fluid Intake Recommendations for Before, During, and After an Event or Mission

	TYPE OF FLUID	FREQUENCY	VOLUME
Low to moderate intensity activities in the water for less than 3 hours (short dives)			
BEFORE[1]	Water	0–1 hour before	12–16 oz.
DURING - If possible	Water or a 5–8% Beverage with CHO	Every hour	8–16 oz. per hour
AFTER	5–8% Beverage with CHO	0–2 hours after	16–32 oz. per hour - Check your weight since you may need more
Low intensity activities in the water for more than 3 hours (long dives or SDV operation)			
BEFORE[1]	Water	0–1 hour before	12–16 oz.
DURING - If possible	5–8% Beverage with CHO	Every hour	16 oz. per hour
AFTER	5–8% Beverage with CHO	0–6 hours after	16–32 oz. per hour - Check your weight since you may need more

[1] In all cases, you should have had sufficient fluid to produce a clear, pale urine (unless you are taking vitamin B supplements), and you should weigh yourself before and after to monitor fluid losses.
[2] CHO stands for carbohydrate, as found in the beverages already described.

When and How Much to Drink?

Remember: the following recommendations are generally sound for most people. However, everyone is different so you must learn to look for signs alerting you to your fluid needs. Also, you need to make adjustments depending on the temperature outside. If it is very hot, you may need to double the recommendations. Remember, the more active you are the more fluid you need. Be careful not to drink TOO much plain water, especially during prolonged exercise in the heat.

Table 6-3. Typical Fluid Losses for Various Events

Event	Duration of Event (hrs)	Typical Fluid Losses (qts)
Typical Day at BUDs	12	10
Working in the Heat	8	6.3
Diving in Cold Water	6	1.4
Working in MOPP Gear	4	6.4
SDV Operation	3–7	2.1
5.5-Mile Swim Wearing Full-Body Wet Suit	4	3.2
2-Day Hike In Cold Weather	3	2.6
Triathalon	4	3.2
Marathon	3.5	3.7

Table 6-4. Determining Amounts of Fluid and CHO to Drink During Exercise

The approximate number of 8-ounce cups of fluid required to provide varying amounts of carbohydrate (CHO) each hour for a given concentration of CHO in the beverage is presented below. Beverage concentrations are on the left (3% to 12%) and the amount of CHO delivered per hour is across the top (20 to 60 gm). For example, if you want to consume 40 grams of CHO each hour and the weather is hot, you may wish to make up a 5% rather than an 8% solution so you are drinking 3.5 cups instead of 2 cups of fluid. This is important because you need more fluid in the heat.

Concentration of Beverage	Carbohydrate Delivered by Beverage of Given Concentration				
	20 gm/hr	30 gm/hr	40 gm/hr	50 gm/hr	60 gm/hr
	Approximate Volumes (cups) of Beverage Required to Deliver CHO/hr[1]				
3%	3	4	6	7	8.5
5%	2	2.5	3.5	4	5
7%	1	2	2.5	3	3.5
8%	1	1.5	2	2.5	3
10%	1	1.25	2	2	2.5
12%	1	1	1.5	2	2

[1] The shaded section represents the volumes of beverage that are adequate for fluid replacement (2 to 5 cups/hr). The unshaded sections are volumes that are either too low (< 2 cups/hr) or too high (>5 cups/hr) to confer any

Chapter 7
Healthy Snacking

Snacking, "eating between regular meals," can be extremely important when it comes to performing your duties and assignments. Your energy expenditure can be extremely high on given days and during various operations, and it is often difficult to eat enough at meals. Snacking becomes very important during this time. In addition, you probably snack at various times during the day and evening anyway, so it becomes important to look at what constitutes healthy snacks. Most people think snacking is unhealthy and leads to weight gain, but that notion has emerged because most people don't eat healthy snacks! If you don't care about gaining weight, just about any snack will do, but if you want to maintain weight and perform well, then selection of snacks is critical.

Tips for Healthy Snacking

Think through a typical day. How often and where do you usually snack? Are your snacks healthy or loaded with fat? In case you aren't sure, here are some tips to help promote health snacking!

Stock your cupboards and refrigerator with plain popcorn, whole grain crackers, Dutch pretzels, unsweetened fruit juices, fresh fruits and vegetables, and low-fat yogurt and cheeses.

Carry naturally sweet fresh fruits, such as grapes, a pear, apple, or watermelon, for a snack rather than candy or cookies.

Limit the amount eaten so your snack does NOT replace a meal. If it is taking the place of a meal, choose a salad or healthy sandwich.

Choose a snack that provides dietary fiber as well as other nutrients (unless the snack is for a mission). Fresh fruits with edible seeds (berries) or skins (apples, peaches, plums, pears), raw vegetables, and whole grain pretzels or crackers are all good sources of fiber.

Try eating dried apricots, bananas, apples, figs, dates, pineapples, and prunes.

Make a snack mix with wheat, rice, and corn ready-to-eat cereals.

Eat raw vegetables such as celery with low-fat cheese spreads.

Table 7-1. Macronutrient Composition of Selected Snacks

FOOD	Serving Size	Approximate amount per Serving				
		Energy (kcal)	CHO (grams)	Protein (grams)	Fat (grams)	Fiber (grams)
Breads, Cereals, and Other Grain Products						
Angel Food Cake	1 piece	129	29.3	3.0	0.1	ND[1]
Bagel	1 each	200	38.0	7.5	1.1	1.5
Commits®	2 oz.	249	41.6	4.8	8.0	6.9
Crackers, whole wheat	82" squares	70	10.0	1.6	4.0	1
Crackers, Saltines	4 squares	50	8.0	1.0	1.0	0.3
Crackers, Round Snack	4 each	60	7.0	1.0	4.0	0.2
English Muffin with Raisins	1 whole	137	27.5	4.3	1.5	0.9
Fig Newtons	2 cookies	112	23.0	1.2	2.4	1.5
Graham Crackers	2 squares	60	11.0	1.0	1.4	0.4
Granola Bars, plain	1 bar	115	15.8	2.5	4.9	ND
Muffin, Blueberry	2.5" dia	158	27.0	3.2	4.0	2.1
Muffin, Bran	2.5" dia	154	27.5	4.0	6.0	4.3
Popcorn, plain air popped	1 cup	30	6.2	1.0	trace	1.2
Popcorn, buttered	1 cup	55	6.3	1.0	3.1	1.1
Pretzels Dutch, hard, plain	2 each	130	26.0	4.0	1.0	ND
Pretzel Sticks, thin, salted	10 each	210	48.0	6.0	2.0	ND

Table 7-1. Macronutrient Composition of Selected Snacks

FOOD	Serving Size	Approximate amount per Serving				
		Energy (kcal)	CHO (grams)	Protein (grams)	Fat (grams)	Fiber (grams)
Sports Bars						
Pure Power	2.3 oz.	240	42.0	12.0	3.0	2.0
Pro-Sports	2.3 oz.	140	40.0	15.0	2.0	ND
Tiger Sport	2.3 oz.	230	40.0	11.0	3.0	ND
Twin Labs Amino Fuel	2.7 oz.	285	50.0	15.0	3.0	ND
Clif by Avocet	2.4 oz.	250	53.0	6.0	3.0	8.0
Cross Trainer	2.25 oz.	236	46.0	11.0	2.0	ND
Exceed Bar	2.9 oz.	280	53.0	12.0	2.0	3.0
Meal on the GO	3 oz.	290	51.0	7.0	9.0	ND
Power Bar	2.25 oz.	225	40.0	10.0	2.0	2.0
Vegetables						
Carrot Sticks	1 large	30	7.0	1.0	0.0	1.8
Cauliflower	1 cup	25	5.0	2.0	0.0	2.3
Cucumbers	6 slices	5	1.0	trace	0.0	0.2
Potatoes, French Fries	10 fries	110	17.0	2.0	4.0	1.2
Tomato Juice	1 cup	40	10.0	2.0	0.0	ND

Table 7-1. Macronutrient Composition of Selected Snacks

FOOD	Serving Size	Approximate amount per Serving				
		Energy (kcal)	CHO (grams)	Protein (grams)	Fat (grams)	Fiber (grams)
Fruits						
Apple	1 medium	80	21.0	trace	trace	2.8
Apricot, Dried	7 halves	80	20.0	1.0	0.0	ND
Banana	1 medium	105	22.0	0.0	1.0	22.0
Cantaloupe	1 half	95	22.0	2.0	0.5	1.8
Orange	1 medium	60	15.0	1.0	trace	2.4
Raisins	1/2 cup	218	57.0	2.5	0.5	2.6
Fruit Cocktail in Juice Pack	1 cup	115	29.0	1.0	trace	ND
Fruit Leather	1 bar	81	18.0	0.4	1.2	ND
Watermelon	1 cup	50	11.0	1.0	trace	0.6
Sweets And Other Snacks						
Beef Jerky	1 large piece	280	2.9	7.9	2.6	ND
Fruit Shake (see recipe at end)	1 serving	330	60	15.0	3.0	ND
Fruit Yogurt, low-fat	1 cup, 8 oz.	230	43	10.0	2.0	ND
Popsicles	1–3 oz.	70	18	0.0	0.0	ND

[1]ND = No Data

What Snacks Are Best for Different Occasions?

In the following charts, examples of snacks are provided. Some of the snacks are part of military rations, and should (could) be used during training or mission maneuvers. Other snacks may not be realistic in the field, but are good choices if you are able to be more selective in what you choose.

Operations at Night

If you need to stay up at night you should select a snack that is *low in fat, high in carbohydrate (CHO), and provides some or a moderate amount of protein.* You want to avoid foods that are 100% CHO. Sports bars would be ideal snacks for night operations. Also, crackers (or other forms of bread) with egg salad, mashed beans, jelly, tuna, or low-fat cream cheese would be suitable. Finally, some of the protein/CHO beverages described in Chapter 6 would be suitable for nighttime operations.

Table 7-2. Snacks to Eat During Nighttime Operations

Sports Bars	**Fruit Bars**
Oatmeal Cookie Bars	**Protein/CHO Beverage**
Trail Mix	**Crackers with Jelly or Cheese**

Exercises in the Heat

The ideal snacks consumed during strenuous activities in warm to hot environments are those which provide the body with fluid. As such, fruits, especially watermelon and oranges, are great snacks for hot weather. Otherwise, the fluid replacement beverages described in Chapter 6 are preferred. Avoid high-fat and dried foods which can make you uncomfortable and thirsty.

Table 7-3. Snacks to Eat During Exercises in the Heat

Watermelon	Oranges
Applesauce	Fruit Popsicles
Grapes	CHO Beverages with Electrolytes

Exercises in the Cold

When working in cold weather, snack on foods that are high in CHO. CHO foods produce more heat when digested than either fat or protein. To go along with your food snack, a hot beverage, like cocoa or soup, would be great.

Table 7-4. Snacks to Eat During Exercises in the Cold

Granola/Sport Bars	Fig Newtons
Hot Chocolate	Crackers/Bread with Jam
Fruit Bars	Chicken Noodle Soup
Trail Mix	Hot Apple Cider

Sustained Operations

By definition, SUSTAINED OPERATIONS are those missions or training sessions where you must work continuously for over 24 hours with minimal sleep, and few rest periods. During these times it is important to receive adequate amounts of CHO to maintain your "blood glucose" and fluid to maintain "hydration status." The specific types of snacks will depend on the temperature and how long you have been working, but in general avoid high-fat foods since they take longer to digest than CHO foods. Also, eating CHO with some protein will help you stay awake when you are feeling drowsy. A combination of the recommendations already made in this chapter would be best, depending on the environmental conditions.

Table 7-5. Snacks to Eat During Sustained Operations

Granola/Power Bars	**Oatmeal Cookies**
Hot or Cold Protein/CHO Beverage	**Cracker/Bread with Jam**
M & M's	**Trail Mix**
Tootsie Roll	**Dried Fruit**

Snacking On Occasion

There comes a time when you just don't want to be healthy—you want to get some quick energy and nothing else. In that case it is still wise to be selective, so if you must have a candy bar or other sweets, choose one that is high in CHO and as low in fat as possible: like Peppermint Patties and 3 Musketeers. Remember, these foods are not encouraged because they provide ONLY energy - no vitamins or minerals, which you must have to process the energy. BUT sweets now and then will certainly NOT hurt you.

Table 7-6. Macronutrient Composition of Some Sweet Snacks

Candy Bars and Sweet Items	ENERGY (kcal)	CHO (grams)	FAT (% of Energy)	CHO (% of Energy)
Almond Joy, 1.76 oz. bar	232	29	51	45
Baby Ruth, 2.1 oz. bar	277	37	40	52
Butterfinger Bar, 2.16 oz. bar	266	41	36	58
Chocolate Coated Raisins, 1.58 oz. pkg	188	32	33	61
Gumdrops, 10 small	135	35	0	100
Jelly Beans, 10 small	40	10	0	100
Kit Kat, 1.625 oz. bar	235	28	49	46
Milky Way Bar, 2.1 oz. bar	251	43	32	64
3 Musketeers, 2.13 oz. bar	249	46	27	70
M & M's Plain, 1.69 oz. pkg	229	33	40	54
M & M's Peanut, 1.74 oz. pkg	242	29	47	45
Peppermint Pattie, 1 large	149	34	22	74
Snickers, 2.16 oz. bar	277	37	42	51
Tootsie Roll, 1 oz.	112	23	19	78

Snack Recipes

Fruit Shake

1 cup ice cubes
1 cup skim milk
1 ripe banana
2 peaches or 1/2 to 1 cup of any fresh fruit
2 tbsp almonds
1 tbsp honey
2 tsp wheat germ

Place all ingredients in a blender or food processor and blend until smooth. For extra protein add 1/4 cup of non-fat dried milk. Makes 1 serving.

Nutrition Information: 520 kcal, 70% CHO, 12% Protein, and 18% Fat per serving.

Trail Mix

3 cups seedless raisins
1 cup dried apricots
1 cup dried apples
1 cup almonds
1 cup dry roasted peanuts
1 cup dried pineapple
1 cup dried dates
1/2 cup sunflower seeds

Mix all ingredients together in large bowl or bag. Makes 10 1-cup servings.

Nutrition Information: 560 kcal, 62% CHO, 7% Protein, and 30% Fat per 1-cup serving.

Chapter 8
Restaurants, Fast Foods, and Eating Out

The average American eats one of three meals away from home each day, and it is likely that many of you are eating 5, 6, 7 or more meals a week away from home. Learning how to "eat out" is very important if you want to optimize your performance. You are probably aware that eating out presents different problems than eating at home. When we talk about eating out we mean eating at restaurants, fast food places, on travel, on vacations, and at social events.

Most people love to eat in restaurants or at places away from home. Eating out provides a change in routine, an opportunity to try new foods, a chance to socialize and a break from cooking and washing dishes (for those who do). Restaurant and fast food meals do not have to be unhealthy. By being informed and by asking appropriate questions, you can stay within the guidelines of your nutrition program and still enjoy the benefits of eating out.

Fast Food Restaurants

Although we don't encourage you to get your meals from fast food establishments, we know fast foods are a way of life. If you can learn to select the types of foods that will suit your activity patterns and performance requirements, then fast food restaurants are OK. Below are selected foods typically available at different fast food places, and the energy, carbohydrate (CHO), and fat contributions of those foods. After providing you with this information, sample breakfasts and lunch/dinners that maybe considered nutritionally adequate in terms of their CHO and fat content are presented.

Table 8-1. Caloric Values of Selected Fast Foods

Breakfast Items	Energy (kcal)	CHO (grams)	Fat (% of Energy)	CHO (% of Energy)
Hot Chocolate, 6 oz.	103	22.5	9.6	87.4
Orange Juice, 8 oz.	112	26.8	0.0	95.7
Biscuit, 1 plain	276	34.4	43.7	49.9
Biscuit w/egg	315	24.2	57.7	30.7
Biscuit w/egg and sausage	582	41.2	59.8	28.3
Croissant w/egg and cheese	369	24.3	60.2	26.3
Cinnamon Danish, 1 medium	349	46.9	43.1	53.8
Eggs, 2 scrambled	200	2.0	68.4	4.0
English Muffin, 1 plain	137	27.5	6.6	80.3
English Muffin w/butter	189	36.4	27.6	77.0
English Muffin w/cheese and sausage	394	24.2	55.5	24.6
Pancakes w/butter and syrup, 3 medium	519	90.9	27.6	77.0
Potatoes, hash browns, 1 cup	302	32.3	55.5	24.6

Table 8-1. Caloric Values of Selected Fast Foods

Lunch and Dinner Items	Energy (kcal)	CHO (grams)	Fat (% of Energy)	CHO (% of Energy)
Chocolate Shake 10 oz.	360	57.9	26.3	64.3
Cola 12 oz.	151	37.6	0.0	99.6
Burrito w/Beans, 2 each	448	71.4	27.1	63.8
Burrito w/Beef, 2 each	523	58.5	35.8	44.7
Chili Con Carne, 1 cup	254	21.9	29.4	34.5
Cheeseburger, double meat, 1 each	416	35.2	45.6	33.8
Fish Sandwich, 1 each	524	47.6	49.1	36.3
Chicken, breast fried, 2 pieces	494	35.7	65.0	15.4
Hot Dog w/chili, 1 each	297	31.3	40.6	42.2
Nachos w/cheese, 7 each	345	36.3	51.1	42.1
Pizza w/cheese, 2 slices	218	31.9	20.6	58.5
Taco, 1 large	569	41.1	50.0	28.9
Onion Rings, 10 each	332	37.7	50.7	45.4
Potato Chips, 10 each	105	10.4	60.9	39.6
Potatoes, French Fries, 1 order	237	29.3	46.3	49.5
Salad w/out dressing, 1 1/2 cups	32	6.7	0.0	83.8
Potato, baked w/sour cream, 1 medium	394	50.0	49.8	44.4
Corn w/butter, 1 ear	155	32	9.7	82.6
Coleslaw, 3/4 cup	147	12.8	67.3	34.8
Brownies, 1 each	243	39.0	37.4	64.2
Chocolate Chip Cookies, 1 order	233	36.2	42.1	52.8
Hot Fudge Sundae	284	47.7	31.2	78.6
Fried Fruit Pie, 1 each	266	33.1	48.7	49.8

Table 8-2. Sample High-Carbohydrate Fast Food Breakfasts, Lunches, and Dinners

MacDonald's Breakfast	Energy (kcal)	CHO (grams)	Fat (% of Energy)	CHO (% of Energy
Orange Juice, 8 oz.	112	26.8	0.0	93.8
2 English Muffins w/jam or honey	378	72.8	27.6	77.0
Eggs, 2 scrambled	200	2.0	68.4	4.0
Hot Chocolate	103	22.5	9.6	87.4
Total	**793**	**124.1**	**31.7**	**62.6**

Wendy's Breakfast

	Energy (kcal)	CHO (grams)	Fat (% of Energy)	CHO (% of Energy
Orange Juice, 16 oz.	224	53.6	0.0	93.8
Cinnamon Danish, 2 medium	698	93.8	43.1	53.8
Hot Chocolate, 6 oz.	100	22.0	9.0	88.0
Total	**1022**	**169.4**	**30.3**	**66.3**

Anywhere Breakfast 1

	Energy (kcal)	CHO (grams)	Fat (% of Energy)	CHO (% of Energy
Orange Juice, 8 oz.	112	26.8	0.0	93.8
Pancakes w/butter and syrup, 3 medium	692	121.2	25.3	70.1
Eggs, 2 scrambled	200	2.0	68.4	4.0
Hot Chocolate, 6 oz.	103	22.5	9.6	87.4
Total	**1107**	**172.2**	**29.0**	**62.2**

Burger King Breakfast	Energy (kcal)	CHO (grams)	Fat (% of Energy)	CHO (% of Energy)
Orange Juice, 16 oz.	224	53.6	0.0	93.8
Egg Croissantwich, 1 each	369	24.3	60.2	26.3
Hot chocolate, 6 oz.	100	22.0	9.0	88.0
Total	**693**	**99.3**	**33.3**	**57.7**

Anywhere Breakfast 2

	Energy (kcal)	CHO (grams)	Fat (% of Energy)	CHO (% of Energy)
Orange Juice, 16 oz.	224	53.6	0.0	93.8
English Muffin, 2 with 2 pkg jam	342	73.0	5.2	85.3
Eggs, 2 scrambled	200	2.0	68.4	4.0
Hash Brown Potatoes, 1 cup	302	32.3	53.6	42.8
Total	**1068**	**161.0**	**30.0**	**60.3**

Taco Bell Lunch or Dinner

	Energy (kcal)	CHO (grams)	Fat (% of Energy)	CHO (% of Energy)
Taco Bell Nachos, 2 orders	692	75.0	48.1	43.4
Cola, 16 oz.	201	50.1	0.0	99.8
Total	**893**	**125.1**	**36.7**	**56.0**

Anywhere Lunch or Dinner	Energy (kcal)	CHO (grams)	Fat (% of Energy)	CHO (% of Energy)
Chili Con Carne, 1 cup	254	21.9	29.4	34.5
Potato, baked, plain, 1 medium	300	69.0	0.5	92.0
Sour Cream, 1 pkt	60	1.0	90.0	6.7
Green Salad, tossed, 1 1/2 cups	32	6.7	0.0	83.8
Italian Dressing, reduced calorie, 2 tbsp	50	3.0	72.0	24.0
Corn on cob, 2 ears	310	64.0	19.7	82.6
Chocolate Shake, 10 oz.	360	57.9	26.3	64.3
Total	**1366**	**223.5**	**24.8**	**65.4**

Wendy's Lunch or Dinner

	Energy (kcal)	CHO (grams)	Fat (% of Energy)	CHO (% of Energy)
Fettucine, 2 cups	480	60	29.7	48.8
Spaghetti Sauce, 1 cup	120	24	0	77.4
Garlic Toast, 1 serving	140	18	38.6	51.4
Caesar Salad, 1 serving	160	18	45.0	45.0
Lemonade, 16 oz.	200	50	0	100
Total	**1100**	**170**	**24.5**	**61.8**

Hardee's Lunch or Dinner

	Energy (kcal)	CHO (grams)	Fat (% of Energy)	CHO (% of Energy)
Big Roast Beef Sandwich, 1 serving	346	33.5	35.8	38.7
Potato, baked, plain, 1 medium	300	69.0	0.5	92
Sour Cream, 1 pkt	60	1.0	90.0	6.7
Green Salad, tossed, 1 1/2 cups	32	6.7	0.0	83.8
French Dressing, low-fat, 2 tbsp	44	7.0	36.0	63.6
Vanilla Shake, 10 oz.	314	50.8	24.1	64.7
Total	**1096**	**168.0**	**24.7**	**61.3**

Restaurants, Fast Foods, and Eating Out

Pizza Hut Lunch or Dinner	Energy (kcal)	CHO (grams)	Fat (% of Energy)	CHO (% of Energy)
Pizza w/cheese, 8 slices	872	127.6	20.6	58.5
Salad w/out dressing, 1 1/2 cups	32	6.7	0.0	83.8
Italian Dressing, reduced calorie, 2 tbsp	50	3.0	72.0	24.0
Orange Soda, 12 oz.	151	37.6	0.0	99.6
Total	1105	174.9	24.0	63.3
MacDonald's Lunch or Dinner				
Plain Hamburger with ketchup, 2	520	61.2	32.9	47.1
French Fries, regular serving	220	25.6	49.1	46.5
Hot Fudge Sundae, 1 each	284	47.7	31.2	67.2
Vanilla Milkshake, low-fat	290	60.0	3.1	82.8
Total	1314	194.5	28.6	59.1

Recommendations for Selecting High-CHO Foods at Restaurants

PLACING AN ORDER

- Order a clear soup, tomato juice or V8 juice, steamed seafood, or fruit for an appetizer.
- Order a green salad with light dressing on the side. Avoid salads with cheese, eggs, meat, bacon or croutons. Avoid cole slaw or potato salad.
- Order broiled, roasted or baked lean meat, poultry or fish—even if the menu does not say broiled. Avoid casseroles and foods with heavy sauces.
- Order baked potato or plain rice—not pasta with sauces or fried or Delmonico potatoes.
- Do not order dessert until you have eaten your main course. If you are still hungry, order sorbet, sherbet, frozen yogurt, ice milk, fruit or angel cake.
- Order juices—they are high in carbohydrates.

DURING THE MEAL

◆ Eat a plain roll, breadsticks or plain crackers rather than biscuits or croissants. Try to avoid spreads completely or use sparingly.

◆ Minimize your nibbling on nuts, buttery crackers, potato and tortilla chips.

◆ Ask the waiter to serve your salad immediately; use the dressing sparingly.

◆ Trim all visible fat off meat.

◆ Limit portions of margarine, butter or sour cream.

◆ Moderate your intake of alcoholic beverages.

Worksheet 8-1. Your Eating Out Checklist

Answer the following questions to see how many foods and food groups your meals usually include. THE MORE OFTEN YOU EAT THESE FOODS, THE HEALTHIER YOUR MEALS ARE.

How Often Does Your Lunch or Dinner Contain	Seldom or Never	1 or 2 Times per Week	3 or 4 Times per Week	Almost Daily
Fruits or fruit juices?	☐	☐	☐	☐
Vegetables or vegetable juices?	☐	☐	☐	☐
Enriched breads, pastas, or other grains?	☐	☐	☐	☐
Lean meat, fish, or poultry?	☐	☐	☐	☐
Beans, peas, lentils, tofu, nuts, or eggs?	☐	☐	☐	☐
Lowfat milk, cheese or yogurt?	☐	☐	☐	☐

Chapter 9
Nutritional Considerations for Endurance Activities

As SEALs you must be in excellent physical condition and be able to endure arduous physical tasks for extended periods of time. Your capacity to endure can be greatly improved by regular physical conditioning and by following special dietary practices. Prolonged running, swimming, load carrying, and/or multiple shorter bouts of higher intensity activity impose significant demands on energy stores and fluid balance. Failure to replace the energy or fluids lost during prolonged operational or training activities can greatly impair your performance in subsequent mission activities. Meeting daily vitamin and mineral needs is also important since these micronutrients play an important part in physical performance (see Chapter 3). In this chapter, information on dietary interventions to enhance endurance performance is provided. It is important to remember that your daily energy intakes will vary according to your activity level.

Glycogen Stores and Meeting Your Energy Needs

During heavy physical training you must increase your caloric intake, especially from carbohydrate (CHO) foods, to meet your energy demands. Failure to do so may result in:

◆ Chronic muscular fatigue
◆ A feeling of staleness
◆ Weight loss
◆ Poor sleep patterns

Liver and muscle glycogen is the primary source of glucose for your muscles during prolonged endurance activities. Therefore, the key to optimal endurance performance lies in maintaining muscle and liver glycogen stores. Once glycogen stores are exhausted, your ability to continue to perform an endurance activity will decrease sharply. When you wake up in the morning, your liver stores are low from not eating for several hours, and your blood glucose may be low. Thus, breakfast is critical to maintaining energy balance and liver glycogen stores.

> ## Keep a weight chart during periods of heavy training and arduous operations to document energy needs

Carbohydrates and Endurance Performance

Liver and muscle glycogen stores are replenished by eating carbohydrate (CHO) foods. Therefore:

> ## CHO is the most important energy-providing nutrient for endurance training

The endurance capacity of an individual on a high-CHO diet is approximately three times greater than when on a high-fat diet. When CHO intake is low, rigorous training sessions over several days will result in a gradual depletion of muscle glycogen stores and eventually impair performance. The figure below illustrates depletion of muscle glycogen over three days of running two hours per day. Note that when subjects ate a low-CHO diet, glycogen stores gradually became depleted over the three-day period. When the high-CHO diet was consumed, glycogen stores were repleted between training sessions. Remember that glycogen is composed of glucose molecules linked together. This figure clearly demonstrates the need to consume foods that are high in CHO.

You should eat 2.5 to 4 grams CHO per pound of body weight each day.

EXAMPLE

You weigh 175 lbs and work out two hours each day

2.5 X 175 lb = 437 grams of CHO

4 X 175 lb = 700 grams of CHO

Your CHO needs are between 437 and 700 grams per day

Worksheet 9-1. Calculating Your Daily CHO Needs

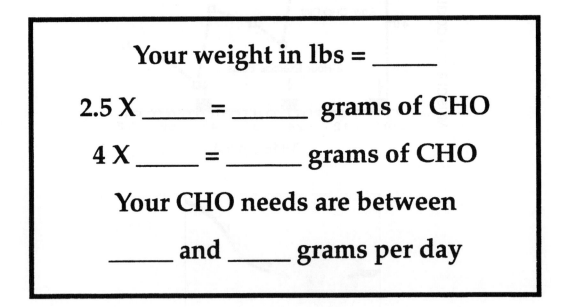

Your weight in lbs = _____

2.5 X _____ = _____ grams of CHO

4 X _____ = _____ grams of CHO

Your CHO needs are between

_____ and _____ grams per day

Another way to think about CHO needs is in terms of energy intake. Ideally, *60 to 65%* of your daily energy should come from CHO. When energy intake is greater than 4,000 kcals then 60% is the proportion of CHO kcals to strive for. Since each gram of CHO is 4 kcal, we can calculate the number of grams needed from your energy intake.

Example

You train 3 hours and eat 3,500 kcal per day

60% of calories from CHO =

3,500 X 60/100 = 2,100 kcal from CHO

Amount of CHO =

2,100/4 kcal = 525 grams of CHO

Lists of various high-CHO foods and the grams of CHO provided by each food are provided in Chapters 7 and 12 and Appendix 1. Complex CHO foods are preferable since they also provide vitamins and minerals in addition to CHO (see Chapter 2). Other important recommendations include:

Eat high-CHO snacks in between training sessions to replace your glycogen stores.

Consume at least 50 grams of CHO immediately after completing your training session.

For example, you could eat a banana and drink a cup of orange juice. Commercially available high-CHO liquid supplements may be beneficial during recovery from long training sessions because they supply CHO, water, protein, vitamins, and minerals.

Keep a log of all CHO foods eaten for several days to see if your intake is high enough.

CHO Loading/ Glycogen Supercompensation

What is CHO Loading?

CHO loading/glycogen supercompensation is a regimen that combines diet and exercise to "pack" more glycogen into muscle and liver. It is used by endurance athletes to optimize physical performance during prolonged endurance events. Although well-trained muscles have the capacity to store 2 to 3 times more glycogen than untrained muscles, CHO loading allows you to store 2 to 4 times the usual amount of glycogen in liver and muscle. CHO loading may be useful for long duration missions and extended water operations.

CHO loading involves tapering or reducing the number, duration, and intensity of your training sessions the week prior to an event. As shown in the figure below, 5 days before the event (on day 2), be it an extended dive, land, and water mission, or a sports competition, your training is tapered such that on days 2 and 3, no more than 40 minutes is spent on physical activities (solid line). CHO intake (dotted line) would be approximately 50% of your total energy intake. On days 4 and 5 the time spent exercising should be no more than 20 minutes, and your CHO intake should be increased to 70% of the total energy intake. Note day 6 is a rest day and CHO intake remains at 70% of the energy intake.

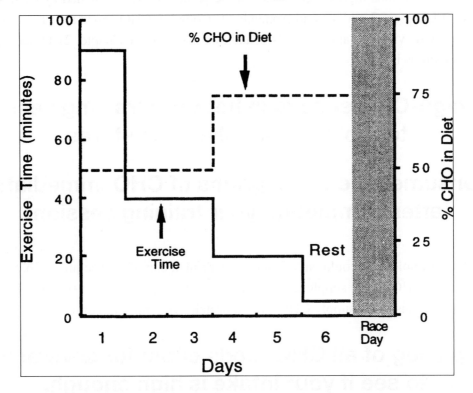

An accurate body weight should be obtained for reference purposes prior to modifying CHO intake and decreasing the intensity of training because 2.7 grams of water are stored with every gram of glycogen. Thus, on the day of the competition, if an additional 200 grams of glycogen have been stored, body weight should have increased by 0.54 kg or 1.2 pounds.

Who Should (and Shouldn't) CHO Load?

For most regimens of intense physical training, a daily diet that provides 2.5 to 4 grams of CHO/lb body weight and adequate calories is sufficient to maintain muscle and liver glycogen reserves. However, for SDV operations, extended load-bearing marches, and other training scenarios with extremely high energy demands, CHO loading may prove to be very useful. Remember that CHO loading is not useful for events lasting only 60 minutes or less, and may in fact impair performance in activities requiring short bouts of maximal effort as you will weigh more from the additional water stored.

Protein Needs

Endurance training increases protein needs, and to meet the increased needs:

Protein intakes should range from 0.6 to 0.8 grams per pound body weight per day.

You calculated your protein requirements in Chapter 2 so refer back to that chapter for more information. It is likely your regular diet provides what you need because rarely do American men have protein intakes below the recommendations. Most men, including athletes, typically consume protein in excess of their actual needs.

Vitamin and Mineral Needs

Currently, the micronutrient requirements of people engaged in endurance activities are not well-defined. Because of the nature of your training, your daily overall needs may be 1.5 to 3 times greater than those of the average man. If you eat a healthy diet, your daily vitamin and mineral needs should be met from a variety of different foods (see Appendixes 5 and 6 for information on food sources of various vitamins and minerals). Because endurance exercise may increase your need for antioxidants, it is recommended that each day you should eat several foods rich in antioxidants (vitamin C, vitamin E, and beta-carotene), as shown in the table below.

Table 9-1. Some Good Food Sources of Selected Antioxidant Nutrients

Vitamin C	Vitamin E	Beta-carotene
Orange juice	Sunflower seeds	Carrots
Grapefruit juice	Almonds	Spinach
Broccoli	Peanuts	Cantaloupe
Orange	Spinach	Broccoli
Strawberries	Olive oil	Winter squash
Cauliflower	Tomato	Dried apricots

Pay close attention to your electrolyte (sodium and potassium) needs when training in hot weather. You should get more than enough sodium in the foods you eat, whereas potassium requires a more careful selection of foods. See Appendix 6 for good food sources of potassium.

Fluid Requirements

Ingesting fluids at regular intervals and eating foods with a high water content are important for maintaining hydration and fluid status during training. Chapter 6 provides a thorough overview of fluid requirements and different types of beverages. In general:

Drink 1-2 cups of water 60 minutes before
a training session.

Drink a cup of 5–8% CHO drink every
30 minutes during prolonged exercise.

During exercise, do not drink anything with a
CHO content greater than 8% or you are likely to
get stomach cramps.

Commercial fluid replacement beverages or
diluted juices are recommended.

Consume beverages with a higher percentage (>8%) of
CHO after exercise to replace glycogen stores and
fluids lost during exercise.

The beverages you drink during and after
prolonged exercise should contain
sodium and potassium.

Nutritional Interventions During Training Sessions

Nutritional manipulations/interventions can delay fatigue and prevent conditions such as low blood sugar, dehydration, and low blood sodium that are detrimental to performance. These interventions include:

> ## Drink 1 to 2 cups of a beverage supplemented with CHO (5–8%) and electrolytes every 30 minutes throughout exercise to extend your endurance.

When an activity has been maintained for 2 to 3 hours without a CHO source, blood glucose levels may fall and cause fatigue. Ingestion of CHO beverages will prevent the fall in blood sugar (glucose) and delay fatigue. Although providing a CHO beverage 15 to 30 minutes before the anticipated onset of fatigue may extend performance for a short time, ingesting CHO after exhaustion will not allow you to immediately resume your activities.

> ## Consume CHO beverages at regular intervals during prolonged exercise.

Solid CHO foods, such as fruits and sports bars, are acceptable as CHO sources provided you are able to tolerate them during the activity and drink fluids with them. Food selections are personal choices and dietary manipulations should be tested during training and omitted if they prove troublesome to you. Some foods may cause stomach cramps and diarrhea if eaten during exercise. Dietary fiber intake should be limited during exercise to avoid gastrointestinal problems.

Summary

- Maintain energy balance by repleting glycogen stores between training sessions.
- Eat at least 2.5 grams of CHO per lb body weight or at least 400 grains of CHO per day to maintain your glycogen stores.

- Maximize glycogen stores before an event by ingesting 4 to 5 grams of CHO per lb body weight (or 70% of calories from CHO) for 2 to 3 days before the event.
- Drink at least 250 to 300 ml of a CHO-supplemented (5–8%) beverage containing electrolytes every 30 minutes throughout prolonged training sessions.
- Consume at least 50 grams of CHO within 30 minutes of completing an extended training session and continue to eat/snack on high-CHO foods every 2 hours for at least 6 hours to rapidly replace your glycogen stores.

Chapter 10
Nutritional Considerations for Strength Training

SEAL missions and training require strength. Thus, a strength training program will enhance your physical conditioning and ability to perform and complete strenuous mission tasks. In addition, it will keep you "looking" fit! In this chapter information on strength training and the unique dietary requirements for strength training will be provided.

Benefits of Strength Training

Strength training should complement endurance training workouts. The specific benefits of strength training include:

- ◆ Increased muscle strength and endurance
- ◆ Increased muscle fiber size
- ◆ Increased ligament and tendon strength
- ◆ Greater protection against "overuse" injury

Because strength training makes you stronger, it will also reduce your risk for injuries that typically accompany endurance training. Finally, strength training can make you faster at tasks that require quick, short bursts of activity (such as a running from a boat to land).

Factors Determining Muscle Mass

The various factors that "regulate" the size of the muscle are shown below. Some factors, such as genetics, we can't control. Often we have no control over environmental factors, either. Factors that we can control and that play major roles in determining muscle mass are physical exercise and nutritional status.

Protein Requirements for Strength Training

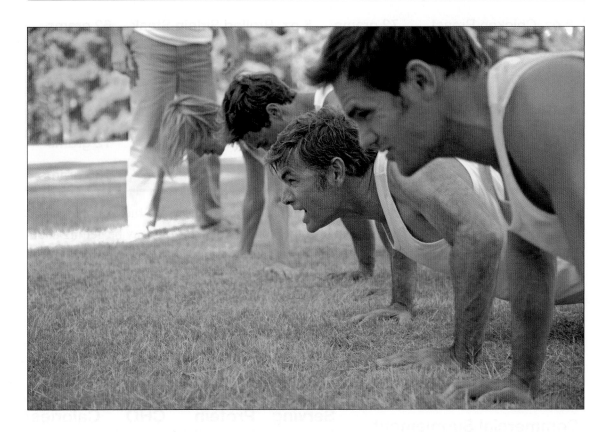

Research has shown that the protein needs of strength athletes and endurance athletes are quite similar: *You should eat 0.6 to 0.8 grams of protein per pound body weight each day to meet your daily protein requirements.*

Worksheet 10-1. How Much Protein Do I Need?

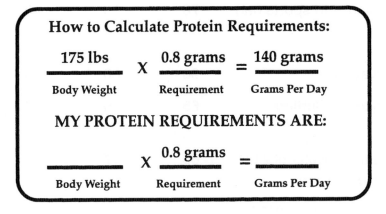

How to Calculate Protein Requirements:

$$\frac{175 \text{ lbs}}{\text{Body Weight}} \times \frac{0.8 \text{ grams}}{\text{Requirement}} = \frac{140 \text{ grams}}{\text{Grams Per Day}}$$

MY PROTEIN REQUIREMENTS ARE:

$$\frac{}{\text{Body Weight}} \times \frac{0.8 \text{ grams}}{\text{Requirement}} = \frac{}{\text{Grams Per Day}}$$

Table 10-1. Examples of Where You Get Protein

Monday		Tuesday	
8 oz. Chicken Breast	72 grams	8 oz. Broiled Sirloin Steak	62 grams
Subway Roast Beef Sandwich	41 grams	Subway Turkey Sandwich	42 grams
Vanilla Milkshake	9 grams	8 oz. Bowl of Chili	19 grams
1 Egg McMuffin	18 grams	1 Sports Bar	12 grams
TOTAL	138 grams	TOTAL	135 grams

It is likely your diet provides even more protein than shown in the example, since protein is also in milk, cheese, fish, and many other foods. Some of you may be getting additional protein from commercially available sports bars, protein powders or carbohydrate/protein supplements as well as the foods you eat. Commercial supplements often provide considerable protein, as shown in the next table.

Table 10-2. Protein Content of Some Commercial Protein Supplements

Commercial Supplement	Serving (grams)	Protein (grams)	CHO (grams)	Calories/ Serving
SPORTS BARS (see Chapter 7 for others)	ONE BAR			
Hardbody	78	18	45	320
ICO Pro Super Protein™ bar	68	13	45	250
Oroamino (amino acid sports bar)	78	18	40	296
BEVERAGES[1]				
Anabolic activator II	90	60	20	338
Bavarian Chocolate Cutting Advantage	65	25	37	225
Champion Nutrition Metabolol II™ (the metabolic optimizer)	66	17	42	260
Cybergenics Super Infiniti 3000	555	125	370	2400

Table 10-2. Protein Content of Some Commercial Protein Supplements

Commercial Supplement	Serving (grams)	Protein (grams)	CHO (grams)	Calories/ Serving
Exceed Sports Meal	240	14	54	360
Hot Stuff (Advanced formula)	90	60	13	320
Joe Weider's Dynamic Muscle Builder	44	18	27	190
Joe Weider's Performance Muscle Builder	55	18	31	200
Mega Mass 2000	140	27	106	550
Met-Rx	72	37	24	262
Optimum Nutrition Mighty 1 3000	224	22	153	700
Twin Lab Opti Fuel 2	140	20	100	480
Twin Lab Anabolic Pre-Exercise Energy Drink Mass Fuel	183	15	150	660
Victory Anabolic Cuts (low-fat body definition mix)	42	15	24	170

[1]Beverage information is based on reconstituting one serving with water according to the manufacturer's directions. If these beverages were reconstituted with milk, calories and protein content would be higher.

The High Protein Myth

Inorganic Salts, Urea, Lactate 5%

The excess protein in an athlete's diet, not required by the body, is often around 100 grams per day. Because muscle is 20% protein, the additional 100 grams of protein per day should result in a gain of 500 grams of muscle per day

Or about 1 pound of muscle per day.

If we look at what muscle is actually made up of we see that eating a high-protein diet just doesn't add up. Muscle is only 20% protein; the rest is water and minerals, lactic acid, urea, and high-energy phosphates.

If you ate 100 extra grams of protein every day for one week, you should gain 7 pounds of muscle mass! CLEARLY, this is not the case.

The extra protein results in an increase in the formation and excretion of the waste product "urea," increases your fluid requirements, and places a considerable load on the liver and the kidneys.

You should avoid protein supplements that provide excessive amounts of protein or selected amino acids. Although heavily advertised, and in some cases endorsed by celebrities, very high protein intakes from supplements are NOT needed to build muscle. This practice can be very expensive, dangerous to your health, and quite unnecessary. A regular balanced diet can meet your protein needs very effectively.

Concerns with Very High Protein Intakes

◆ Increases the work load of the kidneys and in extreme cases result in kidney failure. In some individuals this practice has resulted in hypertension.
◆ Can be dehydrating especially during endurance events if additional fluids are not consumed.
◆ High intake of free amino acids may cause diarrhea and abdominal cramps.
◆ Creates imbalances of the essential amino acids.

Worksheet 10-2. How Much Protein Do I Eat?

For each weekday over a one-week period, write down all foods you ate that are high in protein. Using food labels and protein values in Appendix 3, record the protein content of each food in grams. For example: if you ate a hard-boiled egg and drank a glass of skim milk for breakfast on Monday, record under Monday those foods in the column labeled FOOD and in the column labeled G for grams enter 6 and 8. Similarly, write down the food or protein supplement and its protein content for each day. Then, add up the numbers to see how many grams of protein you typically eat.

Monday		Tuesday		Wednesday		Thursday		Friday	
Food	**G**	**Food**	**G**	**Food**	**G**	**Food**	**G**	**Food**	**G**
TOTAL		TOTAL		TOTAL		TOTAL		TOTAL	

As you can see it is relatively easy to meet your daily protein requirements from food. You will probably find that your intake is far greater than your actual requirement.

Other Nutritional Requirements

Carbohydrate Requirements

Strength training relies on glycogen stores for energy. Thus, carbohydrates (CHO) are very important.

> # 55 to 60% of your daily energy intake should come from CHO

The CHO recommendations for strength training are somewhat less than for endurance athletes since the overall energy requirements of weight lifting are less. BUT depending on your training schedule and length of your aerobic workouts, you may need 2.5 to 4 grams of CHO per pound body weight per day. For more information on carbohydrates see Chapters 2 and 9.

You may remember the term carbohydrate loading from Chapter 9. This practice is discouraged for weight lifters because of the extra water stored in the muscle. In other words, CHO loading provides no additional advantage in increasing muscle girth.

Fat Requirements

A thorough discussion of fat was provided in Chapter 2. But for fats in general, the recommendation is:

Less than 30% of your energy should come from fat

Remember there are three different types of fat: monounsaturated, polyunsaturated, and saturated fats and each should provide less than 10% of the daily energy.

Vitamins and Minerals

Meeting your daily energy needs from a variety of different foods should enable you to easily meet you vitamin and mineral needs. See Appendixes 5 and 6 for information on food sources of various vitamins and minerals.

Multi-Ingredient Steroid Alternatives—The Bottom Line

Some supplements containing herbs, glandulars, minerals such as chromium or boron, and a number of other compounds are being marketed as "muscle builders." Manufacturers claim that these products are *alternatives to steroids*. The major concerns associated with using such products are:

Not properly tested and absolutely no basis to substantiate the claims.

Potential for harmful side-effects, allergic reactions, and toxicities.

Metabolic pathways and waste products formed from some of these compounds are not known.

Potential for testing positive for banned substances when using such products, especially those that do not reveal their "secret" ingredients.

Expensive and unlikely to replace the benefits of a good diet and sound training program.

If a product sounds too good to be true, it is usually not worth trying. Check Chapter 15 for more information on selected products or contact a sports nutritionist to verify the claims being made.

Summary

◆ Eat a wide variety of foods and match your energy intake to energy output.
◆ Aim for between 0.6 and 0.8 grams of protein per pound per day or between 120 and 150 grams per day.
◆ Drink plenty of fluids.
◆ Don't get trapped into buying so-called "muscle building" powders and potions. Proper training and a good diet will provide the lasting EDGE when it comes to building strength and muscles.
◆ SAVE YOUR MONEY or spend it on "real" foods.

Chapter 11
Nutrition for Optimum Mission Performance

Nutrition is important for maximizing or optimizing mission performance. What you eat or don't eat before a physically demanding event could either "help" or "hurt" you. For example, eating a high-fat meal before vigorous activity can slow you down as fat takes longer to digest than CHO. Knowing when to eat is also important since both fasting or eating a heavy meal shortly before endurance activity can decrease performance. Information to help optimize your performance during simulated and actual missions, including field deployment, is presented in this chapter. Suggestions for maximizing performance during BUDS training are also provided. In some instances you may be unable to control what or when you eat, however, it is important to meet your energy and fluid requirements.

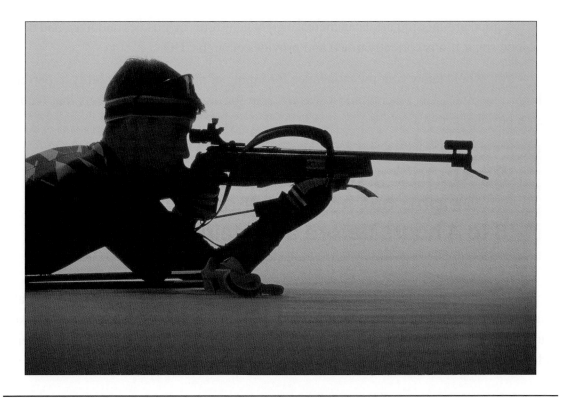

Nutritional Readiness Before a Specific Mission

In this scenario you may already be deployed under field conditions or locked down on base. Regardless of where you are, the two main considerations to nutritional readiness before missions are:

♦ Maximizing glycogen stores
♦ Being well-hydrated

In order to **be ready**, you must consider your pre-mission food and beverages.

Several Days Before a Mission

The average, lean, 175-pound man has approximately 1800 calories of carbohydrate (CHO) stored as glycogen in liver and muscle, and 75,000 to 150,000 calories stored as fat. In spite of these large energy stores in fat, once glycogen stores are exhausted, physical and mental performance will decrease and exhaustion will set in. A diet high in CHO for several days before a mission has the potential to increase liver and muscle glycogen stores, and thereby extend the time to exhaustion during a mission (see Chapter 9). Sample 3-day high-CHO diet menus are provided in Appendix 7.

Timing and Composition of Pre-Mission Meals

A good pre-mission meal can increase glycogen stores in muscles and liver, and delay low blood sugar if it is correctly timed and provides enough CHO.

You should know your own tolerance for timing of meals and your ability to perform endurance activities. In general, allow greater time for digestion before events that require intense physical activity.

> # Eat up to 2 grams of CHO per pound body weight, but no more than 400 grams, 3 to 4 hours before a sustained operation.

This meal should provide a minimum of fat and protein, since these nutrients take longer to digest. CHO beverages and CHO/ protein drinks are excellent choices if taken hours before the start. Avoid a high-protein meal since this can increase fluid requirements and may cause dehydration.

If you weigh 175 pounds
2 X 175 = 350 grams of CHO

You may eat up to 350 grams of CHO
for your pre-mission meal

If this is not possible, eat a small high-CHO meal 2–3 hours before your mission (400–500 calories).

A CHO beverage 1–2 hours before a mission will leave the stomach faster than a solid meal.

Nutrition for Maintaining Performance During Training and Missions

Three major nutrition-related issues encountered in the field are:

- Inadequate ration consumption
- Dehydration
- Gastrointestinal complaints

Inadequate Ration Consumption

One of the biggest problems with eating rations is that it gets boring. Monotony and lack of time to eat contribute to decreased ration intake and weight loss.

Weight loss in the field is common and may impair mental and physical performance.

Therefore, it is important that you continue to consume your daily field ration so you can continue to perform.

Eat at least part of each ration item
to get all essential nutrients

Limit your use of non-issue food items as meal/ration substitutes since they may be lacking in several important nutrients. Use these items as snacks to supplement your daily rations. Also pack high carbohydrate items, such as crackers, dried fruits, trail mixes, sports bars, etc. (see Chapter 7 for snack ideas). Experiment beforehand to see what suits you best. If you are planning to use high-CHO bars, check the fat content because if the fat content is greater than 3 g/100 calories it slows down absorption and can cause cramps.

If possible, drink 25 to 60 g of CHO/hr
to maintain blood glucose.

Dehydration

You will become dehydrated if sweat and urine losses are not replaced by drinking water and other beverages (see Chapters 6 and 14). Dehydration may occur at any temperature and even under conditions of low levels of physical activity. Mild dehydration can decrease appetite and cause lethargy. Moderate dehydration decreases work capacity and severe dehydration could be fatal, as shown in the figure on the next page.

Effects of Dehydration on Body Functions

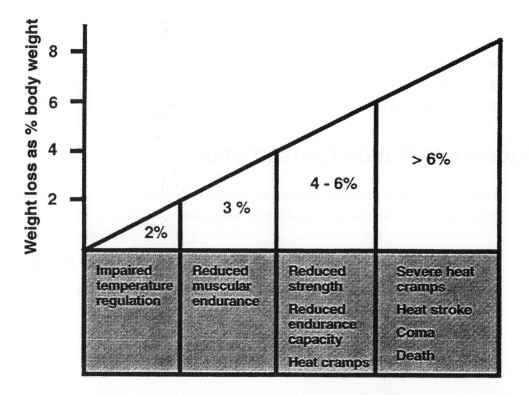

> **Drink water/fluids during water breaks.**
> **You should drink at least 4 canteens per**
> **day, or more if you are in a hot environment.**

See Chapters 6 and 14 for more information on fluid replacement.

Monitor the color of your urine; if your urine is dark, increase fluid consumption until the color becomes pale yellow. If you are taking B vitamin supplements, your urine may not be pale but bright yellow.

Gastrointestinal Complaints

Change in diet, dehydration, too much fiber, poor sanitary conditions or stress may result in diarrhea or constipation in the field. Make sure you are well hydrated at all times, and avoid trying new non-issue foods unless they have passed sanitation inspection.

Dietary Considerations for Selected Training and Mission Scenarios

Developing sound nutritional plans for specific training and mission scenarios should improve your performance. Sample nutrition plans will be provided for the following training scenarios.

- ◆ Platoon/compound work
- ◆ SDV sub trips
- ◆ Typical land warfare
- ◆ Double dive days
- ◆ BUDS Phases 1, 2, and 3

For each scenario, the macronutrient recommendation assumes an energy requirement of 4,000 kcal/day. If your energy requirements are lower or higher, you will need to alter the amounts of CHO, protein, and fat accordingly. **The timing and/or nutrient amount at any particular time can be modified to suit your individual needs based on the scenario and your personal experiences.** Snacks refers to food and beverages that can be carried and consumed while on the go.

Table 11-1. SEAL Team Platoon/Compound Work

This scenario requires small meals throughout the day to help maintain blood sugar and energy levels. Remember to drink fluids regularly.

	CHO	Protein (grams)	Fat
0530 - Wake up			
0600 - CHO/ prot beverage	50	10	-
0700-830 - Work out			
0830 - Breakfast	125	25	25
0900 - Start department/ Platoon work			
1000 - Snack	50	10	10
1130 - Break for lunch	125	30	35
1230 - Return for department/ Platoon work			
1400 - Snack	50	5	10
1600 - End work day			
1700 - Possible second work out			
1830-1900 - Dinner	150	30	35
2200 - Snack	50	10	10
TOTAL	600	120	125
% of 4000 calories	60%	12%	28%

Table 11-2. SDV Sub Trip

These maneuvers can cover 18–20 hours/day for several days; this makes recovery a crucial aspect of continued, optimal performance. Nutritional preparedness for this scenario includes replenishing glycogen stores and being well hydrated at all times.

	CHO	Protein (grams)	Fat
0700 - Breakfast	125	30	20
0830 - Rig Zodiacs for Sub Lock Out			
1000 - Snack	50	10	5
1200 - Lunch	125	30	20
1400 - Brief			
1600 - CHOW	125	25	15
1700 - Jock up			
1800 - Dive			
1900 - Begin Lock Out of Sub op to Beach			
2200 - CHO Beverage	50	10	5
2400 - Beverage	50	10	-
0200 - Beverage	50	10	-
0400 - Dive - Lock In			
0600 - De- jock/ Clean up			
0630 - Snack	75	25	25
TOTAL	650	150	90
% of 4000 calories	65%	15%	20%

Table 11-3. Typical Land Warfare

Typical land warfare operations can continue for 3 to 4 weeks, so it is important to avoid losing weight during this period. Eat CHO snacks with some protein when you feel drowsy (see Chapter 7 for snack ideas).

	CHO	Protein (grams)	Fat
0800 - (PT/ Breakfast)	125	20	15
0900 - Muster			
0930 - Range (Hot environment- 1600 Shooting and moving in combat gear)			
1030 - Snack	50	10	5
1200 - Lunch	125	20	20
1400 - Snack	50	10	5
1600 - Dinner/ rest	125	30	30
1900 - Snack	50	10	5
2100 - Range (Late night fire 2400 and movement)			
2200 - Snack	50	10	5
2400 - Cut loose			
2400 - Snack	75	10	15
2430 - Clean weapons			
TOTAL	650	120	100
% of 4000 calories	65%	12%	23%

Table 11-4. Double Dive Day (for 3 weeks)

Double dive day series which continue for 3 weeks require adequate recovery between dives. Water operations are associated with high energy expenditure and fluid losses, especially when in cold water (see Chapter 14).

	CHO	Protein (grams)	Fat
0600-CHO/prot beverage	50	10	-
0630-0800 - Physical training			
0800- Breakfast	100	20	5
0830-1000 - Classroom/dive prep			
1000-1200 - Dive			
1100- Snack	50	10	-
1200-1330 - Lunch	150	40	40
1330-1600 - Class/gear prep			
1430- Snack	50	10	5
1600-1730 - Dinner	75	20	15
1800-2400 - Brief dive, downstage			
2000-CHO/prot beverage	50	10	-
2200-CHO/prot beverage	50	10	-
2400- Snack	75	20	25
2400-0600 - Personal time			
TOTAL	650	150	90
% of 4000 calories	65%	15%	20%

Table 11-5. Typical BUDs Training Day—1ˢᵗ Phase

Phase I training at BUDs is grueling. Many trainees drop-out because they cannot manage the physical and psychological demands; eating to win may help them succeed. Importantly, the energy expended requires a matching energy input. Some suggestions for timing and distribution of energy are provided in this table.

	CHO	Protein (grams)	Fat
0600-0730 - Breakfast	100	15	10
0745-0930 - Obstacle Course			
0930-CHO/prot beverage	50	10	-
0930-1030 - Classroom			
1030-1130 - Conditioning run			
1130-1300 Lunch	150	40	40
1300-1330 - Classroom - Dive Brief			
1330-1600 - 1 mile Bay Swim without Fins			
1600-1800 - Dinner	150	40	45
2000-2100- Snack	100	15	25
2200-CHO/prot beverage	50	10	-
TOTAL	600	130	120
% of 4000 calories	60%	13%	27%

Table 11-6. Typical BUDs Training Day—2nd Phase

Phase 2 training which involves multiple bouts of physical activity each day makes recovery between bouts an important aspect of optimizing physical performance. Make sure you are well hydrated at all times.

	CHO	Protein (grams)	Fat
0600-0730 - Breakfast	100	20	15
0730-0800 - Pre-Dive			
0800-CHO/ prot beverage	50	10	-
0800-0900 - Dive Brief			
0900-1130 - Dive			
1130-CHO/ prot beverage	50	10	-
1130-1300 - Lunch	125	40	40
1300-1430 - Post/Pre-Dive			
1430-1630 - PT-Run	50	10	5
1630-1800 - Dinner	125	20	25
1800-1900 - Dive Brief			
1900-2130- Dive			
2130-CHO/prot beverage	100	20	-
2130-2230 - Post Dive			
2230-Snack	75	20	25
TOTAL	600	150	110
% of 4000 calories	60%	15%	25%

Table 11-7. Typical BUDs Training Day—3rd Phase

In this situation you would want to eat a light lunch to avoid feeling uncomfortable during the 6-mile run. Instead, drink a CHO-containing beverage or eat a high-CHO snack (see Chapter 7) while at the pistol range. As in every scenario, here too it is important to be well hydrated at all times (see Chapter 6).

	CHO	Protein (grams)	Fat
0600-0700 - Breakfast	100	20	30
0700-1200 - Pistol Range			
0900-CHO/ prot beverage	50	10	-
1000-CHO/ prot beverage	50	10	-
1200-1300 - Lunch	100	20	15
1300-1500 -DEMO classroom			
1500-1600 - Conditioning run (6 miles)			
1600-CHO /protein beverage	100	20	-
1600-1630 - Transit locations			
1630-1730 - Dinner	125	45	45
1730-2000 - Review (classroom)			
2200-Snack	75	25	20
TOTAL	600	150	110
% of 4000 calories	60%	15%	25%

Other Considerations

For all of the sample scenarios, the following recommendations apply:

◆ Eat a variety of foods
◆ Maintain energy balance
◆ Maintain hydration status
◆ Include high-CHO snacks in between meals to replenish/maximize glycogen stores (especially if there are two periods of high activity)
◆ See Chapter 14 for additional considerations about training or operating in the heat, cold, and other adverse conditions.

Dietary Composition

The breakdown of energy from CHO, protein, and fat should be 60 to 65% from CHO, 10 to 15% from protein, and 20 to 30% from fat. When energy requirements are above 4000 kcal, more fat may be required since it is difficult to get sufficient calories from CHO alone. Recommendations for the approximate gram amounts of CHO, protein, and fat for various energy levels are shown in the following table.

Table 11-8. Recommended Grams of CHO, Protein, and Fat for Various Energy Levels

Energy Level (kcal)	CHO (grams)	Protein (grams)	Fat (grams)
3000	500	110	65
3500	550	115	90
4000	650	125	100
4500	700	135	125
5000	700	160	170

Vitamins and Minerals

As of now there are no definitive recommendations. If you meet your energy requirements from a variety of foods, by including fruits and vegetables, you should be able to meet your vitamin and mineral requirements (see Appendixes 5 and 6). Selected recommendations would be to:

◆ Include foods that are good sources of antioxidants in your daily diet.
◆ If you feel you need to take vitamin and mineral supplements follow the guidelines presented in Chapter 4.
◆ During extended dive series you may want to consider taking a multi-mineral supplement.

Immersion in water, especially cold, can increase urinary losses of magnesium, calcium, zinc, and chromium (see Chapter 4 for safe amounts).

Fluid and Electrolytes

All of the scenarios require adequate fluids. Immersion increases fluid losses and operations in a warm/hot environment deplete body water. Replace electrolytes lost through sweating by consuming a fluid replacement beverage that contains electrolytes or by eating foods that contain these nutrients (see Chapter 12 and Appendix 6).

Forced drinking is highly recommended for all environments since normal thirst mechanisms cannot keep up with increased requirements. See Chapter 6 for the ideal composition of fluid replacement beverages.

Chapter 12
Nutritional Interventions for Mission Recovery

After a mission it is important that you recover quickly and continue to train and prepare for the next mission. A quick recovery will enhance preparedness, boost morale, and help protect you from training injuries. Both rest and nutrition play an important part in the recovery process. In this chapter information about nutritional measures that can help you speed up your recovery after a mission is provided.

Glycogen Restoration

Glycogen depletion is common following prolonged events requiring sustained physical activity. For example, an extended dive, sustained efforts on land, and prolonged shivering can deplete muscle glycogen stores. During recovery it is critical that these stores be repleted, and nutritional interventions can accelerate the process.

Glycogen repletion in muscles takes place at a relatively constant rate as long as blood glucose remains elevated. In other words, blood glucose must be high for it to be made available to muscle for storage.

To optimize glycogen restoration consume 50 grams of carbohydrate (CHO) soon after the completion of the mission, and 50 grams of CHO every two hours for six hours after the mission.

Ingestion of greater amounts of CHO will not further increase the rate of glycogen resynthesis.

Not all CHO foods are equally effective in restoring glucose. Certain foods are better at raising blood glucose concentrations and promoting glycogen synthesis. The term *Glycemic Index* is used to describe how high a particular food will raise blood glucose levels; foods with a high glycemic index (*GI*) are the most effective for glycogen restoration. Thus, after a mission, consume foods and beverages that have a moderate to high *GI*. A list of foods classified according to their *GI* is provided on the next page.

GLYCOGEN REPLETE MUSCLE

GLYCOGEN DEPLETED MUSCLE

Table 12-1. A Selection of Foods with a High, Moderate, or Low Glycemic Index

Foods	Amount of Food Required for 50 grams of CHO
Highly Glycemic Foods	
Bagel	1.3 bagel
Bread (white or whole wheat)	4.2 slices
Cornflakes	2.5 cups
Honey	2.9 tbsp
Maple syrup	3.1 tbsp
Potato, baked w/skin	1 medium
Raisins	0.4 cup
Shredded Wheat Cereal	1.4 cups
Sweet Corn, cooked	1.5 cups
Watermelon	4.5 cups
Moderately Glycemic Foods	
Baked Beans	1.0 cup
Banana	1.8 medium
Grapes	55 grapes
Oatmeal, cooked	2.0 cups
Orange Juice	2.0 cups
Rice, cooked	1 cup
Sweet Potato, boiled	0.8 cup

Foods	Amount of Food Required for 50 grams of CHO
Low Glycemic Foods	
Apple	2.5 medium
Peaches	5 medium
Pear	2 medium
Green Peas, cooked	2.2 cups
Ice Cream	1.6 cups
Spaghetti and Other Pasta, cooked	1.4 cups
Yogurt, nonfat plain	2.9 cups

Rehydration

Begin rehydrating immediately after the mission.

After a mission, forced fluid ingestion is essential because the sensation of thirst may be blunted. **Typically, voluntary consumption of fluids will restore only half of the fluid lost.** If possible, weigh yourself after the mission and compare this weight to your usual weight. Over a period of several hours you should:

Drink at least two 8 oz. cups of fluid for every pound of body weight lost.

Fluid replacement beverages ingested during exercise are also appropriate for rehydration. Fluids used for rehydration after a mission can contain a higher percentage of CHO than those used during exercise. A list of various fluid replacement beverages and more information on fluid replacement techniques is provided in Chapter 6.

Sodium/Electrolyte Replacement

Sodium and potassium losses in sweat can be quite high during prolonged physical activity, especially in warm weather. Replacing these electrolytes is an important part of the recovery process. Most commercially available fluid replacement beverages contain electrolytes. Also, sodium is widely present in a variety of foods, but if the weather is warm:

Each quart of fluid should contain about one quarter teaspoon of salt.

A little bit of salt will speed up rehydration better than plain water. Typically, commercial fluid replacement beverages contain both sodium and potassium, but your recovery foods should also include foods rich in potassium. Some excellent food sources of potassium are listed below and additional information is provided in Appendix 6. You will notice that these foods are also good sources of CHO and most have a moderate to high glycemic index.

Table 12-2. Good Sources Of Potassium

Foods	Beverages
Banana	Orange juice
Apricots, dried	Tomato juice
Dates	Pineapple juice
Dried peaches	Grapefruit juice
Melons	Skim Milk
Baked potato	
Yogurt	

NOTE: 1 cup of orange juice or tomato juice will replace the potassium, calcium, and magnesium lost in 3 quarts of sweat.

Summary

- High-CHO foods and beverages are ideal recovery foods
- Consume 50 grams of CHO as food or drink immediately after mission completion and 50 grams every 2 hours for 6 hours
- Choose foods and drinks with a moderate to high glycemic index to accelerate glycogen repletion
- Drink plenty of fluids after a gruelling mission, even if you are not thirsty
- Your fluid replacement beverages should contain sodium and potassium

- Fruit juices are excellent recovery fluids as they provide CHO, vitamins, minerals, sodium, and potassium
- If you can't tolerate solid foods after intense physical exertion, drink a CHO-containing beverage (see Chapters 6 and 9 for additional information on CHO-containing beverages)

Chapter 13
Food for the Field: Military and Other Rations

Field rations are designed to supply adequate energy and nutrients for a particular type of mission. Since the duration and environmental conditions of missions vary, different types of operational rations have been developed. For example, there are cold-weather rations for frigid conditions, and lightweight rations for missions lasting no longer than 30 days. These rations have different caloric contents with varying proportions of fat, protein, and carbohydrate to meet the nutritional demands of the various conditions. This chapter describes what rations are available and compares some military and commercially prepared foods. You can decide where your money would best be spent after comparing their distribution of calories.

The Meal, Ready-to-Eat, Individual (MRE) Menus

Many people think that military rations are sub-optimal: Not enough calories, too much fat, bad taste, and too much salt are some claims leveled against military rations. The revised Meal, Ready-To-Eat, Individual (MRE) ration consists of 12 meals (see next page for menus); each meal, or menu, contains an entree, crackers, a spread (cheese, peanut butter, or jelly), a dessert, beverages, and an accessory package. No rehydration of these meals is necessary. This ration will certainly keep you going and based on your energy requirements you will need to eat 2 to 4 MREs per day.

Each menu provides 1300 Calories
49% CHO, 15% protein, 36% fat
Supplemental Bread Pouch: 200 Calories
55% CHO, 12% protein, 33% fat,

It is also important to note that some components of the MRE have been supplemented with selected vitamins (A, B_1, B_2, niacin, B_6, and C) and minerals (calcium). Fortified items include cocoa beverage powder, cheese spread, peanut butter, crackers, oatmeal cookies coating, and brownies coating.

Table 13-1. MRE Menus

MENU 1	MENU 2	MENU 3	MENU 4	MENU 5	MENU 6
Pork W/Rice In BBQ Sauce	Corned Beef Hash	Chicken Stew	Omelet w/Ham	Spaghetti w/ Meat & Sauce	Chicken A La King
Apple sauce[1]	Fruit[2]	Fruit[1]	Potato Au Gratin	Fruit[2]	
	Oatmeal Cookie Bar		Oatmeal Cookie Bar	Maple Nut Cake	
Jelly	Jelly	Peanut Butter	Cheese Spread	Cheese Spread	Peanut Butter
Crackers	Crackers	Crackers	Crackers	Crackers	Crackers
				Candy[3]	Candy[3]
Cocoa Beverage	Cocoa Beverage	Cocoa Beverage	Cocoa Beverage		Cocoa Beverage
Beverage Powder	Beverage Powder	Beverage Powder	Beverage Powder	Beverage Powder	Beverage Powder
Hot Sauce	Hot Sauce	Hot Sauce	Hot Sauce	Hot Sauce	Hot Sauce
Packet B	Packet B	Packet B	Packet B	Packet A	Packet A
Spoon	Spoon	Spoon	Spoon	Spoon	Spoon

MENU 7	MENU 8	MENU 9	MENU 10	MENU 11	MENU 12
Beef Stew	Ham Slice	Meatballs & Rice in Spicy Tomato Sauce	Tuna w/ Noodles	Chicken w/ Rice	Escalloped Potatoes w/ Ham
	Potato Au Gratin	Fruit[2]			Apple sauce[1]
Cherry Nut Cake	Brownie, Chocolate Covered	Cookie, Chocolate Covered	Chocolate Nut Cake	Cookie, Chocolate Covered	Brownie, Chocolate Covered
Peanut Butter	Jelly	Peanut Butter	Cheese Spread	Cheese Spread	Jelly
Crackers	Crackers	Crackers	Crackers	Crackers	Crackers
				Candy	Candy
	Cocoa Beverage				Cocoa Beverage
Beverage Powder	Beverage Powder	Beverage Powder	Beverage Powder	Beverage Powder	Beverage Powder
Hot Sauce	Hot Sauce	Hot Sauce	Hot Sauce	Hot Sauce	Hot Sauce
Packet A	Packet A	Packet A	Packet A	Packet A	Packet A
Spoon	Spoon	Spoon	Spoon	Spoon	Spoon

Packet A: Coffee, Cream Substitute, Sugar, Salt, Chewing Gum, Matches, Toilet Tissue, Towelette

Packet B: Coffee, Cream Substitute, Sugar, Salt, Chewing Gum, Matches, Toilet Tissue, Towelette, Candy (Vanilla Caramels, Tootsie Rolls, or Heat Stable Chocolate Bar)

[1]Thermostablized;

[2]Freeze-Dried Fruit: Peaches, Pears, Fruit Mix, or Strawberries

[3]Charms or Heat Stable M&M's

Ration, Cold Weather (RCW)

The Ration, Cold Weather (RCW) was designed to sustain individuals during operations in cold conditions. The six menus should provide sufficient calories to meet energy requirements during strenuous exercises in extreme cold. The ration is high in carbohydrate (CHO) since this macronutrient generates more heat, and comes as two meal bags, Bag A and Bag B. Each menu is sufficient for a 24 hour period, but more can be eaten when energy needs are higher. The RCW is also lower in salt and protein than the MREs to reduce daily water requirements and lessen the possibility of dehydration. If consumed hydrated, one day's ration requires 90 ounces (about 9 cups or 3 canteens) of water. Although it could get very boring, it will definitely help maintain your performance.

Each menu provides 4500 Calories

60% CHO, 8% protein, 32% fat

Sodium content: 5 grams

Table 13-2. Ration, Cold Weather Menus

	MENU 1	MENU 2	MENU 3	MENU 4	MENU 5	MENU 6
BAG A	Oatmeal, Strawberry & Cream	Oatmeal, Apple & Cinnamon	Oatmeal, Apple & Cinnamon	Oatmeal, Maple & Brown Sugar	Oatmeal, Strawberry & Cream	Oatmeal, Maple & Brown Sugar
	Nut Raisin Mix	Nut Raisin Mix	Nut Raisin Mix	Nut Raisin Mix	Nut Raisin Mix	Nut Raisin Mix
	Cocoa Beverage Powder (2)	Cocoa Beverage Powder (2)	Cocoa Beverage Powder (2)	Cocoa Beverage Powder (2)	Cocoa Beverage Powder (2)	Cocoa Beverage Powder (2)
	Apple Cider Mix	Apple Cider Mix	Apple Cider Mix	Apple Cider Mix	Apple Cider Mix	Apple Cider Mix
	Chicken Noodle Soup	Chicken Noodle Soup	Chicken Noodle Soup	Chicken Noodle Soup	Chicken Noodle Soup	Chicken Noodle Soup
	Fruit Bars, (Fig or Blueberry)	Fruit Bars, (Fig or Blueberry)	Fruit Bars, (Fig or Blueberry)	Fruit Bars, (Fig or Blueberry)	Fruit Bars, (Fig or Blueberry)	Fruit Bars, (Fig or Blueberry)
	Crackers (2)	Crackers (2)	Crackers (2)	Crackers (2)	Crackers (2)	Crackers (2)
	Spoon	Spoon	Spoon	Spoon	Spoon	Spoon
	Accessory Packet	Accessory Packet	Accessory Packet	Accessory Packet	Accessory Packet	Accessory Packet

Table 13-2. Ration, Cold Weather Menus

	MENU 1	MENU 2	MENU 3	MENU 4	MENU 5	MENU 6
BAG B	Chicken Stew	Beef Stew	Chili Con Carne	Chicken A La King	Chicken & Rice	Spaghetti w/ Meat Sauce
	Granola Bars (2)	Granola Bars (2)	Granola Bars (2)	Granola Bars (2)	Granola Bars (2)	Granola Bars (2)
	Oatmeal Cookie Bars (2)	Oatmeal Cookie Bars (2)	Oatmeal Cookie Bars (2)	Oatmeal Cookie Bars (2)	Oatmeal Cookie Bars (2)	Oatmeal Cookie Bars (2)
	Chocolate Covered Cookie or Brownie	Chocolate Covered Cookie or Brownie	Chocolate Covered Cookie or Brownie	Chocolate Covered Cookie or Brownie	Chocolate Covered Cookie or Brownie	Chocolate Covered Cookie or Brownie
	Orange Beverage Powder	Orange Beverage Powder	Orange Beverage Powder	Orange Beverage Powder	Orange Beverage Powder	Orange Beverage Powder
	Tootsie Rolls	Tootsie Rolls	Tootsie Rolls	Tootsie Rolls	Tootsie Rolls	Tootsie Rolls
	M&M's	M&M's	M&M's	M&M's	M&M's	M&M's
	Lemon Tea (2)	Lemon Tea (2)	Lemon Tea (2)	Lemon Tea (2)	Lemon Tea (2)	Lemon Tea (2)
	Spoon	Spoon	Spoon	Spoon	Spoon	Spoon

Accessory Packet: Coffee, Cream, Sugar, Chewing Gum, Toilet Paper (2), Matches, Closure Device (2)

Ration Lightweight - 30 Days (RLW-30)

This ration was designed for individuals of the Special Operation Forces who might participate in reconnaissance missions of up to 30 days. Thus, it is as it's name: a low-weight, low-volume ration. There are six menus, each consisting of dehydrated, compressed, and "low water containing" foods. The foods may be eaten dry or reconstituted with water.

Each menu provides 2132 Calories

52% CHO, 18% protein, 30% fat

Sodium content: 5 grams

If this ration is used during extended operations, more CHO would be needed to obtain the recommended amount (at least 400 grams); it provides only 277 grams as is.

Table 13-3. Ration Lightweight Menus

MENU 1	MENU 2	MENU 3	MENU 4	MENU 5	MENU 6
Chicken A La King	Beef Stew	Pork with Rice	Chicken w/ Rice & Ham	Spaghetti with Meat & Sauce	Chili Con Carne
Cheese Bread Crisp	Tamale Bread Crisp	Pizza Bread Crisp	Cheese-Bacon Bread Crisp	Coconut Bread Crisp	Orange-Nut Bread Crisp
Almond Dairy Bar	Strawberry Dairy Bar	Pecan Dairy Bar	Orange Creamsicle Dairy Bar	Mixed Nut Dairy Bar	Maple Walnut Dairy Bar
Blueberry Dessert Bar	Chocolate Chip Dessert Bar	Apple Cinnamon Dessert Bar	Pecan Dessert Bar	Chocolate Halva Dessert Bar	Graham Dessert Bar
Shredded Wheat Cereal Bar	Wheat Flake Cereal Bar	Bran Flake Cereal Bar	Oat Cereal Biscuit Bar	Malted Wheat Granules Cereal Bar	Com Flakes Cereal Bar
Tropical Punch Bar	Lemonade Beverage Bar	Orange Beverage Bar	Lemon-Lime Beverage Bar	Strawberry Beverage Bar	Raspberry Beverage Bar
Cocoa Beverage Bar	Cocoa Beverage Bar	Cocoa Beverage Bar	Cocoa Beverage Bar	Cocoa Beverage Bar	Cocoa Beverage Bar
Beef Snacks	Beef Snacks	Beef Snacks	Beef Snacks	Beef Snacks	Beef Snacks

Accessory Packet (5/case): Instant Coffee (6), Cream Substitute (3), Sugar (3), Chewing Gum (6), Instant Tea (6), Matches (2), Toilet Tissue (6), Plastic Picnic Spoon (2), Closure Device (1).

Food Packet, Long Range Patrol, (Improved) (LRP[I])

This ration was designed for special operations and initial assaults and has a shelf life of 10 years. The eight menus, which have been revised significantly since the ration was used during the Vietnam war, consist of dehydrated entrees, cereal bars, candy, and instant beverages. Each menu requires approximately 28 oz. of water to prepare, although some of the foods may be eaten dry. It is lightweight, has proven acceptance, and is relatively inexpensive.

> ## Each LRP[I] menu provides 1570 Calories
> ## 50% CHO, 15% protein, 35% fat
> ## Sodium content: 2.6 grams

To obtain adequate CHO and calories during extended operations, at least two menus would need to be eaten; one menu provides only 195 grams of CHO as is.

Table 13-4. Long Range Patrol (LRP[I])

MENU 1	MENU 2	MENU 3	MENU 4
Chicken Stew	Beef Stew	Escalloped Potato &Pork	Chicken in White Sauce w/ Vegetables
Cornflake Bar	Granola Bar	Cornflake & Rice Bar	Cornflake Bar
Oatmeal Cookie Bar	Chocolate Covered Cookie	Fig Bar	Chocolate Covered Cookie
Tootsie Rolls (4)	Caramels	Chocolate Bars w/ Toffee (2)	Chuckles
Apple Cider Drink	Cocoa Beverage	Apple Cider Drink	Orange Beverage
Spoon	Spoon	Spoon	Spoon
Accessory Packet	Accessory Packet	Accessory Packet	Accessory Packet

MENU 5	MENU 6	MENU 7	MENU 8
Chicken & Rice	Spaghetti w/ Meat Sauce	Chili Con Carne	Beef & Rice
Granola Bar	Cornflake & Rice Bar	Granola Bar	Cornflake Bar
Chocolate Covered Brownie	Oatmeal Cookie Bar	Chocolate Covered Brownie	Fig Bar
Chuckles	Tootsie Rolls (4)	Charms	M&M's
Lemon Tea (2)	Beverage Base (MRE)	Orange Beverage	Lemon Tea (2)
Accessory Packet	Accessory Packet	Accessory Packet	Accessory Packet
Spoon	Spoon	Spoon	Spoon

Accessory Packet: Coffee, Creamer, Sugar, Chewing Gum, Toilet Paper (2), Matches, Salt

Commercial Freeze-Dried Products

Lightweight, freeze-dried foods are commercially available from a number of manufacturers. Two of the most popular manufacturers are Mountain House and AlpineAire. As with any food manufacturer, their products differ in terms of taste, caloric distribution, protein, and sodium content. Many of the items from both companies have been tested under field conditions for up to 30 days, and the acceptability varied from person to person. Choose a ration that will provide adequate calories and CHO to fit your requirements.

Table 13-5. Here's a Look at Two Similar Dinner Entrees from the Two Companies:

Menu: Chili

Macronutrients	Mountain House	AlpineAire
Total Calories	220	340
% Fat	25%	5%
% Protein	22%	28%
% CHO	55%	64%

Menu: Beef Stroganoff

Macronutrients	Mountain House	AlpineAire
Total Calories	250	306
% Fat	43%	18%
% Protein	14%	29%
% CHO	43%	59%

Note the differences in total calories and the distribution of calories. For example, Mountain House Beef Stroganoff provides 8.8 grams of protein whereas AlpineAire's Beef Stroganoff provides 22 grams. This shows how important it is to check the nutritional listing on the package label. A variety of other meals and their macronutrient distribution is provided on the following pages.

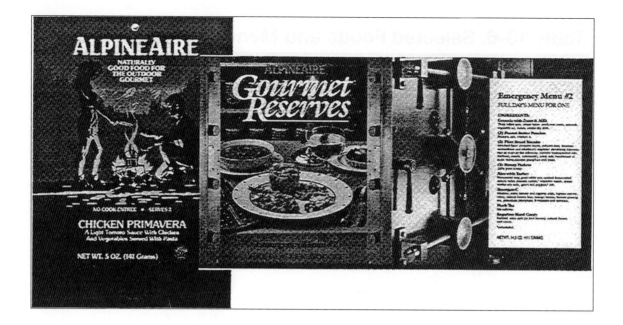

Table 13-6. Selected Foods and Menus from AlpineAire

Items	Serving Size	Calories per Serving	CHO (grams)	Protein (grams)	Fat (grams)	Sodium (mg)
	ENTREES					
MOUNTAIN CHILI	3.5 oz.	340	54	24	2	1,334
LEONARDO DA FETTUCINE	2.75 oz.	295	45	15	3	686
CHEESE NUT CASSEROLE	3.25 oz.	372	62	16	16	1,073
SPAGHETTI w/ MUSHROOMS	2.75 oz.	257	50	18	1	746
PASTA ROMA	3 oz.	328	47	18	1	686
WHOLEWHEAT PASTA STEW	3 oz.	275	57	10	1	652
MUSHROOM PILAF W/ VEGETABLES	3.5 oz.	373	77	41	2	2,196

Table 13-6. Selected Foods and Menus from AlpineAire

Items	Serving Size	Calories per Serving	CHO (grams)	Protein (grams)	Fat (grams)	Sodium (mg)
WILD RICE PILAF W/ALMONDS	3 oz.	291	89	10	6	1,233
SHRIMP NEWBURG	3 oz.	318	49	16	6	538
SHRIMP ALFREDO	2.75 oz.	300	44	18	3	641
TUNA & NOODLES W/CHEESE	2.75 oz.	325	39	23	7	1,129
CHICKEN ROTELLE	3 oz.	311	63	25	3	875
SIERRA CHICKEN	3 oz.	297	50	18	2	671
ALMOND CHICKEN	3.5 oz.	395	59	21	7	930
CHICKEN PRIMAVERA	2.5 oz.	266	43	17	2	924
BROWN RICE & CHICKEN W/ VEGETABLES	3.25 oz.	318	52	17	4	1,230
WILD TYME TURKEY	3.25 oz.	346	51	18	6	864
MASHED POTATOES & GRAVY W/ TURKEY	2.8 oz.	284	54	11	1	745
TERIYAKI TURKEY	2.75 oz.	279	46	16	2	929
BEEF STROGANOFF W/NOODLES	2.75 oz.	306	45	22	6	858
COUNTRY BEAN & BEEF CASSEROLE	3 oz.	282	40	24	4	1,184
BEEF ROTINI	2.75 oz.	357	58	21	5	466

SIDE DISHES

Items	Serving Size	Calories per Serving	CHO (grams)	Protein (grams)	Fat (grams)	Sodium (mg)
VEGETABLE MIX	0.75 oz.	71	16	3	0.4	65
GARDEN VEGETABLES	0.75 oz.	79	17	4	0.5	20

Table 13-6. Selected Foods and Menus from AlpineAire

Items	Serving Size	Calories per Serving	CHO (grams)	Protein (grams)	Fat (grams)	Sodium (mg)
POTATOES & CHEDDAR W/ CHIVES	2 oz.	232	35	8	7	207
PEAS	0.75 oz.	81	14	6	0.4	2
SWEET CORN	0.75 oz.	85	20	3	1	
PINTO BEANS	1.25 oz.	97	18	6	0.4	3
BROCCOLI	0.25 oz.	25	5	3	0.2	12
CARROTS	0.8 oz.	71	17	2	0.3	58
WILD RICE	1 oz.	106	22	4	0.3	1
BROWN RICE	1 oz.	77	17	2	0.4	0.5
MASHED POTATOES	1.75 oz.	181	42	3.5	0.3	5.25
DICED TURKEY	0.5 oz.	80	-	13	1	-
DICED CHICKEN	0.5 oz.	80	-	13	1	-
DICED BEEF	0.5 oz.	106	-	15	5	30
TOMATO DICES	2 oz..	43	10	2	1	18
MUSHROOMS	0.5 oz.	28	4	3	-	15
SWEET BELL PEPPER COMBO	1 oz.	45	55	2	0.5	23
ONIONS	1.5 oz.	74	17	2	-	19
TOMATO POWDER	2 oz.	104	22	5	1	14
CHEDDAR CHEESE POWDER	2 oz.	164	1	11	14	397

SOUPS

Items	Serving Size	Calories per Serving	CHO (grams)	Protein (grams)	Fat (grams)	Sodium (mg)
ALPINE MINESTRONE	1.75 oz.	159	33	7	2	629
MULTI BEAN SOUP	1.75 oz.	140	27	9	0.5	823

Table 13-6. Selected Foods and Menus from AlpineAire

Items	Serving Size	Calories Per Serving	CHO (grams)	Protein (grams)	Fat (grams)	Sodium (mg)
CREAMY POTATO CHEDDAR SOUP	2 oz.	225	33	9	7	864
CREAM OF BROCCOLI SOUP	1.25 oz.	143	19	6	5	861
BREAKFAST ITEMS						
BLUEBERRY PANCAKES	3.25 oz.	369	63	6	8	0.2
PURE MAPLE SYRUP GRANULES	1.25 oz.	95	24	—	—	1
RANCH OMELET W/BEEF	2.25 oz.	399	12	2	25	542
SCRAMBLING & OMELET EGGS	2 oz.	308	10	20	21	433
BLUEBERRY HONEY GRANOLA & MILK	3.25 oz.	367	54	15	11	2
STRAWBERRY HONEY GRANOLA & MILK	3.25 oz.	367	54	15	11	2
FRUITS AND DESSERTS						
APPLE ALMOND CRISP	2.5 oz.	275	44	6	10	2
APPLESAUCE W/ CINNAMON	1.25 oz.	125	33	0.5	0.8	3
REALAPPLE-BLUEBERRY FRUIT COBBLER	2 oz.	210	46	2	2	2
STRAWBERRIES	0.5 oz.	55	-	1	0.6	30
BLUEBERRIES	0.5 oz.	60	15	0.7	0.5	1

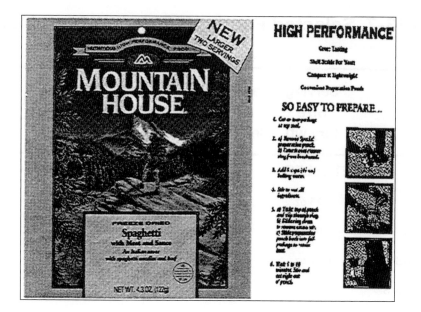

Table 13-7. Selected Foods and Menus from Mountain House

Items	Serving Size (dry wt)	Calories per Serving	CHO (grams)	Protein (grams)	Fat (grams)	Sodium (mg)
BREAKFAST ENTREES						
PRECOOKED EGGS W/BACON	1.3 oz.	190	6	12	13	920
GRANOLA W/ BLUEBERRIES & MILK	2.0 oz.	270	38	8	10	60
CHEESE OMELETTE	1.2 oz.	180	8	13	9	600
EGGS W/BACON	1.1 oz.	160	6	10	11	750
HASH BROWN POTATOES	2.5 oz.	150	36	2	0	80
BEEF SAUSAGE PATTIES	0.55 oz.	80	0	8	5	250

Table 13-7. Selected Foods and Menus from Mountain House

Items	Serving Size (dry wt)	Calories per Serving	CHO (grams)	Protein (grams)	Fat (grams)	Sodium (mg)
VEGETABLES						
CORN	0.75 oz.	90	18	2	1	1
GREEN PEAS	0.55 oz.	70	12	4	1	90
GREEN BEANS	0.21 oz.	35	6	1	0	1
FRUIT & SNACKS						
NUT CHOCOLATE LURPS	1.5 oz.	250	18	6	17	75
FRUIT CRISPS-STRAWBERRIES	0.5 oz.	60	13	1	1	0
FRUIT CRISPS-PEACHES	0.55 oz.	60	15	0	0	5
FRUIT CRISPS-MIXED FRUIT	0.55 oz.	60	15	0	0	5
FRUIT CRISPS - PEARS	0.5 oz.	60	14	0	0	0
MAIN COURSE ENTREES						
CHICKEN POLYNESIAN	1.75 oz.	210	33	10	4	810
GREEN PEPPER & ONION SAUCE W/ BEEF & RICE	1.9 oz.	230	32	10	7	1200
LASAGNA W/ MEAT & SAUCE	1.8 oz.	240	23	14	10	630
CHILI MAC W/ BEEF	1.8 oz.	220	30	12	6	540
BEEF STROGANOFF	1.8 oz.	250	27	9	12	750
BEEF BOURGUIGNON	2.0 oz.	280	20	20	13	880
BEEF STEW	1.68 oz.	260	26	16	9	820

Table 13-7. Selected Foods and Menus from Mountain House

Items	Serving Size (dry wt)	Calories per Serving	CHO (grams)	Protein (grams)	Fat (grams)	Sodium (mg)
SPAGHETTI W/ MEAT & SAUCE	1.7 oz.	220	27	10	8	940
CHICKEN STEW	1.8 oz.	230	30	9	8	1200
TURKEY TETRAZINI	1.6 oz.	210	21	13	8	1150
CHICKEN A LA KING	2.38 oz.	300	33	18	10	1350
SWEET & SOUR PORK W/RICE	2.3 oz.	270	44	12	6	730
VEGETABLE STEW W/BEEF	1.7 oz.	230	27	11	7	580
BEEF & RICE W/ ONIONS	2.4 oz.	330	42	11	12	1300
RICE & CHICKEN	2.4 oz.	400	41	13	13	1170
CHILI W/BEANS	2.3 oz.	310	30	16	14	950
NOODLES & CHICKEN	1.75 oz.	200	28	13	4	970

What Do You Choose?

The next question you should ask is: Given this information, which is the best product for me to eat during a particular mission scenario? What foods will most impact my performance? The best way to answer that question is to figure out what your expected caloric expenditure will be and what kinds of foods you like! The ration for any mission that involves high activity should provide at least 400 grams of CHO.

Look over some of the food selections provided. What is important is that you eat and drink. Compare the military and commercial foods, and try setting up a menu plan that fits both your personal tastes and energy requirements. The military RCW caloric distribution is a good model to follow, and is an acceptable alternative to store-bought lightweight foods.

The Table below provides sample menus for two days; each menu supplies about 4,500 kcal. Use these menus as a template. Other food choices in the preceding tables can be substituted accordingly. There are many types of soups, breakfast products, and dinner entrees to chose from. The important points to remember are:

◆ Get enough CHO

◆ Drink lots of fluid (preferably low caffeine)

◆ Limit sodium and caffeine intake

Table 13-8. Two Sample Daily Menus for High Activity

DAY 1	DAY 2
Breakfasts - ~1500 kcal, 250–270 grams of CHO	
Oatmeal, 3 pkg	Cream of Wheat, 3 pkg
Raisins, 1/2 cup	Honey, 2 tbsp
Cashews, 1/2 cup	Ranch Omelet w/ Beef, 2.5 oz.
Honey, 2 tbsp	Applesauce w/ Cinnamon, 1.25 oz.
Cocoa, 2 cup	Cocoa, 2 cups
Orange Drink, 1 cup	Grapefruit Drink, 2 cups
Lunches - ~ 1600 kcal, 235–250 grams of CHO	
Power Bar, 2.25 oz.	Granola Bars, 1 pkg
Raisins, 1/2 cup	Fig Newtons, 6 each
Peanuts, 1/2 cup	Creamy Potato Cheddar Soup, 2.5 oz.
Minestrone Soup, 3.5 oz.	Beef Jerky, 4 oz.
Exceed/Glucose Polymer Beverage, 1 quart	
Dinners - ~ 1500 kcal, 300 grams of CHO	
Chicken Primavera, 5 oz.	Spaghetti with Mushrooms, 11 oz.
Garden Veggies, 1.5 oz.	Triscuit, 10 each
Apple Almond Crisp 2.5 oz.	Apple/Blueberry Cobbler, 4 oz.
Apple Cider, 2 cups	Apple Cider, 2 cups
Fig Newtons, 6 each	Granola Bars, 1 pkg

An advantage to the military rations is that you don't have to count calories on labels to get the desired caloric distribution. For example: If you are training in a cold weather environment, you know that the RCW has 4,500 kcal/day with an appropriate distribution of calories. There's no need to look at labels three times a day to figure out what you are eating. The time saved by not counting calories may or may not be important to you. However, if you don't like military rations, spend some time developing a meal plan that suits your taste buds, as indicated above. You need to eat on your missions!

Other Ration Information

How Long Will Rations Keep?

As long as the package is left unopened, stored properly in a fairly cool environment (low humidity and less than 80° F), and not handled excessively, most of the military rations will be usable for at least 3 years. The MRE, RLW-30, and RCW all have shelf lives of 3 years. Most commercial foods have expiration dates noted on the packaging, but generally they will also keep for at least 3 years. Mountain House promotes a shelf life of up to 5 years. The ration with the longest shelf life is the improved Long Range Patrol (LRP[I]), which has an estimated life of 10 years at 70 to 80° F.

Rations and Water Requirements

If the rations are prepared as instructed, and you drink fluids as recommended, freeze-dried rations will not increase your need for water. However, if the rations you select contain greater amounts of sodium or protein, you may need additional water.

Chapter 14
Nutritional Considerations for Adverse Conditions

Adverse conditions such as exposure to extreme environments impose considerable physiological demands. The human body responds to adverse conditions by increasing energy expenditure and water losses. If energy and fluid balance is not regained, then performance and perhaps mission integrity can be at stake. In this chapter, information on nutritional interventions that may improve performance or alternatively reduce performance decrements under adverse conditions is presented.

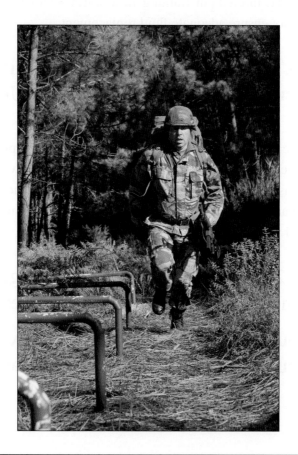

Heat Exposure

Clearly, the major concerns during operations in a warm or hot environment are maintaining fluid and electrolyte balance. Any time you have to work or exercise in the heat, you will lose water and electrolytes through sweating. The amount of sweat produced depends on:

◆ Environmental temperature and humidity
◆ Work rate
◆ Fitness level and acclimatization
◆ Volume and rate of fluid replacement

Working at a high work rate in hot, humid surroundings results in very high fluid and electrolyte losses. You can easily lose one to two quarts per hour and even more when special clothing, such as chemical protective gear, is required. The highest sweating rate ever reported was 4 quarts per hour.

Fluid Needs

Failure to replace fluids lost through sweating will result in dehydration and eventually heat injury (see Chapters 6 and 11 for additional information on dehydration). Forced drinking is recommended throughout training in a warm environment since your normal thirst mechanism will not ensure adequate fluid replacement.

Drink 1 to 3 cups of fluid every 30 minutes.
More than 3 cups per 30 minutes is TOO MUCH to absorb.

It is a good idea to get a body weight prior to starting a prolonged training mission in the heat, and weigh yourself as time permits. This will allow you to determine your sweat rate and help ensure adequate hydration in later training and simulated operations. Remember that your water needs may be higher when you wear chemical protective clothing or other gear when you work in the heat.

Drink 10 to 12 quarts of water per day at regular intervals when working in a hot environment.

One pound of water loss equals approximately 2 cups of water or about 0.475 quarts.

It is estimated that a water loss of 2% body weight can impair physical performance and mood, decrease appetite, and increase the risk of heat injuries. Below is a sample calculation:

If A SEAL weighs 175 pounds
A 2% weight loss would be
175 X 0.02 = 3.5 lbs
Goal: To stay above 171 lbs

A 5% loss of body weight decreases work performance by 30%. This amount of water loss is a serious threat to your health.

Worksheet 14-1. Calculate Your Lower Weight for Fluid Losses

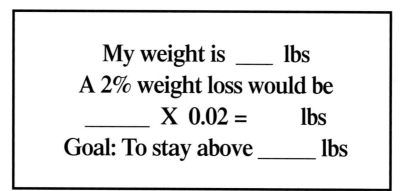

My weight is ____ lbs
A 2% weight loss would be
_____ X 0.02 = ____ lbs
Goal: To stay above _____ lbs

Monitor hydration status by inspecting the color of your urine.

A dark yellow or smelly urine suggests some degree of dehydration; increase fluid consumption until the color becomes pale yellow. If, however, you are taking B vitamins your urine may be not be pale but bright yellow.

Excessive water weight gain can also be a threat to your health. This condition results when individuals drink large amounts of plain water to replace fluid losses during long duration (lasting for 8 or more hours) endurance activities. To prevent overhydration, make sure that you drink beverages that contain electrolytes (sodium and potassium) to replace fluids lost during extended missions.

Electrolyte Balance

It is a fact of life that electrolytes are lost in the sweat, and excessive loss of electrolytes (example: sodium, potassium) can lead to muscle cramping or severe medical problems. However, being in excellent physical condition will help minimize electrolyte losses. The best way to maintain electrolyte balance over prolonged exposure to heat is to drink fluid/ electrolyte replacement beverages.

Table 14-1. Upper Limits for Sodium and Potassium in Fluid Replacement Beverages During Heat Stress

Units	Sodium	Potassium
mg/8 oz.	165	46
mg/L	690	195
mEq/8 oz.	7.2	1.2

Look at the label from the beverage you have selected and be sure it provides no more sodium and potassium than indicated in the chart above. The National Academy of Sciences recommends that chloride be the only "anion" (negatively charged electrolyte) accompanying sodium and potassium, and no other electrolytes are recommended. Typically magnesium and calcium are included, but the amounts are well below recommended upper limits. Finally, after your operations, choose foods that are high in water (Chapter 6 - Fluid Replacement) and foods that are rich in potassium (see Chapter 12 and Appendix 6).

Carbohydrate (CHO) Intake

Fluid replacement beverages with CHO are great during exercises in the heat, but the amount of CHO should be lower than usual so that the fluid/water is rapidly absorbed. Chapter 6 provides a chart showing the concentration of CHO in the beverage to use for maintaining hydration status.

Beverages consumed in the heat should be no more than 8% CHO and 5% CHO is optimal

Energy Intake

Although appetites may be suppressed in hot weather, especially during the first few days after arriving, adequate caloric intake is very important. Inadequate food intake will lead to weight loss which can impair both physical and mental performance. Remember:

Dehydration can result in a loss of appetite.

When you do the same task in a hot environment, energy requirements are slightly increased due to the increased work of maintaining thermal balance. When living/working in temperatures ranging from 86 to 104° F (30 to 40° C) caloric intakes should be increased by 10% as shown below, unless activity level decreases accordingly.

> ## If a SEAL requires 4000 kcal/day
> ## A 10% increase in energy would be
> ## 4000 X 0.10 = 400 kcal/day
> ## Goal: Eat 4400 kcal/day

Worksheet 14-2. Calculate Your Energy Requirements for a Hot Environment

> My energy requirements are: _____
> A 10% increase would be
> _____ X 0.10 = _____
> Goal: To eat _____ kcal/day

TIP: If your activity level decreases you do not need any extra calories.

Other Recommendations:

◆ Eat a high-CHO diet as they are absorbed more readily than fat and protein.

◆ Avoid fatty foods which may not be not well tolerated in the heat.

◆ Avoid high or excessive protein intakes which will increase water loss and can lead to dehydration.

Cold Exposure

Exposure to a cold environment, be it air or water, is a challenge to be taken very seriously; performance decrements are common when you become cold. The body's response to cold exposure is a "tightening of blood vessels" to conserve heat, and shivering to generate heat and guard against hypothermia (a dangerously low core body temperature). Side effects of these responses are an increase in urine output and an increase in energy metabolism. Therefore, the most important aspects of nutrition in a cold environment are:

◆ Energy intake

◆ Fluid status

◆ Vitamin and mineral needs

Energy Intake

Energy requirements can increase 25 to 50% during cold weather operations as compared to warm weather operations.

A 3°F to 4°F decrease in body temperature can result in a two to fourfold increase in resting energy expenditure. That's a huge increase in the body's metabolic rate. Factors that increase calorie needs include:

◆ Added exertion due to wearing heavy gear
◆ Shivering which can increase resting metabolic rate by two to four times above normal
◆ Increased activity associated with traveling over snow and icy terrain
◆ Increased activity to keep warm

Many studies have shown that soldiers tend to progressively lose weight when conducting field exercises in the cold for 2 to 3 weeks. Because significant weight loss can result in fatigue and performance decrements, energy intake must increase to meet the increased energy demands.

Both fats and CHO are used as fuel when exposed to a cold environment. However, a high-CHO diet is preferred as it will replenish glycogen stores that are rapidly being used to maintain core temperature. A high-fat diet is discouraged as it would require a prolonged period of adaptation and may result in gastrointestinal problems. Ideally 60% of your energy should come from CHO, 30% from fat and 10% from protein, with high-CHO snacks eaten in between meals. Protein supplements or high-protein diets are not recommended as they would increase water losses.

Table 14-2. Calculating Energy Requirements for Cold Weather

If a SEAL requires 4000 kcal/day

A 25% increase in energy would be

4000 X 0.25 = 1000 kcal

Goal: Eat 4000 + 1000 or 5000 kcal/day

Eat frequent snacks during the day and a large snack before going to bed

Fluid Status

Becoming dehydrated in cold environments is very easy because of the cold-induced increase in urine output, increased fluid losses through breathing, involuntary reduction in fluid intake, and sweating. Because dehydration will decrease performance and potentially lead to various medical problems, maintenance of fluid status by drinking plenty of fluids and monitoring hydration status is absolutely critical (see Chapter 6).

Tips for Maintaining Fluid Status

◆ Force yourself to drink 2 to 4 cups of warm fluid at hourly intervals.
◆ Avoid alcoholic beverages as alcohol tends to increase heat and urine losses.
◆ Moderate caffeine consumption since caffeine increases fluid losses.
◆ Avoid consuming salty foods that increase fluid needs.
◆ Drink beverages with CHO to increase energy intake.
◆ Don't eat snow without first melting and purifying it.

Vitamin and Mineral Needs

When working in the cold, the requirements for some vitamins and minerals may increase to meet the demands of increased energy metabolism (example: thiamin) or greater urinary losses (example: magnesium, zinc). The amount by which daily vitamin and mineral needs may increase above the RDA (see Chapter 3 for RDAs) during cold weather operations was recently proposed: suggested amounts are shown in the Table below. These amounts are based on intake data from field studies, urinary excretion of nutrients, and other measures of "nutrient status." In most cases, if you meet your energy requirements by eating all ration components you should be able to meet your vitamin and mineral needs.

Table 14-3. Suggested Increases in Daily Intakes of Vitamins and Minerals During Cold Exposure

Nutrient	Suggested Increase	% of RDA
Vitamin B_1 (Thiamin)	3 mg	200
Vitamin B_2 (Riboflavin)	2 mg	118
Vitamin B_3	5 mg	26
Pantothenic Acid	5 mg	100
Folic Acid	200 µg	100
Vitamin B_{12}	1 µg	50
Magnesium	200 mg	57
Zinc	5 mg	33

Sustained Operations

Sustained Operations (SUSOPS) are work periods of 12 hours or more that usually result in physical and mental fatigue and sleep loss. In contrast, Continuous Operations (CONOPS) are periods of uninterrupted activity of "normal shift length" followed by sufficient sleep. Your missions, which usually include both SUSOPS and CONOPS, frequently result in fatigue and sleep loss. Nutritional interventions can partially offset the effects of fatigue and sleep deprivation on physical and mental performance. The most effective nutritional interventions include:

◆ CHO intake
◆ Hydration status
◆ Caffeine intake

CHO Intake

A high-CHO diet is needed for replacing muscle glycogen stores that are used up during prolonged activity and for maintaining a sufficient "blood glucose" level. Thus, your diet during SUSOPS should provide 60 to 65% of energy from CHO, 10% from protein, and the remaining calories from fat.

High-CHO snacks or CHO-containing fluid replacement beverages providing 15 to 30 g of CHO/hour will also help to maintain blood glucose and delay fatigue during strenuous prolonged missions (see Chapters 6 and 9 for additional information). When blood glucose levels fall, your performance will drop rapidly, and you will become unable to continue working.

Table 14-4. Symptoms of Hypoglycemia (Low Blood Sugar)

Headache	**Blurred vision**
Weakness	**Confusion**
Dizziness	**Unconsciousness**
Fatigue	**Sweating**

CHO loading can be useful when preparing for missions that require continuous movement such as snow shoeing, skiing, swimming, trekking over difficult terrain etc. for a few hours in order to reach the objective (see Chapter 9 for information on CHO loading).

Caffeine

If you are a regular user of caffeine, it will not do much to "pick you up" but if you discontinue caffeine use, it may cause discomfort. In general, caffeine increases urine output and could cause dehydration. However, you may want to try some caffeine to see if it increases your alertness and delays fatigue during extended operations. See Chapter 15 for the caffeine content of various beverages and medications.

Fluid Intake

On some training and actual missions water may not be available. Thus, prior hydration will assume a greater importance. When water or beverages are available it is important to remain well hydrated given that dehydration can decrease both mental and physical performance (see Chapter 6).

Forced drinking of 1 to 3 cups per 30 minutes, depending on the temperature, is recommended.

Beverages containing 5 to 8% CHO and some electrolytes are best.

Nutritional Considerations for Adverse Conditions

Diving and Immersion in Water

Like exposure to altitude and a cold environment, water operations, especially cold water operations, are associated with increased energy expenditure and fluid losses. Thus nutritional concerns for diving are maintenance of:

- ◆ Energy intake
- ◆ Fluid intake
- ◆ Replacing mineral losses

Energy Intake

When working at the same rate in water as on land, the energy expenditure to accomplish the same task is greater in water. The reasons for this increased energy expenditure during water operations include:

- ◆ Greater resistance offered by water
- ◆ Decreased efficiency of movement when thermal protective clothing is worn

This is especially true in cold water. To meet the increased energy requirements you may need to increase your intake of CHO. If the water is cold, this is very important.

Tips for maintaining performance in cold water

- ◆ Eat a high-CHO diet (see Chapters 2, 9, and 11).
- ◆ Consider CHO loading for extended dives

Glycogen stores are rapidly used when performing hard work in cold water. These stores must be replaced between operations to prevent performance decrements (see Chapter 9). CHO loading before an anticipated dive has been shown to improve and extend exercise performance during prolonged dives and has been discussed in Chapter 9.

Fluid Intake

Immersion in water increases urinary output by 2 to 10 times above normal. Without adequate hydration a diver can quickly become dehydrated and suffer performance decrements. For example, immersion during a single dive for 3 to 6 hours can result in a 2 to 8 pound loss in body weight by urination; this is equivalent to losing 1 to 3 quarts of fluid.

Although fluid ingestion during immersion has not been found to improve hydration status during short term dives (less than 3 hours), attempts to drink fluids with CHO should proceed whenever possible to maintain blood glucose. A decline in blood glucose is known to adversely affect performance.

Mineral Needs

Immersion in water, especially in cold water, can increase urinary losses of magnesium, calcium, zinc and chromium; see Chapter 3 and Appendix 6 for good food sources and recommended intakes.

Altitude

Ascent to altitude can cause a variety of disturbances, and adequate nutrition can play a crucial role in maintaining performance. The major nutritional concerns at altitude are:

◆ Weight loss
◆ CHO intake
◆ Dehydration
◆ Disturbances in digestion
◆ Vitamin and mineral needs

Weight Loss

Virtually all persons who go to altitude experience weight loss and loss of lean body mass. At altitudes below 5000 m weight loss can be prevented by increased caloric intake, whereas above 5000 m, a 5 to 10% weight loss is almost inevitable. Some reasons for weight loss at high altitude are:

◆ Energy requirements are increased 15 to 50% above sea level
◆ Decreased sense of taste causing a reduction in food intake
◆ Loss of body water from increased breathing rate and dry air
◆ Impaired absorption of nutrients
◆ Acute Mountain Sickness (AMS) which can result in nausea, vomiting, headache, and decreased appetite

The only way to minimize weight loss is by increasing your energy intake.

Energy requirements can increase 15 to 50% above requirements at sea level.

Recommended caloric intakes range from 3500 to 6000 calories per day; this is equivalent to eating at least four MREs or one Ration, Cold Weather daily.

Table 14-5. Calculating Energy Requirements at Altitude

If a SEAL requires 3000 kcal/day
A 50% increase in energy would be
3000 X 0.50 = 1500 kcal
Goal: Eat 4500 kcal/day

Tips for Maintaining Energy Balance

◆ Eat small, frequent meals.
◆ Protein should constitute no more than 10% of the daily caloric intake. Higher intakes will be excreted along with water.
◆ Fatty foods may not be well tolerated at altitude and may exaccerbate AMS.

CHO Intake

High-CHO foods are the preferred energy source at altitude because they:

◆ Replete glycogen stores—glycogen stores are depleted in a couple of hours by strenuous physical activity
◆ Require less oxygen (which is decreased at altitude) than fat to burn and are therefore the more efficient energy source.
◆ Can blunt and delay the progression or severity of symptoms of AMS (nausea, vomiting, headache).

You should derive 60% of calories or at least 400 g from CHO diet. This can be accomplished by eating high-CHO snacks (see Chapter 7) between meals and drinking CHO- containing beverages during strenuous activity and recovery (see Chapter 6 for recommended rehydration practices).

Dehydration

Water losses are increased at altitude and if these losses are not replaced dehydration results. As stated several times before, dehydration impairs physical and mental performance and increases the risk of cold injury. Dehydration occurs at altitude for several reasons:

◆ Increased respiratory losses due to increased ventilation
◆ Increased urine output due to altitude and cold temperatures

- ◆ Possible diarrheal fluid losses
- ◆ Failure to drink water
- ◆ Meeting the increased fluid needs can be a challenge since thirst does not always keep pace with needs

---

Fluid requirements may be 4.25 quarts or more per day at high altitude

---

A drinking schedule must be established and hydration status should be monitored daily.

Vitamin and Mineral Needs

As discussed in the section on cold, vitamin and mineral needs are likely to be increased at altitude where it is cold and oxygen availability is decreased. In particular, increased metabolic rate and hypoxic conditions at altitude can increase the production of harmful free radicals which may slow blood circulation and impair physical performance. Preliminary findings indicate that taking vitamin E (400 IU/day) at high altitude reduces free radical production, and helps maintain blood flow and aerobic energy metabolism in men.

Summary

Energy and fluid requirements are higher than normal during all the scenarios described in this chapter (see each section for estimated increases). Importantly, weight loss due to inadequate energy intake and/or dehydration can result in fatigue and impaired performance. Therefore, keys to being nutritionally prepared during training and missions in adverse environments are:

- ◆ Meet energy needs preferably by **eating a high-CHO diet**. Eat high-CHO snacks to meet increased energy needs.
- ◆ **Be well hydrated.** Follow a forced fluid replacement schedule since thirst is not a good indicator of fluid needs.
- ◆ Avoid protein supplements as the extra protein is excreted along with water and can be dehydrating.

Chapter 15
Ergogenic Agents—Looking for "The Edge"

Ergogenic agents are by definition, substances or techniques that enhance performance. Because SEALs are required to perform at a high level both mentally and physically, many are looking for substances or techniques to improve performance and provide "an edge." To perform longer, to be faster, to be stronger, and to be leaner, if not a mission goal, are personal goals of many SEALs and elite athletes. People have been trying to accomplish these goals for centuries through the use of ergogenic agents. It is the goal of this chapter to present information and comments about certain products commonly found in retail stores or by mail order, that claim performance-enhancing effects.

The comments in this chapter are based on the most up-to-date objective scientific information, although in some cases limited information is available, and most have not been tested for their ability to enhance SEAL or Special Operations mission-related performance. Some products are unlikely to hurt you, and you will have to decide if you want to try them, whereas other products may be harmful and you may be strongly discouraged from trying them. In many cases you may be using supplements that are a waste of money. This chapter will assist you in making good decisions.

Nutritional Products Advertised as Ergogenic Agents

This section lists many of the nutritional ergogenic agents sold by manufacturers with claims to "enhance performance" or have "muscle building" properties. Some have valid claims whereas others do not. It is often difficult to differentiate false claims from valid ones if you haven't carefully researched each product individually. Many claims sound very scientific and convincing but, unfortunately, they are often false or unproven. For each agent described below, the claims, the usual dose used, and a comment are provided. Remember, if the comment is NO, the product may be harmful.

Table 15-1. Nutritional Ergogenic Agents

AGENTS	CLAIMS	DOSE	COMMENT
Arginine, Lysine, and Ornithine	Stimulate growth hormone release.	Variable. Arginine - 500 mg. one hour before meals and/or before workout. Ornithine - 500 mg. a day or 250 mg. one to three times a day. These items are sold separately or in combinations with varying amounts of amino acid content.	Ornithine - No. Gastrointestinal disturbances are common. Arginine, Lysine - Some benefit reported.
Sodium Bicarbonate, ("Bicarb loading," "Soda loading")	Enhances anaerobic performance during high intensity exercise lasting 1 to 5 minutes.	0.3 grams of Sodium Bicarb per kg body weight mixed with 1 liter of water 1 to 2 hours before exercise.	Some benefit reported - Be careful...harmful if taken in large amounts. Discontinue use if abdominal cramps or diarrhea occurs.
Branched Chain Amino Acids (BCAAs) - Leucine, Isoleucine, Valine	Anabolic and growth hormone stimulator; may protect against mental fatigue of exercise.	There are various products with different amounts of BCAA in them. Here's an example: Leucine 800 mg. daily. Isoleucine 300 mg. Valine 200 mg. These are usually consumed prior to working out. Foods rich in BCAAs include turkey, chicken, navy beans, and other meats.	Some benefits reported.

Table 15-1. Nutritional Ergogenic Agents

AGENTS	CLAIMS	DOSE	COMMENT
Caffeine	Delays fatigue, enhances performance, "burns" fat.	4 to 9 mg/kg 30 minutes to one hour prior to exercise. Look at the caffeine levels in some common beverages.	Some benefits reported, but discontinue use if side effects (stomach pain, tremor) interfere with concentration or steadiness.
L-Carnitine	"Fat burner," delays onset of fatigue.	500 mg daily. Foods rich in Carnitine include beef (average content equals 50 mg/100 grams of edible portion).	Little to no benefit reported - not harmful at recommended doses. AVOID D-carnitine - a carnitine deficiency may occur.
Choline	Enhances endurance performance	400 to 900 mg daily as choline bitartrate. Foods rich in choline include meat, liver, and peanuts.	No benefit reported - not known to be harmful at above doses. Most claims based on theoretical possibilities.
Chromium Picolinate	Increases muscle mass, growth stimulating.	50 to 1000 µg/day as a dietary supplement. Foods rich in chromium include beer, brewer's yeast, oysters, mushrooms, meats, and whole grain cereals.	Some benefit reported.
Coenzyme Q10	Increases energy and cardiac performance. Potent antioxidant.	1.0 mg three times a day. Foods rich in CoQIO include beef, eggs, and spinach.	No benefit reported in athletes.
Dibencozide or cobamamide - Coenzyme forms of B_{12}	Anabolic and growth promoting.	500 mg daily in tablet form.	Little or no proven benefit - no harmful effects at recommended doses.
λ-Oryzanol and Ferulic Acid	Increases testosterone and increases lean body mass.	Variable, but commonly found in 50 mg per day doses.	Little or no proven benefit - no harmful effects at given doses.

Table 15-1. Nutritional Ergogenic Agents

AGENTS	CLAIMS	DOSE	COMMENT
Glandulars (ground up animal organs usually testes, pituitary, or hypothalamus)	Will elevate your testosterone levels. This "extra" testosterone will make you more anabolic (build up) and get bigger.	As a dietary supplement mixed with protein/carbohydrate powders.	Truly not worth the money!
Inosine	Energy enhancer; Increases endurance, strength, and recuperation.	500 to 1000 mg 15 minutes prior to exercise.	No. People with gout should avoid inosine. Dubious effects not worth the risk.
Octacosanol - Wheat Germ Oil	Improves endurance capacity.	100 to 6000 mg daily with expected results in 4 to 6 weeks.	Some benefit reported.
Sapogenins - Smilax, Diascorea, Trillium, Yucca, or Sarsaparilla	Increases muscle mass and lean body weight by increasing testosterone levels. A testosterone precursor.	Sublingual or capsular as directed. Use prior to workout and before bed.	Little benefit reported. Some products suspended in 18% alcohol. READ the label.
Tyrosine	Reverses cold-induced working memory deficit. Positive impact on stress-induced cognitive performance degradation.	75 to 150 mg/kg of L-tyrosine 1 to 2 hours prior to exposure.	Some benefits reported in SEAL cold weather operations. Branch chained amino acids should not be taken with tyrosine since they will interfere with tyrosine's action.

Table 15-2. Caffeine Content of Selected Beverages, Products, and Medications

Coffee (8 oz.)	mg	Soda (12 oz.)*	mg
Percolated	102–200	Mountain Dew	55
Drip	176–240	Coke	46
Instant	64–176	Dr. Pepper	40
Decaffeinated	3.2–8	Pepsi	38
Tea (8 oz.)		Mellow Yellow	52
3-Minute Brew	32–74	Mr. Pibb	50
Instant	24–45	Chocolate (1 oz.)	25
Iced	35–58	Pain Relievers (1 tablet)	
Stimulants (1 tablet)		Anacin	32
No Doz	100	Excedrin	65
Vivarin	200	Dristan	0

*Sugar-free and diet versions of above sodas have same caffeine content as original.

Table 15-3. Summary of Ergogenic Agents

Agent	Comment
Delays Fatigue/Increases Energy Levels	
Caffeine	Some benefits reported
Choline	No benefit reported
Coenzyme Q_{10}	No proven benefit
Inosine	No proven benefit
Octacosanol	Some benefit reported
Sodium Bicarbonate	Some reported benefit
Tyrosine	Some benefits reported during SEAL cold weather ops

Agent	Comment
Fat Burners/Lean Body Mass Increasers	
Carnitine	Little or no benefit reported
Chromium	Some benefit reported
λ-Oryzanol/Ferulic Acid	Little or no benefit reported
Testosterone Enhancers	
Glandulars	Not recommended
Hot Stuff	Possible adverse effects
Smilax	Little or no benefit reported
Growth Hormone Releasers	
Arginine	Some benefit reported
Branch Chain Amino Acids	Some benefit reported
Dibencozide	Little or no proven benefit
Lysine	Some benefit reported

Protein-Carbohydrate Supplements

Go into a retail or specialty store that caters to athletes and you may become overwhelmed by the number of different products available. One of the most highly visible and advertised group of products are the powdered protein and carbohydrate beverages. "Weight gaining," "anabolic," "muscle building"—these are just a few of the various claims made by manufacturers. They do share one thing in common however: they are sold as supplements to your diet. These products are intended to fortify your diet to meet the nutrient demands of your body. In general, there are three basic reasons why people supplement:

◆ Compensate for less than adequate diets or life-styles
◆ Meet unusual nutrient demands induced by heavy exercise and/or
◆ Produce direct positive effects on performance.

Your profession and life-style impose unique physical demands that require stamina, power, and strength. Consequently, your caloric (energy) expenditure is greater than the average person.

In Chapter 1 you calculated your REE and then, based on your activity level, your total daily caloric expenditure. Do you think your caloric intake supports your activity level? If not, you have two methods to increase your energy intake:

◆ You can eat more (which can be difficult based on your daily schedule)
◆ You can use a supplement to make up for the extra calories you need.

Supplements are a quick and convenient means for obtaining the nutrients you need. For example, some people find that after eating a normal breakfast they feel ill or nauseous during morning PT. If you can't tolerate exercising on a full stomach, then a powdered beverage may be the answer for your breakfast. You get the calories you need in the morning, but don't have that heavy feeling in your stomach. Remember that you may not need the full recommended serving size. Count the calories to suit your own energy requirements and goals.

It is also important to realize that it is not the supplement alone that leads to better performance. Success lies in addressing your goals and analyzing and adapting your diet to meet those goals. It will take some work on your part to calculate how much supplement, if any, you need to use. Read the labels and figure out how many calories you will expend before your next meal. Also, make sure you add up the vitamins and minerals you are getting from all the different supplements you are taking. Many products provide similar nutrients and you may be taking TOO much of one or several nutrients.

Another decision to make is whether or not to use a protein, carbohydrate, or combination beverage. Once again, it all depends on your goals. If you want to increase lean body mass through resistive training, then some protein may be the way to go. Remember:

All you need is 0.6 to 0.8 grams of protein per pound body weight per day

If you need more than you can eat, then a supplement with protein may be for you. Many powders contain both protein and carbohydrate in a good ratio. Find the one that has the most appropriate amount of each to augment your diet (Refer to Chapter 10 for a list of Protein and Carbohydrate Supplements).

Here is an example: The goal of a 24-year-old SEAL who weighs 175 lbs is to increase his lean body mass through weight training. He knows that he needs between 0.6 and 0.8 and NO MORE than 1.0 grams of protein per pound to achieve this goal. He decides to eat 0.8 grams of protein per pound to see if he'll achieve his goals. His protein requirements are calculated as shown:

---

175 X 0.8 grams protein = desired protein intake
175 lbs X 0.8 = 140 grams of protein daily.
NO MORE THAN 175 X 1 or 175 grams of protein.

Now let's see how much protein he eats on an average day

Breakfast		Afternoon Snack	
Sausage McMuffin	23 g	2 Sports bars	20 g
10 oz. milk	12 g		
1 bagel	6 g	**Dinner**	
		11/2 Chicken Breast	80 g
Mid-morning Snack		Broccoli	3 g
1 Yogurt	8 g	Baked Potato	2 g
Lunch			
Big Mac	25 g	Total Protein Intake	212 g
Cheeseburger	18 g	Calculated Requirements	140 g
Fries	6 g		
Shake	9 g		

MET-Rx

MET-Rx is a nutritional supplement with claims of decreasing body fat and increasing muscle mass, if used in conjunction with a regular exercise program. The exercise program is primarily strength/resistive (weight) training. As with any supplement, it is designed to augment your normal diet to meet the increased nutritional demands of exercise. However, increased nutritional needs can also easily be met by dietary means.

The cornerstone of Met-Rx is that it is a high-protein supplement (see nutritional information below). The protein is in the form of egg whites, whey protein concentrate, and Metamyosin™ which is claimed to be a "unique blend of milk protein isolates."

Table 15-4. Ingredients in One Serving of MET-Rx

Energy-Providing Nutrients

Carbohydrates	24 grams
Protein	37 grams
Fat	2 grams
Total Calories	262 kcal

Selected Vitamins and Minerals (% US RDA)

Vitamin A	40
Vitamin B_6	60
Vitamin B_{12}	50
Vitamin C	60
Vitamin D	60
Chromium	50

Depending on your goals, MET-Rx may or may not be for you. For example, if you are interested in improving aerobic endurance MET-Rx alone is a poor source of the necessary carbohydrates for that kind of activity. If, however, increasing muscle mass is your goal, then this product provides protein for that. Remember that you don't need more than 0.8 grams of protein per pound body weight.

One major drawback of MET-Rx is the cost. Each serving is roughly $3.00 and the directions for use call for 2 to 4 servings a day. That averages to about $9.00 a day! Keep in mind that there are always alternative sources of protein that are very easy to come by and tend to be much less money. For example,

◆ One can of tuna fish has 36 grams of protein,
◆ One 4 oz. breast of chicken has 36 grams of protein
◆ One 8 oz. glass of milk (skim) has 10 grams of protein.

Remember: There is nothing "magical" about this product and all the ingredients are found in nature. Record your intake and see if it is worth your money.

Chapter 16

Ergolytic Agents— "Going Backwards"

After reading about agents that are potentially beneficial to you, its now time to focus on substances that can destroy what you've been trying to build up. Ergolytic agents are those substances which do not enhance, but rather impair, performance, be it physical, mental, or psychological. When using these substances, you may be undoing the benefits and successes gained through training and the use of ergogenic agents. Here's another way to think of it—you may be wasting your money if on one hand you are buying ergogenic agents and on the other continuing to use ergolytic agents. Hopefully, by staying away from ergolytic agents, you can maximally improve your athletic performance.

Alcohol

> ## Heavy alcohol intake can lead to severe dehydration!

Drinking a lot of alcohol in the evening can lead to a state of dehydration the next day if adequate fluid replacement does not occur. There have been incidences during road races and regular training where people have died after a night of heavy drinking, without adequate rehydration prior to and during exercise. Although a rare occurrence, it can happen.

Some athletes believe that drinking a small amount of alcohol prior to an event can be relaxing and instill self-confidence. ***This is completely false.*** In fact, alcohol may compromise physical performance by decreasing the release of glucose from the liver. This will cause a decrease in blood glucose and possibly lead to hypoglycemia.

Numerous studies on young trained athletes have shown that performance decreases after ingestion of alcohol. The myth that alcohol can alter the perception of fatigue is also false. There is generally no effect on perception of performance after drinking.

Smokeless Tobacco

Many SEALs have been or are frequent users of smokeless tobacco. Use of such products has been on the rise in the past 20 years with an annual reported increase of 11% since 1974. Many athletes believe that smokeless tobacco will improve their performance or enhance their reaction time by giving them a quick "rush" during the event. After a brief discussion of what nicotine (the active ingredient in all tobacco products) does to your body, you will understand why performance enhancement and chew don't go together.

Nicotine is the major ingredient of smokeless tobacco and very, very addictive (as addicting as cocaine or heroin). It is termed ***a psychoactive drug*** which means it alters the normal functioning of the brain by stimulating the central nervous system and resulting in the nicotine "buzz" or "high." It is this "mental state" that users claim enhances their reaction time and performance. However, studies have shown no differences in reaction times between users and non-users of smokeless tobacco. Remember: there are NO reaction time improvements with chew.

Nicotine has some very detrimental effects on an athlete. Nicotine is a vasoconstrictor (makes blood vessels tighten). This action on the circulatory system raises blood pressure and heart rate, thereby causing a decrease in cardiac efficiency. In one study of young athletes, two parameters of cardiac performance (stroke volume—the amount of blood pumped out of the heart with each contraction, and cardiac output—the amount of blood the heart pumps in one minute) both showed decreases while using smokeless tobacco. This is very undesirable for an athlete and could cause a severe decrease in performance.

Antihistamines

Antihistamine use is prevalent among all groups of people since it is a common over-the-counter medication. Many types of antihistamines are used, with the most common ones being Benadryl and Seldane. One of the most common side effects of many antihistamines is **drowsiness.** This is not typically seen with many of the newer, "non-sedating" types of antihistamines.

Antihistamines may compromise mental performance

Some of the detrimental mental effects of the sedating antihistamines include:

◆ Decreased ability to concentrate
◆ Increase in reaction time
◆ Sleepiness
◆ Decreased score on rifle target practice—"more misses"

Seldane appears to have the least effects in terms of drowsiness and mental performance decrements, so if you need an antihistamine, it may be best to take this one!

Other Side Effects of Sedating Antihistamines

Dry Mouth	**Increase in Heart Rate**
Blurred Vision	**Constipation**

No clear-cut effects on physical performance have been observed, but caution should be exerted when taking any type of medication.

Appendix 1
Carbohydrate Content of Selected Foods

Food Items[1]	Amount of Food Items (cooked or prepared)	Total Calories	CHO (g)	% Calories from CHO
BEANS/LENTILS/DRIED PEAS				
Baked beans, canned	1 cup	236	52.1	78.0
Black beans	1 cup	225	41	72.9
Chickpeas	1 cup	270	45	66.7
Green peas	1 cup	115	21	73.0
Kidney beans	1 cup	230	42	73.0
Lentils	1 cup	215	38	70.7
Lima beans	1 cup	260	49	75.4
Navy beans	1 cup	225	40	71.1
Pinto beans	1 cup	265	49	74.0
Refried beans	1 cup	295	51	69.2
BREADS and GRAINS				
Bagel	1 each	200	38	76.0
Biscuits	1 each	95	14.	58.9
Bread, cracked wheat	1 slice	65	11	67.7

Food Items[1]	Amount of Food Items (cooked or prepared)	Total Calories	CHO (g)	% Calories from CHO
Bread, mixed grain	1 slice	65	11	67.7
Bread, oatmeal	1 slice	65	12	73.8
Bread, raisin	1 slice	65	13	80.0
Bread, whole wheat	1 slice	70	13	74.3
English muffin	1 each	140	27	77.1
Pita bread, white	80.0"	165	33	80.0
Pasta, egg noodles	1 cup	200	37	74.0
Spaghetti, enriched	1 cup	155	32	82.6
Rice cake cracker	2 each	70	15.2	86.9
Rice, white	1 cup	225	50	88.9
Rice, brown long grain	1 cup	216	44.8	83.0

CEREALS and BREAKFAST FOODS

All Bran	1 oz.	110	21	76.4
40% Bran Flakes	1 oz.	102	22	86.2
Cheerios	1 oz.	110	20	72.7
Granola, Nature Valley	1 oz.	125	19	60.8
Grape-Nuts	1 oz.	100	23	92.0
Oatmeal, nonfortified	1 cup	145	25	69.0
Pancakes from mix, no syrup	3 medium	249	33	53
Raisin Bran	1 oz.	90	21	74.5
Shredded Wheat	1 biscuit	83	18.8	85.0
Special K	1 oz.	110	21	74.5
Total	1 oz.	100	22	88.0
Waffles from mix, no syrup	2 large	410	54	52.7
Wheaties	1 oz.	100	23	92.0

Food Items[1]	Amount of Food Items (cooked or prepared)	Total Calories	CHO (g)	% Calories from CHO
DAIRY PRODUCTS				
Buttermilk	1 cup	99	11.7	48.6
Cottage Cheese, regular	1 cup	232	6.2	10.7
Cottage Cheese, low-fat (1%)	1 cup	164	6.2	15.1
Ice cream	1 cup	264	31	47.0
Ice milk	1 cup	184	30	65.2
Milkshake, vanilla	12 oz.	380	60.4	63.5
Milk, Whole	1 cup	150	11.4	30.4
Milk, 2% low-fat	1 cup	121	11.7	38.6
Milk, skim nonfat	1 cup	86	11.8	54.9
Milk, regular chocolate	1 cup	208	25.8	49.6
Yogurt, regular, plain	8 oz.	139	10.6	30.5
Yogurt, fruit flavored	8 oz.	253	42.7	67.5
Yogurt, nonfat plain	8 oz.	127	17.4	54.8
FRUITS/VEGETABLES				
Apple, raw	1 medium	80	20	100
Avocado	1 medium	306	12	15.6
Banana	1 medium	127	33.0	94.5
Broccoli, raw	1 stalk	32	5.9	75.0
Cantaloupe	1 cup	56	13.3	99
Carrots, raw	1 large	42	9.7	92.3
Cauliflower, raw	1/2 cup	13	2.6	80
Corn, cooked	1 cup	134	33.7	100
Grapefruit	1 medium	78	19.8	90
Grapes, red seedless	1/2 cup	29	7.9	100

Food Items[1]	Amount of Food Items (cooked or prepared)	Total Calories	CHO (g)	% Calories from CHO
Oranges	1 medium	64	16.0	99
Orange juice	1 cup	110	26.1	99
Pear, D'Anjou	1 medium	118	30.1	99
Pineapple juice	1 cup	140	34.5	99
Plum	1 medium	36	8.6	100
Potato, baked	1 large	145	32.8	90.5
Raisins, seedless	1/4 cup	109	28.8	99
Sweet Potato, baked	1 medium	117	27.7	94.7
Tomato juice	1 cup	42	10.3	99
Tomato, raw	1 medium	25	5	80
MISCELLANEOUS				
Angelfood cake	1 slice	129	29.3	90.8
Cheesecake	1 slice	256	20.4	31.8
Doughnuts, plain cake	1 each	198	23.4	47.3
Fig Newtons	2 each	112	22.6	80.7
Popcorn, plain	1 cup	25	5	80
Pretzels, Dutch	2 each	120	24	80

[1]Information for meats, fish, and poultry is not provided since the contribution from CHO is typically < 1% of the energy.

Appendix 2
Fat Content of Selected Foods

Food Items[1]	Amount of Food Items (cooked or prepared)	Total Calories	Fats (g)	% Calories from Fat
BEEF				
Hamburger, lean ground beef, broiled	4 oz.	307	21.3	62.4
Roast Beef	4 oz.	420	34	72.8
Steak, sirloin broiled	4 oz.	320	20.4	57.4
LAMB				
Lamb Chop, loin broiled	4 oz.	336	16	42.9
Lamb Rib roasted	4 oz.	420	34	72.8
PORK				
Bacon, regular	3 strips	110	9	81.8
Bacon, Canadian style	2 slices	85	4	42.4
Bologna	2 slices	180	16	80
Ham, roasted	4 oz.	273	13.8	45.4
Hot Dog	1 each	145	13	80.7
Luncheon Meat	2 slices	140	13	83.6

Food Items[1]	Amount of Food Items (cooked or prepared)	Total Calories	Fats (g)	% Calories from Fat
Pork chop, broiled	4 oz.	392	30.8	70.7
Salami	2 slices	145	11.9	74.5

POULTRY

Chicken, breast roasted w/o skin	4 oz.	187	4	19.3
Turkey, light meat	4 oz.	180	3.7	18.5
Turkey, dark meat	4 oz.	213	8.2	34.6

FISH AND SHELLFISH

Fish Sticks	1 each	70	3.2	40.6
Halibut, broiled	4 oz	187	8	38.5
Oysters, raw	1/2 cup	160	4.4	24.7
Salmon, canned	1 cup	160	6.2	34.9
Sardines, canned	4 oz.	233	13.0	50.2
Tuna, water packed	4 oz.	180	1.3	6.5
Tuna, oil packed	4 oz.	220	9.3	38.0

DAIRY PRODUCTS

Buttermilk	1 cup	99	2.2	20
Cheese, American	1 oz.	105	9	77.1
Cheese, cheddar	1 oz.	115	9.4	73.6
Cottage cheese, regular	1 cup	232	10	38.8
Cottage cheese, low-fat (1%)	1 cup	164	2.3	12.6
Cheese, Swiss	1 oz.	105	8	68.6
Egg, whole, hard boiled	1	75	5	60
Egg yolk	from 1 egg	60	5.1	76.5
Ice cream	1 cup	264	14.6	49.8
Milkshake, vanilla	12 oz.	380	10.3	24.3

Food Items[1]	Amount of Food Items (cooked or prepared)	Total Calories	Protein (g)	% Calories from Fat
Milk, low-fat 1%	1 cup	102	2.6	22.9
Milk, low-fat 2%	1 cup	120	4.7	35.3
Milk, whole	1 cup	150	8.2	49.2
Milk, regular chocolate	1 cup	208	8.5	36.7
Yogurt, regular, plain	1 cup	139	7.4	47.9
Yogurt, fruit flavored	1 cup	253	4.0	14.2

BREADS/CEREALS

Biscuits	1 each	104	5.1	44.1
Bread, cracked wheat	1 slice	65	1	13.8
Bread, mixed grain	1 slice	65	1	13.8
Bread, oatmeal	1 slice	65	1	13.8
Bread, raisin	1 slice	65	1	13.8
Bread, whole wheat	1 slice	70	1	12.9
English muffin	1 each	140	1.0	6.4
Granola, Nature Valley	1 oz.	125	5	36

MISCELLANEOUS

Avocado	1 medium	306	30	88.2
Butter	1 tbsp	102	11.3	99
Cheesecake	1 slice	256	18	63.3
Cookies, chocolate chip	2 each	160	8	45
Doughnut, plain cake type	1	198	10.8	49.1
Margarine	1 tbsp	102	11.3	99
Mayonnaise	1 tbsp	100	11.2	100
Mixed nuts, dry roasted	1 oz.	170	5	11.8
Peanut butter	1 tbsp	95	8	75.8

Food Items[1]	Amount of Food Items (cooked or prepared)	Total Calories	Protein (g)	% Calories from Fat
Peanuts, oil roasted	1 oz.	165	8	43.6
Pecans, roasted	0.25 cup	188	19.6	93.8
Salad dressing, Italian	1 tbsp	69	7.1	92.6
Sunflower seeds, dried	1 oz.	161	14	78.3
Tofu	0.5 cup	183	11	54.1

[1] Information for most fruits and vegetables is not provided since the contribution from fat is typically < 1% of the energy.

Appendix 3
Protein Content of Selected Foods

Food Items[1]	Amount of Food Item (cooked or prepared)	Total Calories	Protein (grams)	% Calories from Protein
BEEF				
Hamburger, lean ground beef, broiled	4 oz.	307	28	36.5
Roast Beef	4 oz.	420	25.3	24.0
Steak, sirloin broiled	4 oz.	320	30.7	38.4
LAMB				
Lamb Chop, loin broiled	4 oz.	336	31.4	37.4
Lamb Rib roasted	4 oz.	420	24	22.9
PORK				
Bacon, regular	3 strips	110	6	21.8
Bacon, Canadian style	2 slices	85	11	51.8
Bologna	2 slices	180	7	15.6
Ham, roasted	4 oz.	273	24	35.2
Hot Dog	1 each	145	5	13.8
Luncheon Meat	2 slices	140	5	14.3

Food Items[1]	Amount of Food Item (cooked or prepared)	Total Calories	Protein (grams)	% Calories from Protein
Pork chop, broiled	4 oz.	355	31	34.9
Salami	2 slices	145	8	22.1
POULTRY				
Chicken, breast roasted w/o skin	4 oz.	187	36	77.0
Turkey, light meat	4 oz.	180	33.3	74.0
Turkey, dark meat	4 oz.	213	32	60.1
FISH AND SHELLFISH				
Fish Sticks	1 each	70	6	34.3
Flounder, baked	4 oz.	160	21.3	53.3
Halibut, broiled	4 oz.	187	26.7	57.1
Oysters, raw	1 cup	160	20	50.0
Salmon, canned	4 oz.	160	22.7	56.8
Sardines, canned	4 oz.	233	26.7	45.8
Shrimp, canned	4 oz.	133	28	84.2
Tuna, water packed	4oz.	180	40	88.9
Tuna, oil packed	4 oz.	220	32	58.2
DAIRY PRODUCTS				
Buttermilk	1 cup	100	8	32.0
Cheese, American	1 oz.	105	6	22.9
Cheese, cheddar	1 oz.	115	7	24.3
Cottage cheese, regular	1 cup	232	28.1	48.4
Cottage cheese, low-fat (1%)	1 cup	164	28	68.3
Cheese, Swiss	1 oz.	95	7	29.5
Egg, whole, hard boiled	1	75	6	32.0

Protein Content of Selected Foods

Food Items[1]	Amount of Food Item (cooked or prepared)	Total Calories	Protein (grams)	% Calories from Protein
Egg white	from 1 egg	15	3.8	100
Egg yolk	from 1 egg	60	3	20.0
Instant breakfast	1 pkt	130	7	21.5
Ice cream	1 cup	264	4.6	7.0
Ice milk	1 cup	184	5	11.0
Milkshake, vanilla	12 oz	380	13.2	13.8
Milk, skim	1 cup	85	8.0	37.6
Milk, low-fat 1%	1 cup	100	8	32.0
Milk, low-fat 2%	1 cup	120	8	26.7
Milk, whole	1 cup	150	8	21.3
Milk, regular chocolate	1 cup	208	8	15.4
Yogurt, low-fat fruit flavored	8 oz.	230	10	17.4
Yogurt, low-fat, plain	8 oz.	145	12	33.1
Yogurt, nonfat plain	8 oz.	125	13	41.6

BEANS/LENTILS/DRIED PEAS

Baked beans, canned	1 cup	236	12	20.3
Black beans	1 cup	225	15	26.7
Chickpeas	1 cup	270	15	22.2
Green peas	1 cup	115	8	27.8
Kidney beans	1 cup	230	15	26.1
Lentils	1 cup	215	16	29.8
Lima beans	1 cup	260	16	24.6
Navy beans	1 cup	225	15	26.7
Pinto beans	1 cup	265	15	22.6

Food Items[1]	Amount of Food Item (cooked or prepared)	Total Calories	Protein (grams)	% Calories from Protein
Refried beans	1 cup	295	18	24.4
Tofu	1/2 cup	183	19.9	43.6

BREADS AND GRAINS

Bagel	1 each	200	7	14.0
Biscuits	1 each	95	2	8.4
Bread, cracked wheat	1 slice	65	2	12.3
Bread, mixed grain	1 slice	65	2	12.3
Bread, oatmeal	1 slice	65	2	12.3
Bread, raisin	1 slice	65	2	12.3
Bread, whole wheat	1 slice	70	3	17.1
English muffin	1 each	140	5	14.3
Muffin, Blueberry or Bran	1 each	140	3	8.6
Pancakes, plain	1 each	60	2	13.3
Pita bread, large, white	6.5" round	165	6	14.5
Pasta, egg noodles	1 cup	200	7	14.0
Spaghetti, enriched	1 cup	155	5	12.9
Rice, white	1 cup	225	4	7.1
Rice, brown long grain	1 cup	216	5	9.3

CEREALS

All Bran	1 oz.	70	4	22.9
40% Bran Flakes	1 oz.	90	3.6	14.1
Cheerios	1 oz.	110	4	14.5
Granola, Nature Valley	1 oz.	125	3	9.6
Grape-Nuts	1 oz.	100	3	12.0

Protein Content of Selected Foods

Food Items[1]	Amount of Food Item (cooked or prepared)	Total Calories	Protein (grams)	% Calories from Protein
Oatmeal, nonfortified	1 cup	145	6	16.6
Raisin Bran	1 oz.	90	3	13.3
Shredded Wheat	1 biscuit	83	2.6	12.0
Special K	1 oz.	110	6	21.8
Total	1 oz.	100	3	12.0
Wheaties	1 oz.	100	3	12.0
MISCELLANEOUS				
Peanut butter	1 tbsp	95	5	21.1
Brewer's yeast	1 tbsp	25	3	48.0
Sunflower seeds	1 oz.	160	6	15.0
Peanuts, oil roasted	1 oz.	165	8	19.4
Mixed nuts, dry roasted	1 oz.	170	5	11.8

[1] Information for cookies, crackers, cakes, fruits, and vegetables is not provided since the contribution of protein is typically less than 1% of the total energy.

Appendix 4
Energy Expenditure for Various Activities

Activities	kcal/min	kcal/hr
Archery	5	273
Badminton	7	407
Basketball - Half Court	4	256
Basketball - Full Court	7	433
Bowling	4	252
Boxing - Sparring	10	580
Calisthenics, Strenuous	9	540
Canoeing - Leisure	3	185
Canoeing - Racing	7	433
Card Playing	2	105
Carpentry - General	4	218
Carpet Sweeping	3	189
Climbing Hills - No Load	8	508
Climbing Hills - Loaded 5 Kg	9	546
Climbing Hills - Loaded 10 Kg	10	588
Climbing Hills - Loaded 20 Kg	11	630

Activities	kcal/min	kcal/hr
Cycling - 5 To 10 MPH	6	336
Cycling - 10 To 15 MPH	8	504
Cycling - 15 To 20 MPH	11	672
Cycling - Racing	14	848
Dancing - Rock	5	273
Digging Trenches	10	609
Dips - 20 per minute	4	261
Eating	2	97
Electrical Work	4	244
Fishing	4	260
Football	9	546
Gardening - Raking	4	227
Gardening - Planting By Hand	8	462
Gardening - Hedging	5	323
Gardening - Mowing By Hand	8	462
Gardening - Digging	9	529
Golf - 2some	6	340
Golf - 4some	4	248
Grocery Shopping	4	252
Handball	11	659
Judo/karate	14	819
Lying At Ease	2	92
Mopping Floor	4	252
Obstacle Course	10	600

Energy Expenditure for Various Activities

Activities	kcal/min	kcal/hr
Outdoor Work - Sawing By Hand	8	504
Outdoor Work - Carrying Logs	13	756
Outdoor Work - Sawing By Power	5	315
Outdoor Work - Barking Trees	8	504
Outdoor Work - Weeding	5	302
Outdoor Work - Chopping Wood	21	1,260
Painting Inside	2	143
Painting Outside	5	323
Playing Ping Pong	5	286
Playing Pool	3	176
Push-Ups - 20 per minute	6	341
Reading	2	105
Rockclimbing	7	420
Roller Blading - Moderate	6	349
Roller Blading - Vigorous	11	638
Rowing - 15 To 20 Strokes/min	9	546
Rowing - 20 To 25 Strokes/min	12	714
Rowing - 25 To 30 Strokes/min	14	848
Rowing - 30 To 35 Strokes/min	16	937
Rowing - 35 To 40 Strokes/min	20	1,172
Rugby/Soccer	9	554
Run - 5.5 Min Per Mile	19	1,134
Run - 6 Min Per Mile	18	1,058
Run - 7 Min Per Mile	16	958

Activities	kcal/min	kcal/hr
Run - 8 Min Per Mile	14	811
Run - 9 Min Per Mile	12	714
Run - 10 Min Per Mile	11	651
Run - 11 Min Per Mile	9	567
Scraping Paint	4	265
Scrubbing Floors	8	462
Scuba Diving, Leisurely	14	865
Scuba Diving, Vigorous	19	1,159
Sit-Ups - 20 per minute	5	330
Sitting in the Cold	3	180
Sitting Quietly	1	88
Skiing, Downhill - Moderate Speed	8	500
Skiing, Downhill - Leisurely (M)	7	420
Skiing, Crosscountry - Uphill	19	1,151
Skiing, Crosscountry - Walking	10	601
Skipping Rope	12	739
Sleeping/napping	1	42
Snowshoeing - Soft Snow	12	697
Squash - Doubles	7	445
Squash - Singles	15	890
Stairclimbing - Slow	9	538
Stairclimbing - Moderate	11	659
Stairclimbing - Fast	15	874
Standing Quietly	2	109

Energy Expenditure for Various Activities

Activities	kcal/min	kcal/hr
Swimming - Treading Fast	12	714
Swimming - Treading Slow	4	260
Swimming - Breaststroke	11	680
Swimming - Backstroke	12	710
Swimming - Crawl Fast	14	840
Swimming - Side Stroke	9	512
Swimming - Crawl Slow	9	538
Tennis, Singles	8	458
Tennis, Doubles	6	336
Video Games, Watching	2	105
Volleyball	4	210
Walking with 70 lb pack - 3 MPH at 2.5% grade	7	439
Washing Dishes	3	155
Watching TV/movies	1	88
Weight/Circuit Training - Nautilus	11	630
Writing/Drawing	2	122

Note: The energy expenditure values in this appendix are for a 70 Kg (155 lb) man and are intended to provide you with an estimate. Your values may be lower or higher depending on your body weight.

Appendix 5
Good Food Sources of Vitamins

Nutrient	Vitamin Food Sources	Nutrient Content in Selected Food	
Vitamin A	green and yellow fruits and vegetables, milk, milk products, fish liver oil, liver	beef liver broiled, 4 oz.	40,900 IU
		sweet potato baked, 1 med	24,880 IU
		carrots raw, 1 med.	20,250 IU
		spinach cooked, 1 cup	14,740 IU
		apricots dried, 7 halves	2,350 IU
Vitamin D	egg yolks, organ meats, bone meal, fortified milk, salmon, sunlight	salmon/tuna canned, 4 oz.	568 IU
		sardines canned, 4 oz.	340 IU
		milk 2%, 1 cup	100 IU
		chicken liver, 4 oz.	60 IU
		egg yolk, 1 each	25 IU
Vitamin E	seed oils, dark green vegetables, eggs, nuts, liver, organ meats, wheat germ, milk fat, desiccated liver	wheat germ oil, 1 tbsp	52 IU
		sunflower oil, 1 tbsp	13 IU
		milk nonfat, 1 cup	11.3 IU
		avocado Florida, 1 whole	6 IU
		peas cooked, 1 cup	3.4 IU
		salmon broiled, 4 oz.	2.5 IU

Nutrient	Vitamin Food Sources	Nutrient Content in Selected Food	
Vitamin K	green and/or leafy vegetables	parsley, 10 sprigs	70 µg
		spinach raw chopped, 1 cup	192.5 µg
		kale cooked, 1 cup	975 µg
		broccoli cooked, 1 cup	310 µg
		brussels sprouts cooked, 1 cup	341 µg
Vitamin B$_1$ Thiamin	blackstrap molasses, brewer's yeast, whole grains, legumes, pork, nuts, organ meats, wheat germ	brewer's yeast, 2 tbsp	1.25 mg
		sunflower seeds, 2 tbsp	1.3 mg
		pork chop broiled, 4 oz.	1.1 mg
		pecans, 2 tbsp	0.5 mg
		black beans cooked, 1 cup	0.4 mg
		brown rice cooked, 1 cup	0.2 mg
Vitamin B$_2$ Riboflavin	milk and dairy products, green leafy vegetables, black strap molasses, nuts, organ meats, whole grains	beef liver broiled, 4 oz.	3.5 mg
		corn grits cooked, 1 cup	2.0 mg
		yogurt nonfat, 1 cup	0.5 mg
		almonds, 2 tbsp	0.4 mg
		spinach cooked, 1 cup	0.4 mg
Vitamin B$_3$ Niacin	brewer's yeast, seafood, lean meats, milk, milk products, poultry, desiccated liver	beef liver broiled, 4 oz.	12 mg
		chicken breast roasted, 4 oz.	15.7 mg
		hamburger broiled, 4 oz.	5.5 mg
		peanut butter, 2 tbsp	4.4 mg
		mushrooms raw, 1 cup	2.9 mg
		tomato juice, 1 cup	1.6 mg
Pantothenic Acid	Present in all plant and animal foods, brewer's yeast, legumes, organ meats, salmon, wheat germ, whole grains	beef liver broiled, 4 oz.	6.7 mg
		corn cooked, 1 cup	1.4 mg
		salmon baked, 4 oz.	1.3 mg
		milk 2%, 1 cup	0.8 mg
		wheat germ toasted, 2 tbsp	0.6 mg
		orange juice fresh, 1 cup	0.4 mg

Good Food Sources of Vitamins

Nutrient	Vitamin Food Sources	Nutrient Content in Selected Food	
Vitamin B$_6$	blackstrap molasses, brewer's yeast, meat, organ meats, poultry, wheat germ, whole grains, and yeast	beef liver, 4 oz.	1.6 mg
		banana, 1 med	0.7 mg
		sunflower seeds, 2 tbsp	0.5 mg
		brussels sprouts cooked, 1 cup	0.3 mg
		brown rice, 1 cup	0.3 mg
		wheat germ toasted, 2 tbsp	0.3 mg
		prunes dried, 10 each	0.2 mg
Vitamin B$_{12}$	cheese, fish, milk, milk products, organ meats, shellfish and eggs	beef liver broiled, 4 oz.	127 µg
		tuna canned, 4 oz.	3.7 µg
		hamburger broiled, 4 oz.	2.8 µg
		cottage cheese creamed, 1 cup	1.3 µg
		milk lowfat, 1 cup	0.9 µg
		yogurt nonfat, 1 cup	0.6 µg
		egg cooked, 1 med	0.6 µg
Biotin	legumes, whole grains, organ meats, and eggs	brewer's yeast, 2 tbsp	120 µg
		beef liver, 4 oz.	112 µg
		wheat germ, 2 tbsp	14 µg
		peanut butter, 2 tbsp	12 µg
		egg cooked, 1 med	121 µg
Folic acid folacin	dark green leafy vegetables, milk, milk products, organ meats, oysters, salmon, whole grains	brewer's yeast, 2 tbsp	626 µg
		spinach steamed, 1 cup	448 µg
		beef liver broiled, 4 oz.	249 µg
		orange juice, 1 cup	109 µg
		wheat germ toasted, 2 tbsp	100 µg
		broccoli cooked, 1 cup	78 µg
		romaine lettuce, 1 cup	76 µg
		cottage cheese creamed, 1 cup	26 µg
		egg hardboiled, 1 med	24 µg
Vitamin C Ascorbate	citrus fruits, other fruits and vegetables	cantaloupe, 1/2 melon	113 mg
		grapefruit, 1 med	100 mg
		broccoli cooked, 1 cup	97 mg
		peppers green, 1 med	95 mg
		strawberries, 1 cup	90 mg
		orange, 1 med	70 mg
		watermelon, 1 slice,	46 mg
		white potato baked no skin, 1 med	26 mg
		sweet potato baked, 1 med	28 mg

Appendix 6
Good Food Sources of Minerals

Nutrient	Food Sources of Minerals	Nutrient Content in Selected Food	
Boron	fruits, leafy vegetables, nuts, lentils, bean and legumes	pear, 1 med	420 µLg
		dates, 5 each	400 µg
		apple, 1 med	153 µg
		peach, 1 med	119 µg
		peanuts, 2 tbsp	100 µg
		carrot, 1 med	78 µg
Calcium	milk, cheese, yogurt, green leafy vegetables, beans and legumes	Swiss cheese, 4 oz.	520 mg
		low-fat milk, 1 cup	297 mg
		spinach cooked, 1 cup	245 mg
		black beans cooked, 1 cup	140 mg
		broccoli cooked, 1 cup	71 mg
Chromium	whole grains, cheese, brewer's yeast and beer	broccoli steamed, 1 cup	22 µg
		ham cooked, 4 oz.	4.8 µg
		turkey breast baked, 4 oz.	2.3 µg
		green beans cooked, 1 cup	2.2 µg
		banana, 1 med	1 µg
		beer, 12 oz.	0.17 to 20 µg

Nutrient	Food Sources of Minerals	Nutrient Content in Selected Food	
Copper	nuts, organ meats, whole grain cereal, legumes, dried fruit	beef liver broiled, 4 oz.	3.2 mg
		black-eyed peas cooked, 1 cup	1.4 mg
		cashews, 2 tbsp	0.8 mg
		blackstrap molasses, 2 tbsp	0.6 mg
Iron	meat, liver, blackstrap molasses, dark green vegetables, enriched grains, legumes	beef liver broiled, 4 oz.	7.0 mg
		blackstrap molasses, 2 tbsp	5.0 mg
		hamburger broiled, 4 oz.	2.7 mg
		oatmeal, cooked, 1 cup	1.6 mg
		raisins, 1/2 cup	1.5 mg
		apricots dried, 7 halves	1 mg
Magnesium	nuts, wheat germ, whole grains, seafood, fruits, and green leafy vegetables	tofu firm, 1 cup	236 mg
		Swiss chard cooked, 1 cup	150 mg
		wheat germ toasted, 2 tbsp	90 mg
		cashews roasted, 2 tbsp	89 mg
		brown rice, 1 cup	86 mg
		potato baked with skin, 1 med	55 mg
		green peas cooked, 1 cup	46 mg
Manganese	nuts, legumes, whole grain cereals	wheat germ toasted, 2 tbsp	5.7 mg
		brown rice cooked, 1 cup	2.1 mg
		oatmeal cooked, 1 cup	1.4 mg
Phosphorous	milk, milk products, meats, poultry, fish, legumes and nuts	lentils cooked, 1 cup	356 mg
		wheat germ toasted, 2 tbsp	325 mg
		salmon canned, 4 oz.	325 mg
		milk 2%, 1 cup	232 mg
		almonds, 2 tbsp	184 mg
		oatmeal cooked, 1 cup	178 mg
Potassium	fruits such as bananas, watermelon, oranges and dates, bran cereals and vegetables	baked potato w/ skin, 1 med	844 mg
		lima beans cooked, 1 cup	694 mg
		watremelon, 1 slice	600 mg
		banana, 1 med	569 mg
		cantaloupe dried, 8 halves	490 mg
		oranges, 1 med	311 mg

Nutrient	Food Sources of Minerals	Nutrient Content in Selected Food	
Selenium	meats, seafood and cereals	Brazil nuts, 2 tbsp	380 µg
		salmon baked, 4 oz.	93 µg
		hamburger broiled, 4 oz.	29 µg
		wheat germ toasted, 2 tbsp	28 µg
		blackstrap molasses, 2 tbsp	25 µg
		egg boiled, 1 each	12 µg
Sodium	widely present in all foods (especially processed foods) except fruit table salt	table salt	
		cottage cheese 2%, 1 cup	918 mg
		cheddar cheese, 2 oz.	352 mg
		ice cream, 1 cup	166 mg
		milk 2%, 1 cup	120 mg
Zinc	animal and seafood, eggs and dairy products, whole grain breads, cereals, legumes, peanuts	oysters, Eastern, 1 cup	226 mg
		hamburger broiled, 4 oz.	6.2 mg
		turkey dark meat baked, 4 oz.	5 mg
		wheat germ toasted, 2 tbsp	4.7 mg
		pecans, 2 tbsp	1.6 mg
		peanut butter, 2 tbsp	1.4 mg
		salmon baked, 4 oz.	0.5 mg

Appendix 7
Sample High-Carbohydrate Menus

Sample Day One

BREAKFAST

Orange juice	1 cup
Hard cooked eggs	2 eggs
Whole wheat toasts	2 each
Margarine	1 pat
Blueberry muffin	1 each
Banana	1 each
Coffee w/milk & sugar	1 cup

MORNING SNACK

Bagel	1 each
w/jam & peanut butter	1 tbsp ea
Apple	1 each
Instant breakfast	1 packet
w/skim milk	1 cup

LUNCH

Turkey sandwich	
Turkey breast sliced	4 oz.
Whole wheat bread	2 slices
Lettuce, iceberg	1/4 cup
Tomato	1/2
Mustard	1 tsp
Miracle whip	1 tbsp
Carrot	2 med
Chocolate milk, low-fat	1 cup

AFTERNOON SNACK

Orange juice	1 cup
Granola bar - Oats n honey	1 bar

DINNER		DINNER continued	
Spaghetti, cooked	2 cups	Carrots, grated	1/4 cup
Spaghetti sauce w/mush-rooms	1/2 cup	Low-fat salad dressing	2 tbsp
Parmesan cheese	1 tbsp	Hot fudge sundae	1 serving
French bread w/	1/4 loaf	Orange juice	1 cup
Garlic butter	2 pats	**BEDTIME SNACK**	
Salad w/		Ovaltine (malt flavored)	1 cup
Lettuce	1/2 cup	Oatmeal & raisin cookies	4 each
Tomato	1 each		
Cucumber	1/2 cup		

Macronutrient Analysis of Day One

Protein = 140 grams

CHO = 624 grams

Fat = 97 grams

Total Energy = 3,850 kcal

Sample Day Two

BREAKFAST

Cranberry juice	1 cup
Pancakes	3 each
Maple syrup-lite	3 tbsp
Butter	2 pats
Milk, skim	1 cup
Apple	1 each
Coffee (w/milk & sugar)	1 cup

MORNING SNACK

Bran muffin	1 each
Banana	1 each
Low-fat chocolate milk	1 cup

LUNCH

Tuna salad sandwich	
Tuna packed in water	1 oz.
Celery, diced	1/8 cup
Miracle Whip	2 tbsp
Pumpernickel bread	2 slices
Lettuce, iceberg	1/8 cup
Tomato	1/2 each
Mustard	1 tsp
Yogurt, low-fat, fruit flavored	1 cup
Orange juice	2 cups

AFTERNOON SNACK

Apple juice	12-oz. can
Milky Way bar	1 bar

DINNER

Roasted chicken breast w/out skin	1 breast
Steamed vegetable	
Broccoli	1/3 cup
Carrots	1/3 cup
Cauliflower	1/3 cup
Baked potato	1 each
Sour cream	2 tbsp
Whole wheat dinner rolls	2 rolls
Butter/margarine	1 pat
Brownies w/nuts	2 each
Strawberries	1 cup
Orange juice	1 cup

BEDTIME SNACK

Ovaltine malt flavor	1 cup
Whole wheat crackers	3 each
Cheddar cheese	0.5 oz

Macronutrient Analysis of Day Two

- Protein = 156 grams
- CHO = 646 grams
- Fat = 99 grams

63% 22% 15%

Total Energy = 3,990 kcal

Sample Day Three

BREAKFAST		MORNING SNACK	
Apple juice	1 cup	Banana	1 each
Wheaties	1 bowl	Orange juice	1 cup
Milk, skim	1 cup	**LUNCH**	
Whole wheat toasts	2 each	McDLT sandwich	1 each
Peanut butter	1 tbsp	Apple	1 each
Grape jelly	1 tbsp	Orange juice	1 cup
Coffee (w/milk & sugar)	1 cup		

AFTERNOON SNACK		DINNER continued	
Apple juice	12 oz can	Carrots, grated or chopped	1/4 cup
Fruit bar—oat bran & nuts	1 each	Broccoli	1/3 cup
DINNER		Non fat salad dressing	2 tbsp
Pizza—combination supreme—medium	6 slices	Peach cobbler	1 serving
Salad w/		Orange juice	1 cup
Lettuce	1/4 cup	**BEDTIME SNACK**	
Tomato	1 each	Milk, skim	1 cup
Cauliflower	1/4 cup	Chocolate chip cookies	4 each

Macronutrient Analysis of Day Three

Protein = 173 grams

CHO = 602 grams

Fat = 94 grams

Total Energy = 3,855 kcal

Appendix 8
US Navy Special Warfare 10 Commandments Of Nutrition

1. Don't believe anything you read about nutrition written by someone trying to sell you something.

2. Read the labels on food products. Total calories and weights of carbohydrate (CHO), protein, and fat per serving are usually provided.

3. Most Americans need no supplemental vitamins, but use the inexpensive "one-a-day" type if you want to increase your vitamin intake. Megadose quantities of costly wonder-vitamins serve mainly to increase the vitamin content of your body waste products.

4. Don't take protein and amino acid supplements. One gram of protein per pound of body weight per day is the maximum recommended protein intake, even for weight training and body building. Most non-vegetarian athletes take in more than this in their normal diet

5. Limit fat intake to less than 30% of total calories (1 gram of fat = 9 calories). Items to watch are red meat, peanuts, solid dairy products, and french-fried anything.

6. For specific endurance events such as prolonged missions, long cold dives, or triathalons, CHO load with 1500 extra CHO calories a day for 3 days before the event and decrease fat and protein intake. Cut back on your training schedule and avoid stressful cold exposures during this time.

7. For prolonged intense aerobic training schedules (BUD/s or triathalon training), take in enough extra CHO calories to maintain your desired weight. The best sources are pasta, fruits, breads, potatoes, and rice.

8. Eat fresh fruits, fresh vegetables, and high-fiber cereal products every day.

9. Short-term weight reduction diets are generally useless and occasionally dangerous. Lasting weight modification is accomplished only with long-term changes in your eating and exercise habits.

10. The most common nutrition problem in this country is too much nutrition. Don't eat when you're not hungry and stop eating as soon as you've had enough, not when your plate is empty.

Full Mission Profile, January 1992
Compliments of CAPT Frank Butler

Photo Credits

All photos purchased from Thinkstock.com.

iStockphoto	290, 411, 429, 435, 447, 457
David De Lossy, Digital Vision	292
Stocktrek Images	292, 369, 394, 439, 440
Comstock	325, 339, 359, 389
Goodshoot	337, 381, 442
Ingram Publishing	371

NOTES

NOTES

NOTES

_____

NOTES